Integrated Treatment of Co-occurring Substance Use and Mental Health Disorders

Tore Willy Lie • Lars Lien
Editors

Integrated Treatment of Co-occurring Substance Use and Mental Health Disorders

Springer

Editors
Tore Willy Lie
Department of Health and Nursing Sciences and Section for Mental Health and Rehabilitation
University of Inland Norway
Elverum, Norway

Lars Lien
Department of Health and Nursing Sciences and Section for Mental Health and Rehabilitation
University of Inland Norway
Elverum, Norway

Research Centre for Substance Use Disorders and Mental Illness
Innlandet Hospital Trust
Hamar, Norway

ISBN 978-3-032-20048-8 ISBN 978-3-032-20049-5 (eBook)
https://doi.org/10.1007/978-3-032-20049-5

The original submitted manuscript has been translated into English. The translation was done using artificial intelligence. A subsequent revision was performed by the author(s) to further refine the work and to ensure that the translation is appropriate concerning content and scientific correctness. It may, however, read stylistically different from a conventional translation.

This Springer imprint is published by the registered company Springer Nature Switzerland AG
The registered company address is: Gewerbestrasse 11, 6330 Cham, Switzerland

Preface

Individuals with co-occurring substance use disorders and mental disorders (SUD/MH) are possibly the group in society that to the greatest extent falls outside of the society and has participated least in prosperity development in the last 10–20 years in many Western countries. They have a significantly higher morbidity and mortality than the rest of the population and at the same time receive less treatment for their somatic illnesses than others. On the list of young people who die an unnatural death in the form of suicide, overdoses, and accidents, they rank high. The living conditions among people with SUD are among the lowest, often with huge shortcomings related to housing, employment, social network, and economy. They top the statistics of homelessness, have low education, and contribute greatly to the state treasury in the form of taxes on substances like tobacco and alcohol. In addition, they often experience a high degree of discrimination, lack of social inclusion, and mattering.

Why haven't governmental action plans related to mental health and substance use managed to offer more satisfactory, proper services in the last 50 years for this group? Is it about the services not being juridically organized properly according to actual needs? Have we listened too little to the patients? Is the main reason usually about lack of economic resources or the way we prioritize? Does the lack of treatment studies for SUD/MH make some governments reluctant to develop or offer proper services to this group, or use that as an excuse not to do so? Can private insurance-associated healthcare systems offer proper follow-up to people with severe SUD/MH? Are there many mental health workers who have negative attitudes toward SUD that hugely affect daily follow-up? In summary, there are many challenges woven into each other in this field.

That being said, we also see positive changes. For example, the emergence of multidisciplinary outreach teams that challenge traditional sector-based organization and its bureaucratic limitations, alongside the person-centered recovery movement, indicates that our attitudes and approaches are evolving in a positive direction.

This book aims to describe challenges and opportunities in the field, with the hope of contributing to better living conditions for people with SUD/MH. There is much that can be improved despite the challenging frameworks we work within. We want to give the services something they can be inspired by and strive for, with the aim of providing the best possible comprehensive and integrated follow-up with available resources. The central focus is the emphasis on the person's resources and goals to increase quality of life, including themes like social inclusion. The core elements in integrated treatment consist of coordinating treatment planning where relevant aspects are taken care of simultaneously in the same treatment program, by the same team or group. The personnel and services involved must, attitude-wise, show that they actually want to stand together in the respective cases, and strive for something that needs to be ongoing, maintained, adjusted, or further developed according to each country's legislation (which can be challenged) and an eventual lack of resources. This is also an equally important attitude in future cases you are involved in, as you always will be a part of an ecosystem of relevant parties. This is in most cases not an uncompromising solo service project. Further, with different roles, tasks, and areas of expertise, those involved should be open to contribute beyond their own workplaces' core mandate and legislation: Avoid narrow interpretations of your own juridical, tasks and moral responsibilities, and at the same time be clear and open about what your obvious responsibilities and competencies are.

This book conveys a lot of what we believe is necessary basic knowledge, attitudes, and competence everyone should have, and useful cross-sectorial models and practices. It has a mix of academic and practical content, with a focus on the path toward a better life—with health and social services as a part of the journey. The common thread through the chapters is to point out the necessity of a multidisciplinary, cross-sectorial functional level with a certain attitude: Stand together, especially in gray zone and difficult cases, and signal that you want to contribute to the interwoven, overlapping, simultaneous, and compounded that is called life. This is no easy task for the services, patients, and caregivers, and it poses many challenges which must be met with humility and hard work.

Many thanks to all the authors who have contributed. In the spirit of integration, we invited a lot of skilled and dedicated people to contribute, and together we complemented each other to create a broad, composite presentation about integrated treatment of SUD/MH. A big thank you to Fagbokforlaget, who gave us the opportunity to further develop and publish an international edition of the original Norwegian edition, "*Sammensatte problemer, sammenvevde tiltak. Integrert behandling av rus og psykiske lidelser*" (2022). Finally, we thank Springer Nature and associated services, especially Catherine Mazars and colleagues at Springer, for the trust and freedom we have had as editors and for the collaboration during the process of making the book.

Elverum, Norway
2026

Tore Willy Lie
Lars Lien

Contents

About the Editors and Contributors

About the Editors

Tore Willy Lie has a bachelor's degree in psychology and a master's degree in mental health care. He has worked at several types of inpatient units in the specialist service, at a national helpline for gambling and gaming problems, as an advisor for the Norwegian National Advisory Unit on Concurrent Substance Abuse and Mental Health Disorders, and part-time for the Norwegian Directorate of Health. He is currently an Assistant Professor at the University of Inland Norway.

Lars Lien is a medical doctor and specialist in community medicine and psychiatry. He has led the Norwegian National Advisory Unit on Concurrent Substance Abuse and Mental Health Disorders (2012–2020). He is currently the leader of the Norwegian Psychiatric Association and Professor of psychiatry at the University of Inland Norway.

About the Contributors

Jan Aasen is a specialized mental healthcare nurse and has a master's degree in mental health care. He has clinical experience from inpatient and outreach acute/emergency mental health care. He is currently working with digital therapy at Innlandet Hospital Trust and is a PhD candidate at the Research Centre for Substance Use Disorders and Mental Illness, Innlandet Hospital Trust.

Ole Petter Askheim is Professor Emeritus at University of Inland Norway. His main research interest is service user involvement, empowerment, and co-creation of welfare. His studies are empirically mainly within disability studies and mental health.

Therese Bekkevold is a social worker with specialization in the field of substance use. She has several years of experience with Individual Placement and Support (IPS), both as a job specialist and IPS supervisor. She currently works as an IPS supervisor in the Norwegian Labour and Welfare Administration (Nav).

Anne Kristine Bergem is a medical doctor with an Executive Master of Management and specialization in psychiatry. She has clinical and teaching experience; she has advised the Norwegian Council for Mental Health, the National Network for Children as Next of Kin – BarnsBeste, and The Center for Next of Kin and Carers. Currently she works as special advisor to the Norwegian Psychiatric Association.

Jørgen Gustav Bramness has published more than 250 peer-reviewed scientific articles in international scientific journals and over 20 books and book chapters on substance use and addiction. His research areas include psychiatry, epidemiology, psychopharmacology, pharmacoepidemiology, substance use, and more recently, alcohol use and its somatic consequences, with a particular focus on patients who have undergone bariatric surgery and the significance of presystemic alcohol metabolism.

Grethe Breirem-Sveen is a nurse with extensive experience in helping people return to work. She focuses on strengths and what can be achieved together, rather than on barriers. She is currently the general manager at Fontenehuset Gjøvik and has many years of experience from IPS, where she served as team leader.

Erlend Bugge is head of the Regional Centre for Research and Education in Forensic Psychiatry and Psychology (SIFER) and the Centre of Expertise on Voluntariness and Coercion. He is an MD, a specialist in psychiatry, and a PhD in psychoneuroimmunology, and serves as an Associate Professor at The Arctic University of Norway.

Hanne Clausen, Researcher at the Research Centre for Substance Use Disorders and Mental Illness, Innlandet Hospital Trust, and the R&D Department for Mental Health and Addiction Services, Akershus University Hospital. She is experienced in research and implementation of collaborative service models (ACT, FACT, IDDT) for adolescents and adults with mental health issues and substance use problems.

Ruth Marie Donovan is a writer, teacher, and mental health nurse. She is committed to empowering healthcare professionals to speak out and advocate for patient safety, dignity, and ethical practices within the healthcare system. Through her teaching, writing, and advocacy efforts, she strives to amplify the voices of patients. She fosters a more compassionate and responsible approach to patient care.

Karl Petter Gjeterud has worked with Individual Placement and Support (IPS) since 2014, serving in roles such as employment specialist, supervisor, team manager, and fidelity reviewer. His primary responsibility is facilitating collaboration between Nav and regional hospitals to enhance integrated services.

Julie Granlund Hanssen is a senior advisor at the Regional Centre for Research and Education in Forensic Psychiatry and Psychology (SIFER) and the Centre of Expertise on Voluntariness and Coercion. She is a registered nurse with a master's in health-promoting relational work. Her expertise includes violence risk assessment, leadership, psychotherapy, and psychosocial rehabilitation for psychosis, with clinical experience in forensic psychiatry.

Anne Høye holds a medical degree from the University of Oslo, Norway. She is a specialist in psychiatry with extensive clinical and administrative experience. As a professor of psychiatry at The Arctic University of Tromsø, her primary research focuses on somatic morbidity and mortality in individuals with severe mental disorders.

Mads Kristian Johansen is a national lead for Individual Placement and Support (IPS) at the Norwegian Labour and Welfare Administration (Nav). He has worked with IPS since 2017 and has played a key role in implementing and scaling the approach both across Northern Norway and nationally. He has also contributed to the development of a national IPS data system in Norway.

Anne Landheim, PhD and Sociologist, is Research Director at the Research Centre for Substance Use Disorders and Mental Illness, Innlandet Hospital Trust, and a Professor at University of Inland Norway. She has many years of experience in health services research, with a particular focus on integrated care and the implementation of ACT and FACT teams in Norway.

Torgeir Gilje Lid is a specialist in family medicine and a researcher with extensive clinical experience as a general practitioner, in addition to clinical experience from community medicine, substance use treatment, and mental health services. His research focuses on health problems related to alcohol and substance use.

Lars Linderoth is an MD and specialist in psychiatry and addiction medicine. He has worked in the field of co-occurring substance use disorders and mental disorders since 1990, particularly in outpatient clinics and outreach teams. His main field of work has been with severely impaired patients, usually with psychotic disorders and/or addiction. He has also been involved in service planning, scientific work, lecturing, and writing books.

Linda Nesse is a clinical psychologist with a PhD in public health science. Her PhD project focused on recovery and citizenship among people with co-occurring substance use and mental health problems in the Norwegian context. She currently works as a senior researcher at Innlandet Hospital Trust.

Henning Pettersen, MHP, PhD, is a Professor at the University of Inland Norway, Faculty of Health and Social Sciences. His main research interests are recovery in substance use disorders and dual diagnosis, Citizenship, collaborative research, and qualitative approaches. He has regular teaching responsibilities in user involvement, mental health, and health promotion.

Marianne Silsand is a legal advisor at the University Hospital of North Norway in the Regional Centre for Research and Education in Forensic Psychiatry and Psychology (SIFER) and the Centre of Expertise on Voluntariness and Coercion. She has qualifications in law and has nursing experience in mental health care.

1 Thoughts About Interaction

Tore Willy Lie and Lars Lien

Abstract

This chapter points out that a dynamic, pragmatic and cooperative manner between services and professions are necessary to achieve treatment success, where integrated treatment for co-occurring substance use disorders and mental disorders (SUD/MH) is the go-to approach. These disorders are often interrelated and affect each other in different ways, and an integrative model underlines the importance of addressing all conditions simultaneously, through coordinated and multidisciplinary care. It involves a comprehensive approach that includes psychotherapy, pharmacological interventions, psychoeducation, proper housing and a wide array of psychosocial measures. The goal is to improve overall functioning and quality of life and prevent relapse with a wide array of relevant interventions. Ongoing evaluation and actively considering treatment adjustments are necessary to meet the varied needs of each individual.

Keywords

Integrated treatment · Interaction · Cooperation · Non-integrated treatment · Service delivery · Collaboration · Substance use disorders · Dual diagnosis

---

T. W. Lie (✉)
Department of Health and Nursing Sciences and Section for Mental Health and Rehabilitation, University of Inland Norway, Elverum, Norway
e-mail: tore.lie@inn.no

L. Lien
Department of Health and Nursing Sciences and Section for Mental Health and Rehabilitation, University of Inland Norway, Elverum, Norway

Research Centre for Substance Use Disorders and Mental Illness, Innlandet Hospital Trust, Hamar, Norway
e-mail: lars.lien@inn.no

T. W. Lie, L. Lien (eds.), *Integrated Treatment of Co-occurring Substance Use and Mental Health Disorders*, https://doi.org/10.1007/978-3-032-20049-5_1

Interaction: A Problem for Whom?

It is often mentioned in various contexts, publications and by different institutions that the services must work together across levels and services to achieve a useful and effective follow-up for people with SUD/MH. "Integrated," "comprehensive," "collaborative" and "interaction" are words that often recur in normative descriptions about how it is expected that the services should cooperate. Some will say that the core of this is about having a common understanding, a clear task distribution, achieving and working for an overall common goal, and performing tasks in a coordinated way. But what does this mean in practice? What is the problem with interaction and a comprehensive approach? Is it really a problem, if so for whom? Where and why does it eventually fail? Is any of the various ways of organizing health care the main issue (publicly funded—universal health fare, public insurance, private insurance, out of pocket, foreign aid, etc.)? Is it mainly about the separate service levels, each with their own budget, laws and formal responsibilities? Prejudices or lack of clinical competency? Politicians who don't care enough? Let's take a closer look at this with two cases from Norway as a starting point:

Interaction Case 1

Peter (42 years) has a significant substance use problem, with heavy use of alcohol and cannabis, especially during the last 5 years. In addition, he has had several episodes where health personnel have described that he is impulsive, sometimes appearing erratic, and periodically depressed. On several occasions during the last 15 years, he has had short spans of follow-up by mental health services in the municipality, and once had five sessions with a psychologist at an outpatient specialist service before he dropped out. He lives alone in an apartment in a small town and has little or no contact with health and welfare services. Sometimes, when he seems erratic and influenced by drugs, he has been so noisy that the neighbours on several occasions have called the police. He was once in such a situation brought to the emergency room, where the doctor admitted him involuntarily to an acute psychiatric ward. After 5 days in the hospital, he demanded to be discharged because he had no reason to stay there. The doctor at the unit declared 2 days later that he could be discharged. No one was in touch with the municipality while he was admitted, and no initiative was taken by anyone to establish a binding treatment plan for the services recently involved, even though this was his third admission in the past year. An epicrisis was sent to the general practitioner, who has not seen Peter in 3 years. The diagnosis set was substance-induced psychosis, and it was underlined a worry about a possible bipolar disorder or schizophrenia. A referral was later sent by the general practitioner to the local outpatient specialist clinic, with a request for further follow-up of the patient's severe substance use problems, and assessment of what could be a severe independent mental disorder. Peter did not show up for the scheduled appointment at the outpatient clinic, and after a reminder from them, he was removed from the patient list at the specialist unit.

Peter had been offered to live in municipal housing, but the municipality does not have sufficient resources for follow-up in his residence, which is co-located with other municipal housing known for heavy use of drugs and a variety of instability among the neighbours. Peter's parents live in the same city, and they have helped Peter with practical follow-up, so he receives social benefits, as well as supporting him when things get tough, and try to engage him to get in touch with his small and at the moment socially distant drug-free social network.

Peter's prognosis is not perceived as good by several personnel, and no services seem to take responsibility for giving Peter a type of follow-up that suits the treatment stage he is at (read more about treatment stages in Chap. 2). Could better interaction have solved some of these challenges? An available Flexible Assertive Community Treatment team (FACT team, read about such teams in Chap. 12) could have given Peter a comprehensive treatment package, but he has not been diagnosed with a severe independent mental disorder, and the level of functioning is still not noticeably "low enough," partly because his parents compensate and provide a great deal of important support. In periods when he does not use alcohol or cannabis, he can also manage his daily life on his own.

Is it possible to imagine that the acute ward could have done more to increase Peter's engagement for further follow-up, and that while he was admitted, should he have gotten the opportunity to meet personnel with SUD/MH competence? Would it have been possible to ensure transition to a relevant internal inpatient unit? Or should the acute ward have followed him up more closely further when there's a question of possible serious mental illness, instead of just underlining it generally for someone else to take care of? Admissions can be golden opportunities to motivate for change, not just in terms of mental problems and drug problems, but also related to somatic disease. A somatic examination of Peter was done, showing that he had high blood pressure, high liver enzymes, and that his blood sugar was borderline. This was not followed up afterward, and again the admission could have provided an opportunity to get in position for cooperation (read more about somatic illness and lifestyle habits in Chap. 7).

In the respective country, there might be governmental guidelines and legislation that underline the necessity of integration and shared responsibility between specialist and municipal services during admissions. At a minimum, a message should have been sent to the municipality about when the patient is expected to be discharged, including eventual changes in treatment interventions during the stay, which is necessary information for the municipality to immediately know of. In this case, the municipality's services are little known to Peter. Could a meeting while Peter was admitted have been an opportunity for the municipality, preferably together with caregivers, to tell about their available services and start the process of alliance building? What about inviting the general practitioner to get to know Peter better and talk about further follow-up of medical conditions? At the same time, it is important that all services address and help overcome barriers to follow-up, such as lack of ability to pay for sessions with the general practitioner and specialist services, eventual associated insurance issues, and uncover other needs and expectations, like housing, networking and meaningful activities. As soon as possible, because of implications of long-term cross-sectional needs, a responsibility group should have been established, including a case manager and a treatment plan that the group has an active and binding relation to, which is regularly checked and revised.

Interaction Case 2

This case shows how a lack of interaction and cooperation horizontally and vertically in a hospital trust can have severe consequences. This is an anonymized and somewhat adjusted story from a hospital trust about 25-year-old Jane:

It has been a long-standing suspicion and worry among several services during the past years that Jane might have a psychotic disorder. She also injects heroin, and in rare cases, amphetamine. She is followed up by an outreach specialist team but was admitted to a sub-acute inpatient specialist unit with a need for stabilization. She expressed that she was worn out and had suicidal thoughts. It was also a wish from the outreach team to gain better insight into a tentative consideration of psychotic symptoms. Jane had no history of aggression or acting out during previous admissions or in other contexts. When the personnel checked her luggage upon arrival, an unopened syringe needle in original packaging that she got from a low-threshold street-level municipality service was found. The result on the incoming urine sample was as expected, as it harmonized with her own expressions about recent drug use before admission. This information and the syringe discovery triggered a general suspicion and fear among the staff, associated with risks of overdose and use of illegal drugs during the stay.

Jane was given a written "drug contract" made by the personnel at the unit, which determined the length of admission and thereby an attempt to regulate her juridical rights: She was told that a non-given urine sample within the next 6 h is concluded to be a substance positive sample, a factor supposed to be an argument for discharge. Jane mostly stayed in her own room and participated little in activities at the ward, and the staff did not talk with her about the reason for what they perceived as social withdrawal. They kept questioning the rationale for her stay and argued that she does not participate in the units' "treatment program," and thereby, there is no need to stay there. Jane, on the other side, has expressed a desire and cooperation to be admitted to receive help. She also told her psychologist at the outpatient unit that she is afraid of being discharged and feels unwanted by the personnel.

Just before she was to be discharged, her outpatient therapist contacted the acute ward. He knew Jane over time, was updated on the progress for the stay, and questioned the current follow-up in the unit—especially related to what looked like discharge pressure. This led to a dialogue and conclusion where the discharge was prevented. But the different aspects of interventional malpractice and attitudes related to people with SUD were not further followed up to learn and adjust practice and attitudes among the staff. In a meeting between staff from the acute ward and another inpatient treatment ward in the same hospital, they discussed the possibility of long-term treatment and direct transfer to another internal ward. The representative from the ward that seemed most relevant expressed that the patient was not wanted there unless it was an involuntary admission. It seemed that they wanted some type of control or regulation associated with her SUD. Jane wanted treatment voluntarily, and involuntary admission had not been a relevant theme at any time before.

The disagreements between the units and personnel became quite clear in this case in terms of who should help her. No one wants to take responsibility, even though it was well documented over time that her severe mental and physical health condition was not possible to satisfactorily follow up by the regular available services, without a longer period of admission. Instead, she is met with distance, rejection, and resistance, even without any possibility to give feedback about her own perception of the suggested ward transfer. The fact that she didn't have a formal diagnosis of a severe independent mental disorder and known co-occurring SUD was practically used against her. In short, different services can have very different opinions about what benefits the patient best and on which treatment premises, with their ways of defining themselves in or out of a case, which is not just about following an official treatment prioritization guide about who should have the rights to specialist assessment and treatment.

An Amalgam of Clinical Competence, Leadership, Organization, and Politics

A central question that often shows up is who has the responsibility for the patient? One suggestion is that the municipalities should take it to a greater extent for the treatment and follow-up of patients with SUD/MH. Some of the arguments are to increase available resources/lessen pressure and prioritize the more severe cases in specialist services. At first sight, it might sound like a good idea. But are the municipalities equipped for this transfer of tasks from specialist services and are there available resources (personnel, economy) and competence? Is the "burden" just moved to another service level's budget without money following the patient? Does it actually contribute to better integrated treatment, when a certain number of cases aren't clear cut about when specialist services should be a part of the follow-up and how? Regardless of how the services are organized, there are many complicated and unpredictable conditions related to challenges with, e.g., economy, housing, fluctuating functional level, fluctuating motivation to change pattern of substance use in the initial treatment phase, medical problems, occasional use of emergency services (prehospital or acute wards), and little or no support from a stable, safe social network.

When you have juridical rights for help in a municipality, they cannot reject their inhabitant, per se. They often find that they need contributions from external parties, where a possible rejection from the specialist service about having temporary main or long-term shared responsibility can make the suffering individual feel burdened and, as a result, have a perception of blaming her/himself for lack of treatment progression. Basically, you are adding more demoralization and lack of belief in the health and welfare system for the individual, which makes it more difficult for future services to get an alliance and promote themself as a possible useful piece in the persons' life. Some municipal employees also experience condescending, undervaluing, and arrogant communication from some staff in the specialist service. A former colleague summarized this communication and attitude problem well, after working many years in the specialist service: "It's strange how dumb I suddenly became overnight when I started working in the nearby municipality." There can also be unreasonable expectations from the specialist service or a lack of local knowledge about what the municipalities can do or offer, regardless of the size of the municipality, capacity, geographical challenges, juridical room for specific interventions, and actual available services. When different parties across service levels only communicate with each other for short time spans, now and then, you can also get skewed impressions of a person that is practically supposed to be your teammate. All such local frictions tend to persist if the leaders in the different services do not recognize and address such problems together. Such a culture is hard to change within the service alone and only with leaders across service levels involved. This is a matter of having more reasonable expectations to other parties, building common attitudes, trust, belief and support between the services that follow up the same person.

If a service is economically and persistently operationally pressured, it can become overly concerned with its own mandate and protect themself from grey zone tasks and responsibility related to what an individual actually needs. Then the opportunities to work multidisciplinary and integrate across service levels have a tendency to become quite vulnerable.

But all types of cross-sectional factors cannot take all the blame for the lack of a cooperative and solution-based manner. Improvement is also about the clinical and practical competence among individuals and services. Furthermore, it is the case that employees at different workplaces meet people in different phases, contexts and situations, with different durations. This has a vulnerability to give a skewed or unnuanced impression of someone's needs, and thereby your expectations of other services' actions, especially if you don't know the person or have only met him/her in a short time span or only a few times. This can be combined with a personal or service conviction about one model of how mental suffering in general is supposed to be understood and approached (which has a tendency to co-occur with a model they also somehow dislike/disapprove) and thereby a lack of multidisciplinary and differentiating competency. Such a view and attitude set up a risk of unit and service designs that practically exclude people with severe SUD/MH, eventually offering suboptimal or harmful follow-up.

Some people with poor functional level may not want help, even though, from the perspective of the services or caregivers, it may appear as a matter of time before the person comes into contact with the healthcare system. Where is the limit for the amount of time to be spent on outreach efforts on an individual who does not want contact or help, but whom you hope one day will accept the offer of follow-up? And how should the interaction be related to people who do not want any follow-up?

People with SUD/MH are a group with complex, intertwined service needs at the same time, maybe with interventional varied intensity over time. Some need more robust services and staff than they are offered or that are available locally, such as round-the-clock staffing at an institution or shared housing, long-term admission in the specialist service, or a multidisciplinary outreach team. It can, e.g., be substance use problems combined with moderate or severe personality pathology, violence, severe self-harm, low level of functioning as a result of psychosis, or the person is perceived to have long-term reduced cognitive abilities. The tendency of service rejection is also seen in some places, especially if the person has substance use problems, even when specialist care is formally obliged to offer treatment to people with severe SUD/MH.

Such a culture and organization of health services can threaten the legal rights for some of the most vulnerable patients, and they can fall between services over many years. They might end up as a major challenge for the municipalities, which are left with the main and sole responsibility, without a real and well-coordinated follow-up across service levels that the person should have received and is entitled to. Add the factor that municipalities may lack relevant expertise and desired support from the specialist service, the employees have too huge caseloads, and they are pressured on task prioritization and staffing, which can induce persistent personal moral stress. Then it can be a thankless task for the coordinator to try to invite to cross-sectoral group meetings in each case, where as many services as possible ideally show up at the same time and place, with readiness and surplus to be updated and adjusted for further follow-up.

What Can Be Done to Improve a Collaborative Platform?

It is a societal responsibility to continuously assess the usefulness of the services offered. Patience and endurance are some of the most important factors, and it might take months or, in some cases, years before you can go on with more intensity in the follow-up or specific interventions. You can't unreasonably be questioned for non-effect intervening just because there is a slow, natural progression for a certain time, or label the patient "treatment resistant". Further, not avoiding and rejecting people with severe interpersonal functioning, especially if you feel threatened, or feel met in a less reasonable or respectable way. This requires more competence from you as a service provider to position yourself and get an alliance with a variety of cases and individuals. Another aspect of interaction is cultural sensitivity. It's not just about meeting people with immigrant backgrounds, but there can be large differences in culture between health and social workers and service users, regardless of background, and that can put both individual and cross-sectional collaboration to the test. Culture focus challenges the understanding of how follow-up and rejection are understood, and what is desired, culturally adapted treatment.

It is important that all parties, both service levels and personnel, can step into each other's domains without stepping on certain service-specific responsibilities. There is the greatest potential for treatment success by creating and having a shared sense of responsibility, and being solution-oriented with adaptable, intertwined measures. At the same time, each service must take responsibility for their domain. Such an attitude challenges and points out the need for change in local cooperating culture, methods used and established role and service expectations. The main goal is to create or develop flexible and dynamic systems and flexible helpers for the benefit of the person with SUD/MH and others affected. See Box 1.1 for examples of what can be done to improve collaboration.

Box 1.1: Examples: How to Improve a Collaborative Platform Across Services

- The services should prioritize meetings about people that "no one" wants.
- Avoid contributing to a "non-responsibility game" between services or using various opportunities for disclaiming responsibility, especially in compounded, assumed long term cases with possible high costs.
- Employees need local arenas, organized by the services' leaders, where they can learn to know each other and work on developing cooperation without having specific user/patient-related agendas. This includes knowledge about limitations, vulnerabilities, resources and opportunities, and focus on building and maintaining trust. This is not only a matter of agreement between people in other organizational roles and formalized cooperation between services.

Summarized, this book deals in greater depth with some of the challenges and opportunities we have addressed in this chapter. We hope that everyone who works in mental health-related services and the rest of the health services, as well as policy makers and politicians, finds something to be inspired by and to strive for. We want to inspire better organization of services with regard to interaction, as well as a more holistic, dynamic and multidisciplinary approach across service levels. Those who receive health-related follow-up or are caregivers might also find something useful in this book, considering what they can expect and need from the services.

Reflection Questions

- Do you collaborate well with external service providers, together with the individual and/or caregivers? How do you know that you interact well or badly? Under which circumstances do you eventually reject or, in different ways, back out of a case?
- What can you and your workplace do to work better together with others, both internally and externally?
- Do you talk with the patient about factors that can affect follow-up expectations, but that you can't do anything about (e.g., geographical conditions, opening hours, waiting lists, offers that do not exist locally, etc.)?
- Is there something your workplace can do to improve as a group, related to your services' attitude, competency and operational vulnerabilities, which seems feasible without more financial resources or more employees?

Integrated Treatment in Practice

2

Lars Linderoth

Abstract

It doesn't matter how brilliant a single therapist or service may be if the whole ecosystem of services and professions around a patient does not work well together. Only when we manage to establish cooperation between all the involved parties that work well: the patient, relatives, the municipality-based services, and the specialist care, can we achieve a robust treatment result. This chapter is grounded on that attitude and is primarily based on the author's clinical experience with the treatment of individuals with co-occurring substance use disorder and mental disorders in different services in Norway. It includes practical guidance on how to work according to the integrated dual disorder treatment model (IDDT), how to maintain fidelity to the model, and how to handle various treatment challenges along the way.

Keywords

Integrated treatment · Integrated dual disorder treatment · Collaborative interactions · Treatment perspectives · Dual diagnosis treatment

Having completed my specialist training in psychiatry in 1995, I started working in a general psychiatric outpatient clinic in Oslo (Norway). I had just completed an excellent, but traditional, education to become a psychiatrist. At that time, this

L. Linderoth (✉)
Oslo, Norway
e-mail: post@rups.no

T. W. Lie, L. Lien (eds.), *Integrated Treatment of Co-occurring Substance Use and Mental Health Disorders*, https://doi.org/10.1007/978-3-032-20049-5_2

particular specialist outpatient unit had the most burdened catchment area in Norway; inner east Oslo, with the highest prevalence of severe SUD/MH. Studies showed a triple prevalence compared to Norway in general, and at the same time, poor social conditions such as unstable living environments, poverty, a lot of municipal housing, crime, and poor social networks.

It quickly became apparent that my education fell short in many ways. It was not readily accepted to think outside of traditional psychiatric practice. To be responsible for all assessment and treatment myself, by myself in my office, and use traditional therapeutic methods, quickly proved not to be appropriate for the group of patients who had severe mental disorders. In addition, patients often had co-occurring severe SUD, a number of social challenges, and a broad spectrum of functional losses that worsened the situation further. This was also the group of patients that, over time, should be prioritized the highest, according to guidelines from central authorities in Norway. At the same time, we found ourselves without professional tools and methods that were useful for this group of patients.

In the fall of 1995, Robert Drake from New Hampshire in the USA gave a lecture in Norway. Not long after, I was lucky enough to be able to attend a seminar with Kim Mueser, Drake's colleague, about integrated dual disorder treatment (IDDT), at the time called The New Hampshire model. Their take-home messages became an eye-opener for me, and the treatment method was later published in a manual. They presented a way of working that I immediately understood was sensible and professionally more than good enough for reaching the group of people who have the largest needs, are hardest to reach, are most dependent on treatment in order to improve, and who also had the highest priority.

Together with good colleagues with a variety of education and backgrounds, I have been part of starting several treatment initiatives in Norway based on this treatment model. First, *DD Tøyen*—a city-wide outpatient clinic that was tasked with reaching the people in Oslo with the most severe mental disorders, often with co-occurring severe SUD, and who, for various reasons, did not get treatment or follow-up. At the same time, we started what is now called *the Manifest Center* (personal translation). It was initially an inpatient treatment facility, with no locked doors, for people with co-occurring psychotic disorders and severe SUD—at the time called dual diagnosis patients (DD). Five years later, I was involved in establishing an inpatient ward at *Nordland Hospital Trust*, a DD-ward, for people with experience of psychosis and severe SUD. Later, the low-threshold initiative *24SEVEN* in downtown Oslo, and finally *the Collaboration Team in Bærum* (SiB) in 2012. Very different treatment initiatives, but with the same method of treatment approach: integrated treatment—IDDT. This treatment model was implemented in different kinds of services because it actually worked.

The IDDT Model

Before I delve a little deeper into the various parts of integrated treatment, I will briefly introduce the IDDT model. This model is a compilation of many interventions targeting several important domains for the patient, where as many as possible of their needs from health and social services are met by the same team or cross-sectoral group.

There is a focus on these key elements:

- What stage the individual is in in the process of change ("meet people where they are").
- Specific treatment methods such as motivational interviewing (MI), cognitive behavior therapy (CBT), and trauma-informed intervening—when the patient is ready for it, and the method is adjusted to the patient's actual condition at present.
- Psychoeducation of both patient, family, and network.
- Self-help groups, e.g., Alcoholics Anonymous (AA) and Narcotics Anonymous (NA).
- Recovery, e.g., as in Illness Management and Recovery (IMR).
- Family involvement (read more about caregivers in Chap. 13).
- Robust coordination of services.
- Medication as a part of a larger whole.
- In addition, follow-up related to housing, economy, networking, and filling time with meaningful activities, like education, work, or leisure—over a long period.

The follow-up is best conducted in interdisciplinary teams, preferably organized across primary care (the municipality) and specialist services (outpatient). The way to organize this, of course, differs from area to area and from country to country. Detailed knowledge about the catchment area, organization of existing services, financing, and legislation, therefore, is necessary.

Integrated Treatment: Different from What?

In Norway, it was earlier common to think that only substance-free people should be offered- or could benefit from mental health treatment. That is, people had to become substance-free before they were accepted for treatment in mental health services. This treatment tradition is called sequential treatment (targeting one condition before the other). If there was illegal substance use involved, the treatment should be given in a substance use clinic. And vice versa: substance use treatment was exclusively for people with no severe mental disorders and had very little focus on mental disorders at all. A variety of mental disorders were often overlooked. Therefore, we often got a "push-pull game" between these services that was very harmful to the patients. Sadly, this still occurs.

Another challenge was that in Oslo in the mid-1990s, there were no established treatment programs for all: Special teams treated people with problematic use of illicit substances aged 14–30 years in outpatient clinics. When they turned 30 years, there was little outpatient treatment offered to this group. Problematic use of legal substances, on the other hand, including substitution therapy for opioid addiction (at the time methadone or buprenorphine), you got treatment for in an outpatient clinic, but only if you were over 18 years old. If you started using illicit substances, relapsed, or fell out of opioid agonist treatment (OAT), there was no treatment available if you were over 30 years old. This situation represented a huge challenge for both patients and staff. Fortunately, this is no longer the case, but it shows clearly how organizing services is essential and that a multidisciplinary focus is vital when treating co-occurring conditions. We need to see a longer perspective and a broader picture of the patient, as well as in organizing services. The organizing of services must be thoroughly thought through after having involved all relevant parties in the process. The totality of services must be coherent, and all of the population's needs must be met.

Another challenge in treating co-occurring disorders is that the condition that is not treated reinforces the one you are in treatment for. Professionals had previously usually either expertise in substance use treatment or treatment of mental disorders. In that case, it's easy to overlook one relevant condition and focus on the one you recognize, are comfortable with, and are competent to treat. The result is often poor. At the same time, there was an either/or if clinicians were good at treating psychotic disorders or personality disorders. Competence in all the above is, in my experience, needed to meet the patients' demands. And of course, knowledge about drug effects, signs of abstinence, how medication works, and how these can be confused and interact is important to make a good diagnostic assessment and to decide what treatment may be useful and not harmful.

There are major challenges associated with being in treatment in two different services at the same time—or so-called parallel treatment. Kim Mueser is very clear that the only meaningful thing to do is to focus on all the existing conditions simultaneously. If the therapist does not have such combined competence and focus, the treatment must be supplemented with a therapist who has expertise in the different fields that are crucial. Then again, it is important that these two—or more—therapists work in the same team or group of therapists, and according to the same treatment program. Disagreements and unresolved issues should be discussed in this interdisciplinary team. If not, this will affect the patient negatively. I have seen many sad examples of parallel treatment. The burden of integration should be carried by parties in the treatment system and not by the patient. It is food for thought—that it is a burden for people to deal with different services that are not coordinated, on top of all other difficulties. Therefore, it is crucial that a treatment team deals with a wide range of elements and perspectives—both related to health and social conditions. As wide as possible. This is the essence of integrated treatment.

What Characterizes Integrated Treatment?

Integrated treatment is, as mentioned, a concept that is composed of many elements. First of all, the treatment should be integrated; that is, the substance use disorder(s) and the mental disorder(s) should be treated simultaneously by therapists from the same team, who all work according to the same treatment program. In addition, I would add that this treatment also should be integrated with the treatment of physical conditions (read more about somatic health in Chap. 7). The physical and mental states are closely linked. A malfunctioning body negatively affects the psyche. There are many examples that malnutrition, vitamin deficiency, painful conditions, and physical illnesses directly hinder the improvement of the mental disorder. People with severe SUD/MH often have major health challenges and a shorter life expectancy. A study conducted at the *Field Care* in Oslo (Norway) concluded that [1] you must look to famine-stricken areas in the third world to find a comparable state of malnutrition in a population as in this one. This can be related to many things. But it is clear that when it is more important for a person to ensure that the morning dose is secured than that you go to bed on a full stomach, it is obvious that spending money on food is not an option. Few people have enough money, and the little they have is carefully prioritized. They choose not to spend money on going to a doctor nor on medication. Many say that they do not get what they come to the doctor for anyway. This is despite the fact that many are worried about their physical health. They are just as reluctant to spend money on going to addiction treatment or psychiatric treatment, or buying the non-addictive medications they are prescribed there. Therefore, it is absolutely necessary, in order to ensure that patients receive a realistic offer of assessment and treatment, that the economic consequences of treatment get attention. This has led to some social services covering the costs for all sorts of treatment, including medication. Furthermore, if this is not the case, I have arranged that the special service pays for medication, such as antibiotics and antidepressants, and that using the service is free of charge.

There is an overabundance of many physical diseases among those with dual disorders: stomach ulcers, gastritis and esophagitis, infections—both hepatitis and HIV, but also local infections at injection sites and more generalized infections—chronic obstructive pulmonary disease, poor dental health, and, as mentioned above, various conditions that are caused by malnutrition.

The fact that treatment should be integrated also means that the different parts of the treatment system work in the same way and preferably together as much as possible, whatever the organization or funding. If different parts of the treatment system assess a person differently (what problem areas the person has and what is the preferred intervention for it), we impose a big problem on the patient. Gathering all involved parties when this situation arises, discussing different views and priorities, and, if possible, coming to an agreement on a treatment plan, is important. Many do not receive a realistic offer of assessment, treatment, and follow-up. Despite the fact that all formal matters are in order, or even a diagnosis is given, this often occurs. Often, we see a game of pushing responsibility between the parties involved, and I get the impression that many parties think what is most important is that they should not be responsible when something goes wrong. What becomes important in such demanding situations is that everyone involved meets up and clarifies each person's role and responsibility and that they agree on a common strategy, so that not one party is left with all the blame if, e.g., the patient dies from an overdose, commits suicide, or self-harms severely. If we manage to achieve a mutual understanding, colleagues become more confident, and they dare to take on more severely ill patients and achieve better results. This has a very positive effect on the patient, the results of treatment, and treatment costs. Disagreement and conflict across the different treatment systems or services contribute to exacerbating a crisis; agreement and calm help to dampen it. This is something we all concurrently across sections must take responsibility for.

Different Phases, Different Approaches

Not before I started working with people with SUD did I become aware that it is important to assess what stage in a process of change the patient is in, based on a transtheoretical approach (stages of change) [2, 3]. If we do not clarify this and therefore may implement interventions before the patient is ready for it, we achieve the opposite of what we intend. We push the patient in the wrong direction. If our interventions are implemented too early, the only thing we achieve is increasing resistance, diminished motivation, and drop-out. And if we are not aware of this, we do not discover what causes this resistance and will not be able to do anything about it. What one often spontaneously does when we experience resistance in the patient is to increase the "dose" of what we already have given. This only increases the problem further, and the patient could have had a better outcome without treatment at all. In addition to that, the patient risks being dismissed as unmotivated and/or having too much resistance. Also, the therapist risks becoming burned out. If, on the other hand, we have a clear focus on where the patient is in his process of change, so that we do things in the right order, the result will be far better.

It is my responsibility, as a therapist, to work to enhance motivation in the patient throughout the entire treatment process. We often assume or demand that patients are motivated for treatment and change when they seek treatment and are referred to specialist health services. It is not always so. There can be many reasons why people want treatment. If we start with assessment and treatment without checking that the patient is ready for it, we may risk the condition becomes worsened. It is important to take into account that the patient must go through his/her process of change, step by step, in his/her own time. We can enhance this process and in the worst case, reverse it. The first thing we must explore when we establish contact is where the patient is in the process of change.

Step one is to establish a working alliance, then focus on motivation for change. Only when this is in place, we can start active treatment interventions. How do we achieve this? Let's take a look at the different phases (also see overview of the phases in Table 2.1):

Table 2.1 An overview of the four phases, including keywords and points about signs, methods, traps, and more [4]

Engagement	Motivation	Active treatment	Relapse prevention
Goal: Developing a working alliance	Goal: Motivation/ starting to make a change	Goal: Making the desired change	Goal: Stabilizing and preventing relapse
Signs	Signs	Signs	Remember
I don't have a problem This information is not relevant for me There is no need for change The pros are larger than the cons Others believe I have a problem; I don't Behavioral change can appear when there is an external pressure, but the change is unstable and likely to reverse when the external pressure ceases to exist	Experiences negative consequences but is not certain how big the problem actually is Ambivalence—the current situation has both positive and negative consequences Considering change but is not certain Shifting in behavior and motivation Determination to go through with the change in the near future Making plans, such as setting a date for when to start Making small attempts to change Having beliefs and expectations about life after the change	A positive and optimistic phase The change becomes visible for others Reducing undesirable behavior Significant effort by the patient—a change of behavior, thinking and environment occurs Actively using coping strategies	All change is difficult—for everyone Starting to change does not equal permanent change Relapse is frequent. Try, and try again. Get back up on your feet!
Tools	Methods	Methods	Focus
Assistance and support in practical everyday tasks Offer something the person needs here and now Expect to be tested to see if you have what it takes/are up to the job	Motivational Interviewing The payoff matrix Emphasize the freedom to choose Develop new coping strategies	Stimulus control Replacement of behavior Positive enhancement Planning for possible relapse Active use of previous experiences	Making the change more robust Working on motivation to keep it strong Preventing relapse—identifying triggers Learning from the relapses—revise the plans Making changes in ways of life
Mechanisms/psychological defense	Traps	Traps	Common causes for relapse

(continued)

Table 2.1 (continued)

Engagement	Motivation	Active treatment	Relapse prevention
Goal: Developing a working alliance	Goal: Motivation/ starting to make a change	Goal: Making the desired change	Goal: Stabilizing and preventing relapse
Denial/Hesitation Rationalization/Justification Projection/Protest Introjection/tiredness and despair	Waiting for the magical moment Seeking 100% certainty Wishful thinking Searching for an impossible compromise Acting too early Giving advice/ helping the patient making good choices	Poor planning and preparation Few coping strategies—sticking with one strategy only Little investment in change I do as I have always done, although it was not successful	Social pressure Determination to change challenged by oneself Triggers or demanding situations become too challenging

The Engagement Stage

Without a working alliance, we get nowhere. The best way to establish this is to deliver something the patient is interested in right then and there. Often this is about practical help and support. It can be taking care of their physical health, ensuring that they get what they are entitled to in terms of benefits, helping to provide or maintain a residence or other practical matters, which we often do not define as a specialist service's responsibility at all. While we are performing these tasks, we get to know each other, we are tested by the patient if we measure up and can be trusted, and if we have something to contribute that they are interested in. It is not the level of education that determines whether we pass this test, but largely whether we can tolerate them and what they tell us and show us without going into negative reactions such as criticizing, aggression, moralizing, condemning, or reprimanding.

If I have not shown the patient during our time together that I can be trusted, neither will the feedback or interventions I present be received in a constructive way, but rather be seen as criticism and thus will cause a negative effect. When this turns around, for example, you can say to a patient: "Was it really wise that you had so much to drink before this important meeting today? It led to you not showing up," without it being perceived as offensive, but rather as a thought for reflection, as a constructive input. Then you have developed a working alliance and can continue providing feedback and input that can lead to change and not just result in increasing resistance. This also shows that the patient is in the next stage: the consideration phase (see the next paragraph). I am of the clear opinion that it is my responsability as a therapist to work to engage the patient in the treatment. It is not a given that the patient is engaged, motivated, or at all interested in treatment, even though they have asked for a referral. And if we work low-threshold and come into contact with people who we believe could benefit from interventions and even have a legal right to treatment, it often requires a lot to make the person engaged in the treatment. Many experience a great stigma when walking through the doors of a psychiatric clinic, and we must remember that many may have had negative experiences with various parts of the services. It is not a given that they want anything to do with us at all. It is my responsibility to work in a way that the most severely ill patients are more likely to accept starting treatment. If they should have a wish to start treatment, the application is often rejected. Unlike people with less severe conditions and a sorted life, they often have no one to plead their case in a way that the common pathway to treatment is possible. So that task is one we should take on as well. Acting as a spokesman or an ambassador.

Consideration (Motivation)

This phase is in the model called the persuasion phase, but I have taken the liberty to rename it the consideration phase. The reason for this is that attempts at persuasion can lead to people doing the exact opposite of what we try to persuade them to do. This is completely normal and applies to all of us. What we should practice is consideration; to help weigh the pros and cons of various alternatives and choices, preferably by working with ambivalence, for instance, using the payoff matrix (see Fig. 2.1). Something I am very concerned about is that we should not give advice. It is not my job, even if the patient asks for it. I can give people advice not to make important decisions when they are in the middle of a crisis, but I try to stick to that. "What would you have done, then?" many have asked me. It can be quite satisfying for a therapist to be in a situation where one is asked this question, but it is important not to be tempted to answer. Because I am in a completely different situation in life and make my choices based on completely different premises than the people I work

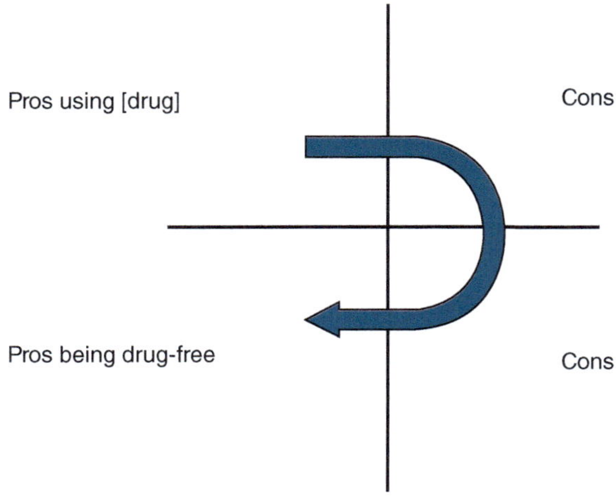

Fig. 2.1 A substance use variant of the payoff matrix

with do. Furthermore, it is the patient who will have to live with the consequences of their choice, and not me. My job is rather to clarify what are the advantages and disadvantages seen from the patient's perspective, and if I can contribute to the patient making a good choice based on their own premises, which they also can stand for later, when they maybe are unsure if it was so wise after all, I am satisfied. It is not uncommon for people to come back to me and believe that the choice they made was not the right one. In that case, it is important that I have not recommended an alternative or told them what to do, but play back that I can vouch for that they made a good choice based on the situation they were in when the choice was made, and that it was not possible to predict which way life has taken later on, which has made the choice later be questioned in doubt. A consequence of this thinking is that people become skilled in making good decisions for themselves and do not become dependent on an advisor. And for me self-help is an important goal in itself.

The goal of the consideration phase is that the patient becomes motivated for change. Many take this for granted when people seek help, and others require the patient to be motivated in a certain way, with little or no ambivalence, at the start of the treatment process. Whatever they mean by that. I believe that it is my job as a health professional to work to promote and enhance motivation in the patients I follow up. And this is something that must be done throughout the entire treatment course. If the patient's motivation declines, it is important that I notice it. And that I respond with motivation-promoting interventions and do not discharge the patient as unmotivated. Unfortunately, this happens not so rarely. But what does it mean to be motivated? And how do I know that it is the case? William Miller, one of the creators of Motivational Interviewing (MI), says that motivation is about something we do, not something we have. It is important to be aware that many of those we work with say what they have to say in order to get what they want. Many who have worked in social services have probably experienced this. It means that a statement from a patient about motivation does not necessarily mean that it is the case. Miller says that we should look for a change in behavior. When the patient actually drinks less before an important meeting, so that the meeting becomes feasible, it is an expression of motivation for change. Once I said to a patient: "If you meet well-adjusted to the appointments with me, you'll get much more out of the sessions," implying: It does not pay for you to be heavily under the influence or in withdrawal because then we do not get a good job done. When he actually did so, he was not visibly under the influence or abstinent, and the mental symptoms that he self-medicated for were not visible either. By doing this, he showed me he was motivated and had moved to the next phase:

Active Treatment

In this phase, you can apply specific treatment interventions, e.g., cognitive behavioral therapy (CBT), MI, and other interventions that are adapted to this stage. If we do this too early, we risk holding the patient back. Our well-intentioned and qualified measures will drive people backward in their process of change if we use them too early, before the patient is ready for them. They will only increase resistance, and we achieve the opposite of what we intended. The term treatment in this context, a range of different interventions and focus areas are included: traditional treatment, such as preferably combining CBT and MI, trauma focused therapy when indicated (e.g., EMDR, if the patient can tolerate this type of intervention), self-help groups, efforts aimed at work, leisure activities and social skills, adapted housing and measures to make everyday life work as well as possible, stress management and other coping strategies, medication for mental disorders and/or SUD and focus on family and network.

Thus, a very broad, multidisciplinary focus that includes both health and social areas and which is significantly broader than we are used to when it comes to treatment, especially in specialist services. It can be challenging but it is always possible if we put our best foot forward. How we can solve this will vary according to where we work. In some areas there are short distances and many residents, then this will not be the challenge. Other places have longer distances, but smaller and more manageable services. There is no guarantee that different services across sectors will see the necessity of working in close cooperation. There are various obstacles to this and uncovering what this is about and doing something about it, is part of the job. Anchoring upward in the management hierarchy and politically will always be a great advantage.

Relapse Prevention

The fourth and last stage is relapse prevention. Many patients have experienced that treatment is finished as soon as they have stopped using. For a lot, if not more or less all, this is when the real challenges begin. Memories come back, as well as nightmares. Feelings that have been masked reappear, and may well be hard to face, as they have no experience in that. The emotional numbness that often is necessary to carry out violent acts or being a sex worker, as well as several other, often antisocial, behaviors, is suddenly gone, and you have to live with your past under totally different circumstances. This is hard to deal with alone.

Everyday actions like making money last the whole month, filling your days with totally different things to do than before and other people to socialize with, managing living as substance free, dealing with psychiatric conditions that are unveiled, mastering being in conflicts and other types of stress, maybe go from a life that you mastered, even had a high status in, to being stigmatized and with a total lack of competence and predictability is a major challenge. And we need to address all these aspects to avoid relapses. If a relapse occurs, the patient will have a far better outcome if they have access to support. This can happen in relapse prevention groups, if possible, with a peer or with a therapist.

Detecting triggers that might lead to a relapse is part of this work. Is it when he/she is in possession of money, is in a conflict, experiences loss or failure, gets ill one way or the other, is exposed to substances, meets people from way back then, or what? Stress and being reminded of the past life have major parts here. What is stressful differs from one person to another, so writing down these individuals' stressors and how they have been dealt with previously is important. Reminding of good and bad outcomes is helpful. To analyze the options when a situation occurs, like using the payoff matrix for the specific situation, can clarify alternatives and consequences, challenge impulsivity, and calm down emotions. Then the way of dealing with difficult situations will be more about will and determination and less about impulsivity.

It is always best to negotiate in peaceful times—when life is less stressful, and thoughts are clearer- than in war, when level of stress is high, and thoughts are blurred and dominated by emotions rather than reason. To be well prepared is a good insurance against relapses.

Central Areas of Focus

Psychiatrist Robert Drake said in a lecture in 2000 that they in connection with the evaluation of the work they had done in New Hampshire came up with a handful of focus areas that are most important in order to get improvement: Working with the family and network of all patients, and if you can do a good job in three or four of the following four areas, the prognosis becomes significantly better: networking, housing, activity, and long-term contact with services.

Family and Network

This is useful. Very useful. It is clearly shown when it comes to young people who are developing schizophrenia, but I dare claim that it is useful for everyone, if it is feasible. Many patients do not want others involved, for example, the family, but that often change over time, so don't take no for an answer; try again later. People with SUD in addition to mental illness are possibly even more keen on keeping distance from others, both therapists, family, and network otherwise. It is important that we do not give up on thematizing this, offering services that are focused on information and education that is general, and that can be provided without hindrance of confidentiality. Again, it is so that knowledge does something with both how we react and how we act. It can reduce the degree of worrying and emotionality in others. And it may reduce the degree of negativity, something people with substance addiction, in particular, are facing.

Social networks are very important. We are all social beings, and living socially isolated is something most of us handle poorly. When the need arises to have someone there, to be with, do something together with, or to talk to, it is important to have a network that does not increase the likelihood of taking drugs when you are in contact with it. It does not have to be a drug-free network; there are many good friends who use drugs, but who do not use in the presence of vulnerable friends or act in another way that increases the risk of relapse.

Work and Leisure

People with substance addiction are often very busy people. It can take all their time to raise money, use, and recover from using drugs. If they manage to stop using drugs or to limit the intake, they get a lot of spare time, and they cannot fill their time the same way as before. Filling their time with something meaningful and constructive is important, but difficult. It can mean leisure activities, exercising, work, or work-like activity, or education. My experience is that establishing a good network and filling their days with meaningful activities are the hardest things to achieve in practice. There is now a lot of focus on providing people with regular work through job specialists who work according to the IPS model (Individual Placement and Support) and other work-oriented measures (read more about IPS and other work-oriented measures in Chap. 5). Being aware of which measures exist for your patients, therefore, becomes very important. An initiative I have particularly appreciated in Norway was a service by the *Church City Mission* in Bodø, where the goal was to provide people with a leisure activity. The first step was to discuss what activity to go for, and conclude with, e.g., judo. Then the local judo club was contacted to find someone who could be a mentor, who the patient could go to judo training together with and practice judo with the others in the local club, not to start an activity for people who had the same challenges. The initiative had a small budget, so they bought a judo suit and paid the membership fee to avoid personal finances as a hindrance to participate. This is one way you can work to integrate people into society and introduce them to arenas where they can build new networks in addition to filling their time with meaningful activities.

Suitable Housing

A proper place to live, where you are not evicted if you use substances, if applicable, or where you are shielded from drugs if that is the right thing, is important for success in change toward improvement. It could be a residence with or without stationary staff, a residence in a regular residential area, or the opposite, a low-threshold residence where people with major problems with drugs, aggression, and other behavioral problems can live. A particular challenge is people with moderate or severe personality disorders, with antisocial traits combined with, e.g., low negative affectivity and disinhibition. They will be able to undermine any living environment and may act destructively in many ways. Individuals with such severely dysfunctional interpersonal styles must be housed outside housing facilities to avoid destroying them.

When people are to be housed, it is important with all the practicalities, such as informing the proper people and services about moving, applying for state and municipal housing support, getting help with the deposit, and practically for the move. If they have the opportunity to get support from the municipality to buy some furniture, it can be very useful that they get assistance both to apply for support and in spending it so that the money lasts as long as possible. There is a lot of usable stuff in second-hand stores, and a lot is given away, often provided you can pick it up. Access to a car is then important. It is also important with janitorial services, among other things, so that the washing machine can be installed according to regulations and other practicalities getting settled. I have met many who never really settled in because these offers do not exist. This can negatively affect people's experience of their own value, and not being able to actually settle in can contribute to the heightened risk of relapses. Other things to consider are: Should my name be on the doorbell? Should my address be visible on the internet? Who should know where I am moving? Should I change my phone number?

It is also an art to follow people up—in a co-located residence and elsewhere. A certain number of individuals say no to most things. That doesn't necessarily mean we should accept that no: It is important to be able to maneuver yourself into position over time, so a collaboration becomes possible. A couple of important clinical points related to this are:

(a) If the individual nevertheless refuses to accept services, it is important to assess the person's ability to consent regarding this specific decision.
(b) If the individual's decision is based on what is considered to be a psychotic belief, it should not be automatically taken literally.
(c) If the individual does not foresee the consequences of their choice when assessed, likewise.

Further, there are several important points related to the capacity to consent according to guidance in Norway [5]:

1. Ability to understand information that is relevant to the decision.
2. Ability to acknowledge this information as relevant in their situation and seeing the consequences of the various alternatives.
3. Ability to resonate with relevant information when weighing various alternatives.
4. Ability to express a choice.

It is, of course, important that one carries out the assistance in a proper and strategic way, but one should, in situations where the individual is not to be taken literally, not let oneself be rejected as easily as I often see. Taking people literally is not taking people seriously when they are not able to make a proper choice. And I am often told that the individual must be motivated and must want the intervention themselves. Such a statement or attitude from the staff tends to act as an excuse or camouflage to not keep on trying or try to find a good strategy to achieve collaboration.

Many are concerned with something they call skills of everyday life. If a person does not have such skills, I often get the impression that the staff means that the patient has to manage themselves as best they can. Many service providers are not willing to compensate for permanently reduced function, only to contribute to training and practice for rehabilitation purposes. What I generally have problems with is that we must be aware that when I define something as not to be my job, I must make sure that someone else is ready to take over, otherwise the individual will suffer. It is not obvious that the municipality will grant help at home if you live in a residence with stationary staff, just as they will deny home nursing, often with the justification that there are nurses employed in the residence. It is often the case that there is not a nurse on all hours who can do advanced wound care or hand out medication. We must remember that it is constantly emphasized by politicians and central authorities in some countries that you should have the same health care no matter where you live in the country. This applies also in residences for people with SUD/MH. So, if you choose to die of cancer at home where you feel safe, it should be obvious that you should get the assistance necessary, in the same way as if you were to live in your own home. This is not always obvious in my experience, and we who work with individuals in this situation often have to fight to get approval for such help. Read more about housing and supported housing in Chap. 4.

Long-Term Contact

The fourth domain, which has a high correlation with good results, is long-term contact.

It is not so important with whom the contact is, as long as it is a steady person who is there over a long time. This can have several functions, including identifying change, which is then held up and clarified for the patient. This person can remember previous coping skills demonstrated, which often go into oblivion for the patient. Change happens slowly and often in bits and parts, and in my experience, it is common that it dawns on the patient and/or me that an important change has taken place when a person suddenly handles a demanding situation in a different and better way than before. When I comment on such a change, I often get the answer: "Oh damn. I had forgotten that." I have experienced the same type of response when someone brought up something they dread or are afraid of not coping with or achieving—and I recall previous experiences where they have indeed managed something equivalent in a good way: "Oh damn. I had forgotten that." This can even happen when the change has been quite extensive, so one would think it was obvious that it was apparent to the patient. An example: A man was denied access to social services because contact with the case worker always ended with him making death threats. After many years of great change, he came to me once after he had had a busy day where he had spoken with many public agencies, including the case worker at social services, face-to-face. He stopped by the office at the end of the day and complained that it had been a tiring day and concluded that he didn't think he could handle this anymore because it was so exhausting. When I reminded him of the situation when we met, he responded that he had forgotten that, was very pleased, and left with a sense of accomplishment.

Other Important Focus Areas

Self-Help Groups

Self-help groups, e.g., Alcoholics Anonymous (AA) and Narcotics Anonymous (NA), are part of the toolbox. Sometimes information and motivation are needed for it to be possible to try out. Different groups can function quite differently, so if you don't find yourself comfortable in one group, you can try another, if there are alternatives nearby. Self-help groups are not for everyone, but everyone should try them, so that they themselves can experience how the groups work for them before they make a decision whether to continue or not.

Medication Treatment

Medication treatment is part of a larger whole. It can provide a significant contribution, but often only marginally, although still helpful. The expectations, on the other hand, for medication can be very high, among patients, family and friends, caregivers, and colleagues. Before starting any treatment, it is important to clarify what realistic expectations can be had for the treatment, that the effect can vary significantly from person to person, and side effects likewise. If the patient uses drugs, even sporadically, it is important to assess the pattern of use, so the choice of medication can be adapted to it. Otherwise, we may risk getting negative consequences of the combination—lethal even—or that the patient discontinues the medication in connection with drug use. If this happens too often, the patient will end up with a mixture of side effects after starting up, after discontinuation, effects of drugs, withdrawal, and no effect of the medication. Often it is helpful to start dosing low and increase slowly, because many people in this group are very sensitive to both the effect and side effects. Following ordinary practice will therefore often lead to negative experiences with the medication in question and thus lead to denying trying it on a later stage. (See more about this later in this chapter.) Likewise, patients, family, other network and/or actual experience in the past may hinder trying out possibly helpful medication. Thus, the matter of medication has to be handled carefully in order not to miss any opportunities.

It is my responsibility as a therapist to achieve as valid answers as possible from the patient. I cannot expect to get more accurate answers on drug use than I deserve. If the patient fears negative consequences of giving accurate information (I try to avoid using words like truthful and honest; they bring in a moral dimension that can have a negative effect in this context), they will of course underreport, as everyone else, and I will be at risk of giving poor and in worst case possibly harmful treatment. It doesn't help that the instruments (screening, diagnostic interview) I use have good psychometric properties, if the result is that the patient risks losing something they want to keep, such as treatment in mental health care and therefore give a response that is tailored and does not reflect reality. It is therefore vital that I take responsibility for the communication; that it is clear, unambiguous and not to be misunderstood, and that all relevant information comes through. And further clarify that they do not risk losing something they want to keep if the answer reflects what actually happened. Furthermore, I will not react with any kind of negative reaction to any information they give. Getting information that reflects reality is my responsibility, and something I must earn.

There is much to be written about medication treatment, but I can only highlight some issues that I have found important:

Physicians who medicate SUD/MH patients must ensure that they have knowledge about how drugs and medications interact with each other and other conditions that affect how the medications work on the patient.

The more severe a mental illness is, the more vulnerable the brain is. That means that the patient often both needs and tolerates medications in lower doses than others. They often get both significant effects and harmful side effects at lower doses than others and also side effects that others rarely get. Other conditions that affect how much the brain tolerates and needs can be brain injuries of various kinds, developmental disabilities, autism spectrum disorders, old age, and the stage of the disease the patient is in. Many are over-medicated because they get a standard dosage, especially at the start of a mental crisis. Many are not tapered down when the crisis is about to subside and remain on too high doses over time. Regarding psychotic disorders, it is recommended that people receive the lowest possible effective dose, and this is often violated. The consequences of overdosing can be misinterpreted as increasing symptoms; hence, the dose is increased instead of decreased, and the condition worsens. When people get too high a dose, also due to medication interaction with drugs, and therefore often get unacceptable side effects, it may lead to them no longer wanting to take the medication in question. For many SUD/MH patients, there are limitations in terms of what medication can be used safely, and it is therefore important that we retain the options that exist and do not make patients unnecessarily dismiss certain medications. It takes away an important room for action later. Something else that is important to consider is that some people have mutations in the enzyme system in the liver that breaks down medications. These mutations can lead to increased or reduced breakdowns and can have a significant impact on whether the medications work or give disproportionately strong side effects.

The Importance of Cross-Sectoral Collaboration

My experience is that the closer we work together between the various services, the easier the collaboration will prove to be. Proximity and familiarity are of great advantage here. We will soon discover that we are not as different as we might think, and we will discover how great the advantage is when different parts of the services collaborate closely. This provides good patient care, a good overview of the available options, and efficient resource utilization. The years I worked in the *Collaboration Team in Bærum (SiB)*, this was shown with all possible clarity. The team was composed of employees from all the outpatient services in the catchment area and all the ambulatory services in the municipality. In addition, we had people from social services and the office responsible for housing in the team. The team was matrix-organized, and all members of the team retained their original employment relationship in the municipality, social services, or specialist health care. Thus, we avoided a long time before startup during hiring, we retained the local anchoring, we achieved a dispersion effect into the different parts of the service apparatus, we avoided undignified pushing between units about who is responsible, and we avoided a long winding-up period when project funding was nearing the end. A general practitioner who came to the team to discuss a difficult case said enthusiastically when he found out who was sitting around the table: This is fantastic! The table catches. The table cannot say no, because all relevant services are represented around the table. This meant that a lot of time and focus were freed up when we did not first have to clarify who was responsible. Ideally, in most cases, responsibility was shared between more services. Furthermore, we could easily and without formalities involve colleagues with different competencies and anchoring in another service when needed. And this was often useful. As a psychiatric nurse working in a municipality said: It is so much easier to work now, because if we need a psychiatrist's assessment, we can just talk to a doctor in the team. Usually, we have to motivate the patient to go to the general practitioner (GP) (read more about the GP role in Chap. 8), we have to work for the GP to write a good application that describes the challenges the patient is facing, then the application must be assessed, and if the patient turns out to have legal right to treatment, it is not certain that it is a doctor who becomes the therapist, or that the doctor who is involved, has sufficient knowledge about what is necessary.

Certain areas in a country may have large distances between services, and the population lives scattered. The work must then be organized in a different way, depending on which resources are available and how they are organized. The principles of treatment are the same, but the way the treatment can be set up will necessarily be completely different and vary from one place to another. The dependence on good anchoring in the management becomes even greater, as more municipalities may become involved, and the dependence on individuals in the services becomes large, and thus the vulnerability increases.

Motivational Interviewing

Motivational Interviewing (MI) and preferably simultaneously or integrated with cognitive behavioral therapy (CBT) is a specific intervention recommended in the treatment of people with SUD/MH in Norway [6]. I myself use MI to a small extent in its strict form as treatment. On the other hand, I have noticed that the longer I have worked in this field, the more this way of communicating influences the dialogue with my patients. I have become more laid back, focusing more on letting the patient come forward; I extract information instead of giving information, and if I want to inform about something, I first ask if it is okay. I am less pushy and insistent, and thus more easily avoid building up resistance. Yes—I avoid building up resistance in the patient. Resistance is something that belongs to both the therapist and the patient; it is not reserved for the patient. It is my responsibility as a therapist to recognize when resistance is building up, in order to try finding its cause and reducing it. Otherwise, the process of change stops. And, yes, I am not perfect, I make mistakes, and I overlook things. And this may have a negative impact on the treatment process. When I notice this, often with the help of the patient, it is my responsibility to do something about it—and it is certainly not to discharge the patient due to resistance or lack of motivation. Ask the patient for an apology and then for permission to try again in a different way. It is never a bad thing to apologize when there is a reason for it. On the contrary, it is correct—not only because there is a reason for it and it is common politeness, but I also show that I am not infallible. I present myself as someone who does not just sit as a know-it-all on my high horse and never make mistakes, but more as an equal person. The goal is not to be error-free, but to make smaller mistakes—a little less often.

We are often seen by the patients we work with as experts, and that may hinder efficient treatment caused by the great difference in status or importance. Good communication and respect develop best between equal parties, and I am therefore aware that I need to tone down my own significance and elevate the patient's. Believing that we become totally equal is not right, but more equality will promote cooperation and development. It can be about, as mentioned above, that I do not let myself be tempted to give advice, that I emphasize when the patient shows mastery and motivation, and remind them of early experiences with this, that I identify and show change to the patient to visualize the development. It can be done through me being clear that self-help is in focus, and that it is not my omnipotent interventions that are decisive for improvement.

In MI, part of the method is to clarify the patient's own goals in life. Not what they think I, the network, or the society around them expects. But the patient's own, egocentric goals. The reason for this is that it has been shown that this is what represents the highest motivation for change. Once this is done, the path to personal goals should be broken down into manageable steps or sub-goals, so that the entire project of change does not become overwhelming. It is important here not to confront the patient about how unrealistic we see these goals. Many have a goal of becoming a therapist. This should not be met with destructive comments about the realism of this but start by asking if the person has the competence to enter university. Or has finished middle school. And then we start, preferably in collaboration with the county school superintendent, to take one subject at a time and work our way from there. Then the goal will often change along the way as the patients have their own experiences. That being said, it is not so rare that the patient can achieve their own goals when it comes to education or other goals, no matter how unlikely I have seen this in advance. It then becomes very clear how important it has been that I have not been an active brake on this path, and that treatment is not time-limited.

The payoff matrix [7] (see Fig. 2.1), a useful way to explore ambivalence, can be a very important tool in decision-making or a change process, regardless of what is relevant to change or make an important decision about. It can apply to all important choices in life for all of us. It's about setting up pros and cons for maintaining the status quo and change.

It is demanding to do such an analysis in a constructive way by only thinking it through. Putting it in writing can be of great help. Many of the patients I work with have challenges with concentration, attention span, memory, and writing down the arguments—pros and cons—to visualize the different arguments, then becomes important in the process of making a valid decision. In addition, the different arguments must be weighed in relation to each other, so this is a demanding process. By using this simple tool, you only need a sheet of paper or a whiteboard. The intention is to empower the patient to make difficult choices and make them more independent of us. We then counteract a common side effect of being in treatment: dependence on a helper or advisor.

This brings me to the next topic.

Psychoeducation

I have a firm belief in competent patients with a competent network around them. The more the individual knows about themselves, their illness, what makes it better, and what makes it worse, the better they can sit at the helm. When a patient comes to me after they experienced early signs of a relapse and reports what has happened and how they managed the situation so that they avoided a full-blown relapse, I am satisfied. It shows that I am becoming redundant. That being said, it does not necessarily mean that the patient should be discharged, at least if that is not what they themselves want. It is important that the "reward for success" is not being discharged—then many will resist improvement, and we will not get any effect from the treatment.

There are many setups for psychoeducation, often group-based. The major point here is that the patients and the network around them learn what is relevant for better disease management and understanding. It is also a point that you get the opportunity to practice difficult situations in a safe setting, for example, initiating a conversation or declining offers of substances. It is, of course, also fully possible to focus on learning and empowerment during consultations under four eyes, so this can also be an element in individual follow-up.

I mentioned IMR earlier in this chapter, which is also related to this topic. This is an approach to recovery that, in my opinion, is very suitable for these patients. It is a concept composed of many modules, a composition that has proven to be both good and effective. The focus is on knowledge about, and management of mental illness and SUD, and the idea is that the better you manage your health issues, the more surplus you get to work with your own life goals, and in that way work on your own recovery.

The Importance of Continuity

The single factor that has the highest correlation with a positive result is long-term contact, Robert Drake said in a lecture in 2000. Not necessarily with a therapist in specialist health services, preferably one from the municipality or an assertive outreach team. A person that is good for you and with whom you have contact over a long period of time. I myself have had contact with—and then I'm not necessarily talking about active treatment—patients for many years; many in a decade, others more. I have found that it takes a long time to build a relationship, especially if a patient has a severe mental disorder and has been in treatment for a long time. It is said that it can take up to a year to develop a relationship with a person with a psychotic disorder. I have heard from environmental therapists in municipal services that building relationships with SUD/MH patients can take up to 3–4 years. I have experienced the same when it comes to building relationships with people who have been in treatment for many years. This again implies that it is important to think about long-term relations, not least when considering applying for a job where you will work with people with long-lasting conditions. When choosing to take people in this population group into treatment, we take on a great responsibility. It's not just about bringing someone in for therapy for a few weeks and then evaluating and ending it if you don't achieve sufficient change. The cost-benefit of the treatment will, in many cases, only show after a long time. In several cases, it will take a long time to develop a working alliance, and it will take a long time to achieve change. Recognizing that something is changing when change happens so slowly is an art in itself. But it's very important to keep up the morale of both the patient and the therapist. This may be particularly true in municipal services, which often offer services to people indefinitely, such as the FACT teams are supposed to do (read more about ACT and FACT teams in Chap. 12). Therefore, it becomes especially important to focus on the evaluation of interventions and their effects. I was taught that a reasonable interval between evaluations could be 6 weeks, both for medical treatment and other interventions. For those with long-term, co-occurring disorders, this is far too short a time to be aware of change. Short intervals between evaluations will lead to change not being detected, giving up, or possibly the staff—and everyone else around—losing motivation. Six months to a year may be a more suitable interval between evaluations. Only after such a long time will we be able to see changes in important areas. And when working with people as long as I have, in many cases, it is striking how much can be achieved. If you just give the patient enough time. There are no quick fixes here: Change takes a long time, so cost-benefit considerations must be made with this in mind. Another important matter is that many of the commonly used assessment scales are not helpful here. They are made for people with much less severe illnesses and loss of functioning. So, if a patient is in the more severe end of the scale, a really significant change must take place before it results in a higher score.

The importance of long-term contact implies that the most important close contact in the services must be in a municipal service or, e.g., an ACT/FACT team. The specialist health service can certainly be nearby—with supervision and maybe a consultation with the patient now and then. In these cases, observations over time and the information I get from colleagues who follow the patient closely over time, for example in a supported housing or an outpatient service, will be the most important factors when I summarize, assess and evaluate a patient. Sessions face to face with the patient will not provide nearly as good information, although this is also important. I have worked closely with community services for many years. Having contact with a patient group "a little at a distance" in this way is in my opinion a very cost-effective way to use my specialist resource. The better I get to know the patient and those who follow up the closest, the better assessments I will be able to make, also with as little use of time as possible. Weekly sessions in my office, as I am trained in, are not a good framework for treating people who have had serious illnesses over a long period of time. Just the fact that I have said hello to people and chatted informally with the residents when I am in a housing facility for meetings and supervision, will often make it much easier for me to position myself if I am to intervene in a crisis. The same is likely to happen if I have a good relation to the staff in the initiative. Accordingly, when it comes to patients in the team I work in; when a colleague has developed an alliance with a patient, much of the relationship building is done for my part already. And not least—if I get a good reputation among the patients, it is very beneficial in building relationships to new patients.

I have experienced more than once that trust that usually takes a very long time to develop, can be established quite quickly if I am recommended by other patients. I recently experienced that an elderly man, who previously has had many negative experiences with the healthcare system, was showing that a working alliance was established after just a short period of trying me out and testing me. We then did a great job focusing on assessment and further treatment in just three sessions. He unexpectedly accepted to take antidepressants that work only after quite some time, which is often a big achievement in itself, and many times is not feasible at all. The SUD consultant for many years was present at the first session, the next two we had alone. This was clearly due to the fact that the patient knows many of my former patients, and that the SUD consultant from the municipality was part of the team and therefore had worked closely with me over time.

I have seen that even in young people, with relatively short experience in the treatment system, change can take a long time. When I worked at the *SUD Psychiatry Ward (Nordland Hospital Trust)*, which started up in early 2006, most of the patients were under 20 years old. What we did was to do a good and thorough diagnostic and functional assessment during hospitalization. Some were readmitted once or twice, but the point here is that we focused strongly on establishing relevant, long-lasting, and robust resources around the patient in the local community after discharge. This led to the admission in our department, which only gave a good start, while the rest—and most—of the further improvement happened locally over several years after discharge. This is a reminder that it is important to educate and support the staff that follow up with patients over time locally, where life is lived, to get the full effect of the treatment.

Health workers in the community, in my experience, do not often have very high thoughts about themselves and their utility, but it is my belief that it is the local services that are of greatest value when it comes to developing the full potential of the individual. Note that the patient has been admitted to a very competent institution or is seeing a specialist for a limited period. As mentioned, they can help give a good start to a positive development, but the greatest and most important job, which releases the greatest potential for improvement, happens locally, where real life is lived, not in an artificial setting in a hospital ward. A solid and close cooperation between these services, and not least with the GP, is of the utmost importance. It doesn't matter how competent the treatment you can get in the specialist health service is, if the services in the municipality are not coordinated and can follow up on the good work over a long time. The demands of all parts of the services are organized for efficiency, productivity, and circulation, also often in the community-based services, and a great focus on cost–benefit is a huge obstacle for people with severe and complex disorders over a long time to get a realistic opportunity for assessment and treatment that works. The paradox is that in my country, it is precisely this group of patients that, according to different types of official country-wise statements in recent decades, should be highly prioritized.

Our Hidden Knowledge

It is important that we acknowledge that everyone who works in the field has relevant and important knowledge and experience, and that we must create professional environments that are broadly composed of people with different educational backgrounds and work experience. The more the merrier. In this way, we will be able to complement each other and not compete with each other, which is absolutely essential to be able to develop robust, qualified teams that provide good services. We have a lot to learn from each other, regardless of background and experience, and to exploit this in the best possible way, it is important that we develop teams with members who feel safe and able. This is a responsibility not only for the team leader, but for all team members. The fact that it is not only allowed for everyone to come forward with their view, but a clear expectation is important. Then it is important that every opinion that comes forward is taken seriously and included as relevant in the discussion. The more views and opinions that come forward, the better. The best view of the patient lies in the sum of everyone's observations and assessments, and it is therefore important that everyone gets to come forward with theirs. Only then do we get access to as many perspectives, possible ways of understanding, and possible ways of targeting treatment as possible. Only then can we create hypotheses and decide on interventions on the broadest possible basis, and these become even better. That being said, it is important to evaluate after a certain time, to then change the hypothesis and strategy if necessary. But in the meantime, it is absolutely vital that everyone adheres to what plans and strategies the team has agreed on and does not go their own way if they have not been heard—in this round. Otherwise, we lose some of the best that teamwork has to offer. And the patient may suffer through the treatment plan being undermined and thus becoming worse.

Another thing that I became very aware of when I started working with SUD/MH patients was that I had much more knowledge than I was aware of. It is so easy to be blind to the differences between us and others, so it is important to focus on what is similar rather than the differences. Then the challenges are not insurmountable. Everyone who works in this field has a background where we know a lot about people; it's just that we have seen people from slightly different angles and with different glasses. This means that we are often more qualified than we first think of. When I was approved as a specialist in psychiatry, I had no knowledge about illegal drugs and drug addictions. But I knew a lot about medication and brain function, and not least about what it is like to be a human being. This was much more applicable working with SUD/MH patients than I was aware of, and after a while, I just had to admit that I knew much more than I was aware of at first.

Over the years, I have been in contact with many competent professionals, and it is so sad to see how many trivialize their own knowledge and their impact on the patients we work with. So not only to help make each other better, but to show each other how competent we actually are, I have become very concerned about. There is enormous potential for change in a well-functioning housing facility and other services, which often are not intended to conduct active treatment; their task is to assist in everyday life. But competent professionals who work under good conditions have a huge influence on the patients they work with. And the potential for change is great. The time horizon is usually significantly longer in a service in a municipality than in a specialist inpatient or outpatient clinic, and it is precisely a long-term perspective that many are dependent on to achieve change. Time is essential. I have worked in inpatient units in the specialist service, and what we achieved there was certainly not to fully treat people. We can do a good assessment and start up treatment, but the patient is usually not fully recovered. There is no time for that, it is not necessary, and long admissions could involve major side effects, such as dependency on services and lack of independence, institutionalization, and loss of function. If we manage to transfer patients from specialist inpatient units to community treatment, which in turn works well, we will often be able to achieve significant change. But it takes time. Often a long time—it can take several years. And with fewer side effects, at a lower cost, and with less use of resources.

Do Not Blame the Patient

Finally, I want to address something that the pioneers of integrated treatment, Robert Drake and Kim Mueser, are concerned about: blaming. There has for many years been a lot of discussion about who is to blame for mental illness in patients, and when people with SUD/MH were also defined as being the responsibility of mental health care, the topic of blaming has not become less. It is still the case that SUD is largely seen as a moral condition. Where one can easily come to believe that the patient is to blame for their own condition and lack of improvement. When the HIV epidemic came, it became very clear to me a distinction between the innocently affected and those who were to blame for being infected themselves. Drug addicts and homosexuals were in the latter group. And that's how many drug addicts are seen even today. They are to blame for the addiction themselves. Drake and Mueser are concerned that we should disregard this tendency of blaming; blaming you for being addicted to drugs, blaming you for relapses, and that you do not stop using. I do not know the evidence for their view, but I am painfully aware that it does a lot with me in the encounter with people with SUD if I manage to meet them like this: without blaming them for that they have a SUD and without blaming them for not being able to benefit from the treatment I provide. Lack of treatment effect is primarily my responsibility and should lead me to reconsider my treatment strategy, seek advice and supervision, or supplement the treatment with another professional—not blaming or discharging the patient.

Summary

Treatment services, policies, and procedures should support an integrated treatment approach, including linkages to complementary services within and outside the health sector. The key elements in integrated treatment (IDDT), an approach that provides a unified message about treatment and recovery, are:

- Simultaneous treatment, where long-term treatment is more the rule than the exception: Address mental health, substance use, and physical health concurrently, including the dynamics between health issues.
- Holistic view: Address the individual's needs, including physical, emotional, and social aspects.
- Comprehensive approach: Consider all factors contributing to the individual's well-being.
- Coordinated care of interdisciplinary teams or cross-sectoral groups.

Reflection Questions

- In what way does the content of this chapter contradict what you have learned and experienced before?
- Is there anything in this chapter that you strongly disagree with or provoke you? Why?
- What are the inhibitors and promoters for it to be possible to work according to the principles described in this chapter (available resources, attitudes, values, willingness to help people with compounded challenges, budget, investment hinders, implementation competency, and more)?

Recommended Literature and Online Resources

- Enhancing Motivation for Change in Substance Use Disorder Treatment (SAMHSA, 2019). Available at https://library.samhsa.gov/sites/default/files/tip-35-pep19-02-01-003.pdf
- Illness Management and Recovery IMR Revised (Hazelden Publishing, 2015).
- Integrated Dual Disorders Treatment Revised (Hazelden Publishing, 2015).
- International Standards for the Treatment of Drug Use Disorders (World Health Organization, 2020). Available at https://www.who.int/publications/i/item/international-standards-for-the-treatment-of-drug-use-disorders
- Practical, printable poster with overview of the Integrated Dual Disorder Treatment (IDDT) phases: https://www.oslo-universitetssykehus.no/4ab147/contentassets/11f9dc10dbf5444c9cc0619491a1f612/iddt-stadieplakat-a3_engelsk_v2.pdf
- Substance Use Disorder Treatment for People with Co-Occurring Disorders (2020, SAMHSA). Available at https://library.samhsa.gov/sites/default/files/pep20-02-01-004.pdf

References

1. Sæland M. Eating on the Edge. A study focusing on dietary habits and nutritional status among illicit drug addicts in Oslo, Norway (Doctoral thesis). Oslo: University of Oslo; 2014. Available at https://www.duo.uio.no/handle/10852/38902.
2. Prochaska JO, DiClemente CC, Norcross JC. In search of how people change: applications to addictive behaviors. Am Psychol. 1992;47(9):1102–14.
3. Prochaska JO, Carlo C, DiClemente CC. The transtheoretical approach. In: Norcross JC, Goldfried MR, editors. Handbook of psychotherapy integration. 3rd ed. New York: Oxford Academic; 2019.
4. Norwegian National Advisory Unit on Concurrent Substance Abuse and Mental Health Disorders. IDDT poster; 2023. https://www.oslo-universitetssykehus.no/4ab147/contentassets/11f9dc10dbf5444c9cc0619491a1f612/iddt-stadieplakat-a3_engelsk_v2.pdf. Accessed 21 May 2025.
5. The Norwegian Directorate of Health. § 4-3 Hvem som har samtykkekompetanse. Helsedirektoratets kommentarer [§ 4-3 Who has the capacity to consent. The Directorate of Health's comments]. 2018. https://www.helsedirektoratet.no/rundskriv/pasient-og-brukerrettighetsloven-med-kommentarer/samtykke-til-helsehjelp/hvem-som-har-samtykkekompetanse. Accessed 21 May 2025.
6. The Norwegian Directorate of Health. Nasjonal faglig retningslinje for utredning, behandling og oppfølging av personer med samtidig ruslidelse og psykisk lidelse – ROP-lidelser. Sammensatte tjenester – samtidig behandling. (IS-1948) [National guideline for the assessment, treatment and follow-up of people with co-occurring substance use disorder and mental illness – dual diagnosis. Compounded services – co-occurring treatment. (IS-1948)]; 2012. https://www.helsedirektoratet.no/retningslinjer/samtidig-ruslidelse-og-psykisk-lidelse-rop-lidelser/Utredning,%20behandling%20og%20oppf%C3%B8lging%20av%20personer%20med%20ROP-lidelser%20%E2%80%93%20Nasjonal%20faglig%20retningslinje%20(fullversjon).pdf/_/attachment/inline/c3cf6958-227f-499a-8f0b-0055dca9fc2c:286222117d81c9f269cddbee85a495a47bf9df29/Utredning,%20behandling%20og%20oppf%C3%B8lging%20av%20personer%20med%20ROP-lidelser%20%E2%80%93%20Nasjonal%20faglig%20retningslinje%20(fullversjon).pdf. Accessed 21 May 2025.
7. Barth T, Näsholm C. Motiverende samtale – MI. Endring på egne vilkår [Motivational Interviewing – MI. Change on your own terms]. Bergen: Fagbokforlaget; 2007.

Screening and Assessment

3

Tore Willy Lie

Abstract

The chapter begins with an introduction to mental disorders, followed by an overview of screening and mapping within primary care services, as well as the referral process. The final and most extensive section delves into various aspects of conducting specialist assessments. This includes recommended instruments, cultural factors, differential diagnosis, the way forward after assessments, and more. It is about what goes on during the assessment, the outcome and usefulness of it, and an ongoing process to re-evaluate. The chapter underlines that assessments should take a wide array of factors and perspectives into account, where the goal is new or updated interventions and treatment plans that are informed by the individual's cultural and social context.

Keywords

Assessment · Differential diagnosis · Substance-induced mental disorders · Mental health screening · Assessment instruments · Substance use disorder · Mental disorder · Diagnostic interviews · Neuropsychological assessment

We usually recognize things that we are used to seeing, hence it can be a short way to conclude that substance use may seem like *the* single problematic factor in a cause-effect explanation for the observable or expressed suffering. Problem areas and symptoms associated with substance use have a tendency to get the most attention. It gives a risk of quick and long-term conclusion (sometimes with a moral

T. W. Lie (✉)
Department of Health and Nursing Sciences and Section for Mental Health and Rehabilitation, University of Inland Norway, Elverum, Norway
e-mail: tore.lie@inn.no

T. W. Lie, L. Lien (eds.), *Integrated Treatment of Co-occurring Substance Use and Mental Health Disorders*, https://doi.org/10.1007/978-3-032-20049-5_3

dimension) by health and welfare services that the current condition is primarily substance use related, where heavy substance use hinders useful interventions, and thereby, nothing or little can be done. The same problem is also noticeable vice versa, when certain mental symptoms are most conspicuous, where we may miss how heavy substance use affects the current condition. Summarized, there are many different stories behind suboptimal assessments. They have in common that it most often leads to treatment planning that is not being adapted according to the individual's needs. This implicates a high risk of personal consequences, with harmful or wrong interventions, worsening of health, repeatedly missed opportunities (which can lessen help-seeking behavior), including persistent and eventually heightened strain, e.g., for caregivers and local communities.

It is important to be aware that approximately half of those who have had a SUD during their lives have also had one or more mental disorders, and approximately half of those who have had a mental disorder during their lives have also had one or more substance use disorders [1, 2]. Another important treatment aspect is that untreated mental disorders can cause substance use relapses. Further, the substance effects can resemble, cover up, or increase many mental disorder symptoms during intoxication and withdrawal. Another point is that substance use can exacerbate other mental disorders, the mental disorders can worsen substance use, or they can mutually worsen each other. There may also be other complicating factors related to social exclusion and conflicts, trouble with housing, and personal finances. This usually contributes to more stress, which characterizes and maintains multifaceted suffering. Substance use can also contribute to or induce medical problems, which in turn can trigger mental symptoms as part of the medical condition. The symptoms can also be secondary to the medical condition, that is, you get mental health problems due to stress related to the medical problem. This, in turn, can reinforce or maintain the substance use problem if the medical problem remains untreated. All this strongly implies that a basic starting point and attitude for all services is that you must maintain curiosity on, treat, and follow-up on all relevant problem areas at the same time.

For various reasons, it can be a very time-and-resource demanding step-by-step process to get an alliance and know a patient, and get an overview and process all the relevant information for both the clinician and the patient. Taking this into account, it is reasonable from a patient's perspective to expect multidisciplinary competence from services that offer assessments, and that the services have enough time and patience for the patients to feel safe and ready to talk about personal themes, and have room for action to continuously handle feasibility-threatening circumstances.

Assessments can be a very important process for the patient in terms of improving quality of life in the short- and/or long-term and trying to stop, avoid, or limit the risk of insufficient or incorrect interventions and cross-sectional dynamics that might already have occurred for a certain time. The word "assessment" in this context can be categorized into at least three variants. The first is the usual time-limited process, which can provide an overview of life history and the current state of physical and mental health, life quality overall, strengths, and needs. A second approach is what can be called an "on and off" assessment process, e.g., by outreach multidisciplinary teams, where an assessment is carried out situationally or periodically over, e.g., a 12-month period, because of feasibility issues. The third variant is that assessment is also a continuous process independent of having a planned, structured specialist assessment, where the treatment plan is re-evaluated and adjusted in the light of how different aspects of the patient's life change over a longer period of time, or more precisely, detailed information becomes available.

What Are Mental Disorders?

All people categorize experiences and phenomena and develop a common language as an attempt to understand the world. Categorization reduces complexity and can provide both rough and detailed overviews. Mental disorders (diagnosis) are descriptive categories, where each diagnosis has a set of criteria that attempt to atheoretically describe separate conditions without providing explanations. Before diagnosing a mental disorder, it must often be assessed whether the symptoms can be better explained by a medical condition, medication, or substance use, and in some cases, cultural aspects. Further, a diagnosis does not have a one-to-one relationship with the need for a specific treatment intervention, and considering the need for a type of treatment and follow-up is a complex decision-making process [3]. You can generally see diagnosis as a pattern recognition model where the main goal is clinical utility, which involves various value judgments about what counts as dysfunctional, harmful, or abnormal. This point was underlined in the revision process for ICD-11, where the highest priority in the construction of the diagnostic guidelines and requirements was to maximize clinical utility [4]. Another point is that assessment is not only about the diagnostic process, but it is a necessary piece. It is also, e.g., about understanding and becoming familiar with the individual's self-concept, underlying and expressed motives, impulse control, defense and coping styles, and cognitive complexity [5]. This is important to bear in mind, as personality style is woven into daily life and the recovery process, with its vulnerabilities and strengths. Further, the criteria for each diagnosis have no intention of embracing all relevant health aspects of a person and the complexity of life. This leads to another important and necessary element in assessments, with varying reliability [6], namely, formulation. That is a collection and synthesis of a wide array of relevant information to get insight into the person's life history and predisposing, precipitating, and perpetuating factors. Given the limitations of each approach, diagnosis, and formulation, it is advantageous to combine and integrate them to get the most out of what can be called a bio-psycho-social-cultural assessment framework.

When diagnosing, mental health professionals worldwide rely on official diagnostic manuals and related instruments, that is to say, the Diagnostic and Statistical Manual of Mental Disorders (current edition: DSM-5-TR) [3] and the International Classification of Diseases (current edition: ICD-11) [7]. The DSM-5 uses operationalized criteria that create sharp dichotomies (criteria are met or not), and in some ways, the descriptions in ICD-11 are more conductive to prototypical application since they often eschew arbitrarily precise thresholds in favor of fuzzy boundaries. The categories in both classifications are prototypical: they are based on the typical or illustrative example of a mental health problem from which real-world presentations will often deviate. From this perspective, a diagnosis is a 'best fit' match between someone's experiences and a prototype, which represents the most specific or notable features of a condition [8]. It is also pointed out that a diagnostic manual is not meant to be used mechanically. Criteria are offered as guidelines for making a diagnosis, and their use should be informed by clinical judgment. That may justify giving a certain diagnosis to an individual even though the clinical presentation falls just short of meeting the full criteria for the diagnosis, as long as the symptoms that are present are persistent and severe. On the other hand, a lack of familiarity with the criteria or excessively flexible and idiosyncratic application substantially reduces its utility. Another associated point is that it has not been possible to completely separate normal from pathological symptom expressions contained in diagnostic criteria. This gap is particularly problematic when symptom expressions, especially in milder forms, are not inherently pathological, where a diagnosis of mental disorder would be inappropriate. Further, this implies that clinicians need to look beyond the prototypical presentations that neatly coincide with the criteria [3].

An often-used criterion for a diagnosis is a requirement for a reduced level of functioning, which indicates that there should be a certain degree of severity related to a specific mental disorder. One could perhaps call it a kind of "decisive" premise for whether to make a diagnosis. This might sound easy to do, but it's not practically obvious: Should it be about the number of symptoms the individual experiences? The intensity of symptoms? The frequency of the symptoms or whether they are persistent? How much do they affect the level of functioning or quality of life? This is not clearly operationalized in diagnostic manuals and varies in several ways when comparing diagnoses, considering how "clinically significant distress or impairment" is described [9]. Further, the validity of diagnoses for mental disorders is questioned and ever-going debated, often with the same themes but with different agendas and rhetoric. This discussion can take different paths, depending on how you define "valid". Anyway, the manuals can make no claim at the moment with regard to "carving nature at its joints" [8]. The same point is also relevant for several medical conditions, where the main focus can be related to reliability and utility [10].

The above-mentioned classifications serve several purposes in health care: They can be both gate-openers and barriers to financial and treatment rights and ideally trigger adjustments in the treatment plan in an ecosystem of case-managed, coordinated services. This is an important theme, related to how diagnosis is used as a resource allocation regulator, where the American Psychiatric Association [3, p. 14] underlines the importance of not justifying limitations of access to appropriate care because individuals do not show all symptoms indicative of a diagnosis. Other purposes are shared language, comparison in research studies, development of interventions for various conditions, in education, forensic evaluations, billing and administrative tasks, and health statistics. It is reasonable to claim that these manuals do an imperfect but good enough job of fulfilling these diverse and at times conflicting needs [11].

Screening and Mapping in Primary Care Services

All services need some type or amount of information in order to consider rights to services, referral, and adjusting follow-up. This implies that screening and mapping are generally as relevant in primary care as specialist services, e.g., for the general practitioner, different community services and health care services in prison. See a selection of recommended instruments for primary care services in the paragraph "Screening instruments" later in this chapter, that can be used at a later, suitable time after initial, general mapping. When caregivers or others are involved in this, obtain information about:

- How do caregivers and other social networks experience the current situation and past level of functioning?
- What is the user or patient like when he/she is well or significantly better than now?
- What has been helpful in past, bad periods/episodes?

Primary services, including general practitioners, that eventually claim that clinical activity, diagnostically oriented screening is only for the specialist services, is wrong for several reasons. Sometimes attitudes like this are locally based, rigid, ideologically oriented beliefs that add trouble to an ecosystem of services that is supposed to develop and maintain a cross-sectoral, dynamic, team-based culture. In other cases, there are tendencies that primary services only use screening instruments to generally map depression and anxiety symptoms, which is a practically insufficient and non-specific screening that doesn't tell you much. All involved services and professions meet the same individual, where all parties might be in possession of, or in a position to collect, a wide array of important information about the patient's health status and life quality that has both separate and cross-sectorial utility. This indicates that all parties should have a minimum competency about mental disorders and how heavy substance use can affect mental and physical health. Some of the most important factors are that the services strive for co-shared understanding about the type of functional level, suffering, level of severity, strengths, and further strive for a multidisciplinary plan that covers the patients' needs and goals.

The Referral Process

The primary care services may feel that they are not getting any further in the follow-up, and much can appear unresolved or on hold. The current state can be experienced as a lack of progress or quality of life that has worsened despite offering the best possible services with the available resources. A typical situation is that the personnel may get a feeling that they over a long period of time only contribute with stabilization or protection, or that problem areas are recurring with a lack of progress over time. An important point is that in the initial phase of the follow-up, the situation may seem partly unchanged over a long time, before the individual moves on to a new phase in the recovery process. In such cases, it is mostly about when the individual is ready to do something more or different, e.g., assessment, in line with the IDDT stage approach (read about the treatment stages in Chap. 2). Regardless of what led to considering referral, the most important point is that the individual and referralist agree about the need to add specialist services or for a period needing inpatient admission for other than emergencies.

In the referral process, the follow-up offered so far from all current service providers should be evaluated altogether, both the interaction between them and the content from each service. Further, an assessment is not something you start with the very beginning of a follow-up, where establishing a working alliance is most often the only or main focus, especially in "hard to reach" cases. Here are a couple of relevant questions to consider related to a possible referral:

- What is the individual satisfied with from the (interaction between the) services?
- Is there something that can be adjusted in the current available services, both from services separately and the services together, which the individual wants to try out for a certain time before a referral is eventually sent?
- Do caregivers have any input about the individual's needs and sufferings, including how themself are affected by it?

A useful approach is to invite the local specialist service for a pre-referral, non-binding meeting, to get a co-shared understanding of the current situation and further implications of how and when the specialist service can be a part of the follow-up. Such meetings can give the specialist services a much better overview and be better prepared in how they can approach specific cases before they get the formal referral. Furthermore, there are several important points to clarify:

- Should it be referred to both assessment and treatment, inpatient or outpatient?
- If a group of health care professionals is established at the time of referral: What can the (cross-sectorial) team do or plan for- and with the individual before, during, and after the planned assessment? Who should be involved in the follow-up in the time period before the start of the specialist assessment?
- What does the individual expect or hope to get out of an assessment? Remember to not express guarantees or promises about what an assessment can trigger afterward, but describe generally possibilities and potential. The

individuals' expectations for the assessment should be described in the referral, and eventually, if they have any thoughts or convictions about a specific diagnosis that they have.

There are many things that should be described in a referral: how the life situation is now (including housing and economy), description of problem areas, family/social (relationships), previous diseases, current service offers, and more. Further, point out eventual former attempts to assess and formally diagnose, and eventual feasibility aspects to take into account in a future assessment. In the process of writing a referral, there must be a dialogue with the patient about the referral content, and caregivers can also contribute with information when needed. In this process, it is also useful, and sometimes absolutely necessary, that the referrer obtains relevant information from other involved services. See "Neuropsychological assessment" later in this chapter for information about cognition that can be gathered.

When Should Screening or Assessment Start?

Some clinicians or specialist services are reluctant to, or refuse to, assess possible mental disorders when the patients have an ongoing substance use problem, where they set strict, unreasonable general rules about the length of cessation of substance use before a patient can get access to a specialist assessment (e.g., 3 months of abstinence). Other times, clinicians are quick to define a person with substance use problems as not motivated, maybe in combination with not taking responsibility to work on increasing the patient's assessment engagement, eventually expecting other services, indirectly or directly, to take that responsibility for the patient. Such an approach will, in most cases, risk worsening the patients' health condition and life quality overall, and hinder progress in the recovery process. It's not the patient's responsibility that you are not motivated to explore their current life quality and suffering because of factors that threaten feasibility. That is solely a responsibility for the services, and at the same time, be open about other practical or organizational factors that might hinder you from making optimal adjustments in order to maximize the potential of the assessment process.

When the patient confirms that he/she is ready to explore their own life history, suffering, and resources, you should start the mapping or assessment process:

1. When there are no serious withdrawal symptoms.
2. When there is no serious intoxication.

If feasible, it can include a period of abstinence, determined by the clinical experience of the diagnostician and considering the setting in which the patient is assessed [12].

Neuropsychological Assessment

Cognitive functions are brain processes that are part of the mental processing of information. It includes both conscious and unconscious mental activities. The individual's utilization of their cognitive potential depends on, among other things, personality characteristics and social conditions. The relative importance of heredity-environment components is different from person to person, where the individual has potential he or she can seek to exploit. In this context, neuropsychological assessment aims to map the entire spectrum of functions, which usually includes processes involved in perception, communication, memory, thinking, and action. Intelligence is the sum of several cognitive functions, i.e., language comprehension, ability for perceptual organization, working memory, and it is important for how a person masters learning. Intelligence in this context provides important information about general cognitive capacity, assumed premorbid functional level, and current or remaining resources [13]. See Box 3.1 about themes that should be covered in a referral.

Box 3.1: Content in the Referral

- Is there information that suggests cognitive impairment? E.g., have changes been observed over time that support the assumption? What does the patient say about this?
- Are there any specific interventions that have helped with the assumed type of cognitive impairment?
- What are the individuals' strengths and weaknesses (according to whom)?

When a neuropsychological assessment does not seem feasible at a given or desired time (not considered useful enough in terms of validity issues), it should not trump the individual's access to assessment and necessary health care. Here is a recommended guide for neuropsychological testing by the Norwegian Neuropsychological Association [14], when heavy substance use or medication use is a part of the clinical picture:

In some cases, a period of abstinence from drugs or the absence of medications that have known cognitive side effects is required before testing. It is the purpose of the assessment to determine which requirements are met. Four factors should be considered in particular:

1. Are the requirements realistic, or do they practically exclude the patient from receiving necessary assessment/health care?
2. What risk does discontinuing medication, ceasing use of substances, or opioid agonist treatment (OAT) entail, in order to have the assessment carried out?
3. Will carrying out an assessment with no or limited requirements related to consuming still provide valuable information for treatment or other follow-up?

4. Will assessment with or without the use of substances and/or medications be most relevant in relation to the purpose of the assessment? This is particularly relevant in situations where the purpose of the assessment is to shed light on everyday functioning, and the patient is assumed to be stably medicated.

If you choose to assess with limited requirements related to the use of medications or substances, it must be clearly stated what uncertainty contributes to the conclusions in the assessment.

The purpose of this assessment is also to detect changes in functional level over time. It can contribute to clarification of whether the difficulties are due to mental disorder or psychosocial stress, or primarily caused by organic disease or injury [14]. E.g., an individual can have attention problems with anxiety disorders, tempo difficulties with depression, and memory and executive difficulties with psychosis [13], and this must be differentiated with regard to whether these challenges, e.g., can be better explained as a result of the individual's substance use.

Furthermore, it is important to be aware of variations in general condition, nutritional status, pain, medications, and, for example, epilepsy, which can affect test results. It is especially important to perform thorough differential diagnostic assessments with a focus on other possible explanations for weak cognitive functioning than mild mental retardation, when it comes to older patients [14]. When mapping this, tests must be chosen that are adapted to the patient's functional level, so that both strengths and weaknesses can be identified. Age is also a significant aspect, considering the lack of standardization in the various tools and the associated interpretation of the results. In the initial phase of an assessment, e.g., the MoCA (available at mocacognition.com.) is used to map attention, concentration, executive skills, memory, language, visuoconstructive skills, abstract thinking, calculation skills, and orientation.

If the cognitive impairment is obvious, and the choice of interventions does not depend on nuances in the functional impairment, then it may be sufficient with simple cognitive function examinations [14]. Another commonly used test is HASI (order at hasi.com.au). If there is an impact on this or on other relevant tests, then a full assessment of IQ and adaptive skills should be done, and, e.g., WAIS-5 (order at pearsonassessments.com) should be conducted. Vineland-3 (order at pearsonassessments.com) may also be relevant. This tool is standardized for people up to 26 years. Experiences suggest that Vineland can be used to test older people, but then you should be more careful with the interpretation. It covers to a small extent conditions that are important for maintaining an independent adult life. This means that one can, for example, get good scores on Vineland even if the patient has great difficulties living an independent life, e.g., related to having a job, handling of finance, responsibility for one's own housing, and having a family life with or without children. In addition, it is necessary to have comparative information to assess whether these problem areas were present before the age of 18.

Intellectual disability, borderline intellectual functioning, and mild intellectual disability in patients with substance use problems is a neglected topic and has been too little assessed in patients with SUD/MH [15]. It can be about the competence of health personnel, but also attitudes. Some clinicians might think that this is an uncomfortable or difficult topic to explore with the patient for various reasons [16]. During the assessment of this, the following specific approaches to people with reduced cognitive level are recommended (partly based on [17]):

1. Common vocabulary: You must map out which concepts and words the patient uses and understands. By establishing a common language, you ensure that both parties agree on what you are talking about. Establishing a common language can also be an important piece in the trust relationship between you and the patient.
2. Use visualizations: Visual stimuli such as pictures and videos can be of great benefit in communication with people with learning difficulties and developmental disabilities. Visual stimuli are concrete, and the patient does not have to search for words that the individual may not be able to name. By using images and other visual stimuli, you can also explore the patient's own choice of words.
3. Let the patient speak: It is important to let the patient have their say. In this way, you can uncover the level of knowledge the individual has in various areas and use this as a basis for further investigation and treatment. It may be important to take your time in the conversations and not confirm/interrupt too early, as some may need more time to express themselves.
4. Adapt interview style: It can be helpful to have a good knowledge of the diagnostic criteria for relevant mental disorders so that you can detach yourself from standard questions in structured interviews, and adapt the questions to the patient in terms of language, follow-up questions, concretization, and more.
5. Obtain comparative information: The patient may have difficulties remembering and explaining information; therefore, information from other close relations can be very useful to get a more comprehensive picture of the patient.

The importance of focusing on this is about facilitating treatment and other aspects for improved quality of life for the individual. Not everyone can manage everything just because they get the same opportunities, due to cognitive prerequisites. For example, methods such as cognitive therapy and motivational interviewing presuppose that the patient has sufficient cognitive functions to be able to benefit from it. In some cases, it may also be necessary to make different arrangements related to cognitive abilities before addressing the substance use problem. Another important aspect in terms of follow-up and adaptation is that some individuals with cognitive disabilities can do fine in an institution, but struggle a lot after the end of the stay [15].

Assessment Process, Context, and Content

Specialist assessments can be done by outreach teams, outpatient clinics, or upon admission, and it might be a relevant measure in municipalities. The different working contexts will affect the available amount of time for assessment, the opportunity to be thorough and systematic, as well as the flexibility in how you carry it out.

Inpatient clinics generally have better conditions in terms of staff resources, available time, practical adjustments of the process, and the amount of information that can be obtained. Dilemma-filled variants are assessments through involuntary admissions (read more about coercion in Chap. 9) or during serving time in prison (read about mental health care in prison in Chap. 11). It will often require an extra alliance-making effort from the staff, sometimes initially with non-motivated patients, to be positioned for dialogue about possible benefits, get started, and get the assessment carried out.

To ensure that the assessment is done systematically, predictably, and targeted within a limited time period, a clear plan is necessary. The content of a feasible assessment plan should, as a starting point when developing and re-evaluating it, be based on the LEAD principle [18], to ensure reliability and the best possible thoroughness and systematicity in information gathering and processing. LEAD is an abbreviation for:

- Longitudinal: Information must be obtained from the entire life course.
- Expert: The assessment is carried out by competent personnel, who discuss the assessment with other colleagues in case of doubt.
- All Data: As much relevant information as possible must be obtained. That is: thorough anamnesis, comparative information (e.g., girlfriend, parents, employer, former teachers, other health services, and more), use of relevant tests and diagnostic interviews, previous journals and epicrisis, as well as observations.

Without such a plan, there's a high risk of more random progress and content, and eventually time-wise drawn far beyond the necessary. In this plan, it should be stated who will contribute to the assessment among the personnel, and what will be done when, in broad terms (e.g., week by week). Evaluate along the way with the patient with regard to how the assessment is carried out, if there is a need, e.g., have shorter and more sessions instead of the typical single 45-min sessions. The clinic should have a thorough standard package that all patients should go through initially. It's better to have a detailed standard plan and, in each case, consider what's not needed, instead of having ongoing speculations during the assessment about what should be assessed. Then you can adjust it in each case if there is something that seems unnecessary to go through, or that is not feasible. Some central principles to follow in assessments are:

- Regularly challenge your own perspectives and hypotheses.
- Take your time. Short assessments have a high risk of being poor assessments or with a lot of tentative considerations. Further, a narrow, criteria-based focus, where the goal is to mainly assess a specific diagnosis in a couple of sessions, has limited value for people with SUD/MH (e.g., "ADHD assessments").
- Get hold of as much relevant data as possible. Triangulation of information from multiple sources provides more reliable information processing and considerations.

- The process should be characterized by empathy and respect, but you must also dare to ask unpopular questions and bring up topics that can be difficult (e.g., cognitive abilities, personality functioning, hygiene).
- Maintain thorough and structured record-keeping during the process; this is often a sign of good assessments.

There is little research that underlines what the minimum standard assessment content should be (instruments, etc.), the setup of the process, and the time allocated for the assessment, which ensures the best possible usefulness of it and reliable diagnostics. What content is chosen to be included as a standard package in assessments also tends to be affected by personal opinions and local preferences, rather than a multidisciplinary and structured approach. The consequence is unreasonable variation in assessment plans, length, type, and amount of information gathering, where the patient practically carries the burden and risk.

Some patients are more eager very early to start specific assessment activities, while others need more time for different reasons to get properly started. There must be time and patience for both. The time aspect is a major vulnerability in outpatient clinics, which cannot be compared with the potential detailed assessments with planned admissions lasting, e.g., 45 days or more. It is also a huge challenge in emergency clinics, where the ordinary length of a stay is usually very short. Some patients are coercively or voluntarily admitted, perhaps repeatedly, and discharged each time with, e.g., a blame-like, moral conclusion that the current type of suffering is "only" substance-induced. These individuals are vulnerable to falling into the category of "hard to reach" or becoming a victim of blame games between services, where they continue to live with untreated and eventually worsening severe mental illness. In cases where it is unclear whether the patient has a psychotic disorder or not, it is important to carefully consider the need and desire for assessment with the patient and other relevant parties. If the specialist service does not manage to offer that with a seamless transmission after an emergency admission, it is very important that this reasonable worry and need for further assessment is pointed out in the epicrisis, and at the same time communicated verbally to the relevant services involved.

Patient-Related Aspects

For various reasons, some patients have few or very variable plans and future visions about how they want to work on changing the course of their own lives and what specific short- and long-term goals they should set. If you have also experienced that most of what you are offered from the health and welfare system over time has been of no or little use, then it is natural that some become demoralized and don't have much belief in new services and personnel that you have to deal with. In addition, the result of an assessment can, depending on the countries' legislation, affect whether the patient is allowed to keep their driver's license, insurance, access to military service, access to certain types of jobs, entry to certain countries, and more. This can be perceived as threatening, where you have to be open about your juridical duties and, at the same time, make it clear that you first and foremost want to offer the best possible assessment.

For some patients, the assessment process itself may be the most meaningful, not necessarily the result of it. Going through one's own life, who you are and have been, can be both meaningful, reassuring, and more. But it can also be perceived as incomprehensible, threatening, or very uncomfortable. It can be useful to express certain things, experience being taken seriously, be in a space to reflect on one's own life, and get a better grip on the previously unclear and chaotic circumstances, in collaboration with the clinician. Or it becomes clearer what you value in life, and how you want to go forward. On the other hand, it can, e.g., be experiences painful, shameful, emotionally overwhelming, you get repeated confirmations of loss and limitations, lack of self-efficacy, and pain or discomfort that one has been inflicted or has inflicted on others. It is natural that an assessment process can be a mix of both something good and painful, and it is important that the clinicians continuously are aware of this, and make any practical adjustments with regard to what is talked about, how, and to what extent certain themes are addressed from time to time. When assessing in an outpatient clinic, it can be useful to have an ongoing dialogue with the rest of the support system around the patient between sessions, with regard to various forms of vulnerability that can be intensified or arise (temporary) as a result of an assessment session. This is to, among other things, take care of the patient's needs, limit or avoid relapse into substance use, or reduce the risk of drop-out from the assessment.

Another factor that can affect the assessment and further treatment plan is internalized stigma. It can be defined as devaluation, shame, secrecy, and withdrawal triggered by attributing negative stereotypes to oneself. This type of stigma can, among other things, be a potent barrier to getting into the workforce and a hindrance to close relationships and social functioning otherwise. Healthcare personnel must explore this with each patient. It is necessary, e.g., to ask the patient directly about the understanding of the diagnoses they got and experience of getting them. This is to try to correct any misconceptions, e.g., that psychosis always has a chronic course with progressive development, or that he/she will never get a job or boy/girlfriend [19].

Cultural Factors

The experience and presentations of mental disorders are affected by culture and the social milieu, not only of patients and families, but also of the individuals and health systems providing care [20]. These cultural views impact what is considered normal or pathological, and influence, e.g., help-seeking behaviors, the expression and course of mental illness [21], and pattern and intensity of substance use can, among other things, be influenced by social mores. The salience of cultural considerations has therefore been increasingly reflected in modern classification systems [3]. See Box 3.2 with a selection of relevant assessment questions [4] that harmonize with this reflection.

Box 3.2: Cultural Elements in Assessments

- What is the role of religion or spirituality in the person's life?
- How might basic cultural factors such as individualistic versus collectivistic values be relevant to the person's experience and their expression of distress and symptoms?
- Are there culturally determined gender role differences (e.g., norms or rules about contact with the other sex or childcare and work outside the home), or identify-forming affiliations with specific ethnic groups or subcultures (e.g., activities/programs to reinforce ethnic identity)?

An assessment should include how an individual's experiences, symptoms, and behaviors differ from relevant sociocultural norms and lead to difficulties in adaptation in his or her current life context. Further, to accurately assess potential signs and symptoms of psychopathology, clinicians should further routinely consider the impact of cultural meanings, identities, and practices on the causes and course of illness [3, p. 16]. The Cultural Formulation Interview (CFI) can be helpful in this process, to contextualize illness experience, maintain person-centered focus, and have a tool to differentiate culture-related factors from mental disorders, e.g., psychosis and personality disorders. Download CFI at psychiatry.org/psychiatrists/practice/dsm/educational-resources/assessment-measures.

There are also general cultural considerations for disorders due to substance use: Use of psychoactive substances is influenced by strong cultural meanings and traditions, which may affect the risk of development of a substance use disorder. The cultural milieu in which the substance is used should be considered when determining risk and the presence or absence of pathology. Cultural values and interpretations related to the use of psychoactive substances in specific communities, and cultural terms used to describe the substance and its effects, vary greatly across cultures. Local availability due to, e.g., the religious prohibitions against alcohol consumption, can affect the prevalence of disorders associated with it. Last, immigration may affect an individual's pattern of substance use as a result of changes in culture, including gender roles [7, p. 441–442].

Imaging Examinations

There are studies that show an increased incidence of traumatic brain injuries in people with SUD/MH [22], which implies the importance of excluding this as a best explanation of certain problem areas, with imaging as one of the assessment interventions. The purpose of imaging examinations is to rule out obvious pathology in the brain. Such examinations should be done if there is suspicion of a severe mental disorder. That is schizophrenia, bipolar disorder, and other severe and long-term mental disorders that do not respond to treatment. It can also be persistent head injuries related to, e.g., overdoses. MR should be the first choice, even though it is only a rough examination that captures larger injuries. It is possible to have minor injuries with significant neuropsychiatric symptoms, where more sensitive examinations can show certain injuries, e.g., positron emission tomography (PET), which can detect changes in smaller areas. Indications for PET examination are [13]:

- Symptoms/signs that implicate a possible neurodegenerative disease
- Symptoms where frontal or temporal forms of epilepsy are a differential diagnosis, and MR/EEG does not provide certain findings
- Symptoms that implicate a possible traumatic brain injury, where MR is unremarkable
- Unusual cases where one of the differential diagnoses is severe mental illness, where altered cerebral metabolism is usually present

Medical Conditions

People with SUD/MH have an increased prevalence of medical conditions compared to the rest of the patient population in specialist health services. It is important that mental health professionals who assess mental disorders are familiar with a range of somatic diseases and injuries, which can manifest as—or trigger—mental disorders or symptoms. An important rule of thumb is always to think that a mental disorder can be an expression of an underlying medical condition. If a mental disorder does not respond as expected to treatment, or there are unusual symptom combinations or unusual courses, it must be considered whether there may be an unrecognized "organic" disease, e.g., psychiatric consequences of head injuries and neurological diseases, as well as conditions characterized by dysfunction of the nervous system, even if the primary disturbance is in another organ. It can also include assessments related to biological aspects of mental disorders. All types of diseases that directly or indirectly affect the central nervous system (CNS) can, to various degrees, trigger mental symptoms. These can be organically caused confusion states, amnestic syndrome (e.g., Korsakoff's syndrome and Wernicke's encephalopathy), epilepsy, psychogenic non-epileptic seizures, Huntington's chorea, viral, bacterial, and parasitic infections in the CNS, and other diseases. All these examples underline that distinguishing medical conditions from mental disorders requires significant clinical and theoretical knowledge in medicine, as well as knowledge in psychology and psychiatry [13].

A Selection of Recommended Instruments

Systematic screening and comprehensive assessment of SUD/MH are essential components in an adequate treatment plan, especially because of the high rates of comorbidity, overlapping symptoms, and the vulnerability of biased (with often substance-associated causal) assumptions by health care professionals. The clinicians who do assessments need to have differential diagnostic competence, where standardized instruments can help ensure consistency and improve accuracy in information gathering and evaluation, specifically in diagnosis, but also in the assessment overall. To facilitate this task, when feasible, several clinically useful instruments are available, and a non-exhaustive list is hereby recommended for a selection of mental disorders and associated themes.

Screening Instruments

Alcohol Use Disorders Identification Test (AUDIT) (available at auditscreen.org) and Drug Use Disorders Identification Test (DUDIT) (available at euda.europa.eu/drugs-library/drug-use-disorders-identification-test-dudit_en) can be used to screen past-year problematic use of alcohol, other substances, and prescription drugs. When the AUDIT or DUDIT score is at a specific level (e.g., at least 7 for AUDIT, 2 for DUDIT), you can use Alcohol-E (available at integrertbehandling.no/forside/kartlegging-og-utredning-av-rus-og-psykiske-lidelser-rop-lidelser/alcohol-e) or DUDIT-E (available at euda.europa.eu/drugs-library/drug-use-disorders-identification-test-extended-dudit-e_en) to systematically map the patients' current view on negative and positive aspects of their substance use and treatment readiness. This information can be a basis, but not the sole source, for further dialogue about substance use-associated treatment planning.

For gambling and gaming screening, instruments like the Gambling Disorders Identification Test (GDIT) (available at gditscale.com) and Gaming Disorder Identification Test (GADIT) (available at integrertbehandling.no/forside/kartleggingutredning/gadit) can be useful. Several mental disorders can be screened with the Dual Diagnosis Screening Interview (DDSI) [23], among them ADHD, psychosis, mania, depression, PTSD, and more. Screening personality difficulties can be done with e.g., Personality Disorder Severity ICD-11 (PDS-ICD-11) (available at personlighed.dk) for level of severity and Personality Inventory for DSM-5 and ICD-11 Brief Form Plus Modified (PID5BF + M) [24] for traits.

DIALOG [25] can be useful for patient-centered communication and feedback-oriented practice, where people rate their satisfaction with eight life domains and three treatment aspects. It provides a score for subjective quality of life and a score for treatment satisfaction (more information at elft.nhs.uk/dialog). At last, the Practical and Social Functioning scale (PSF3) can be used to systematically assess practical and social functioning among patients with severe mental illness in different clinical settings [26].

Diagnostic Interviews

Assessment of personality disorders should be done with the ICD-11 Clinical Descriptions and Diagnostic Requirements [7], with interviews like SCID-5-PD or SCID-5-AMPD, until an ICD-11 interview is available, like Diagnostic Interview for Personality Pathology in ICD-11 (DIPP-11) [27]. Interviews that cover several mental disorders are, e.g., the Structured Clinical Interview for DSM-5—Clinician Version (SCID-5-CV) (available at appi.org/products/structured-clinical-interview-for-dsm-5-scid-5) and Psychiatric Research Interview for Substance and Mental disorders (PRISM-5) [28]. Unlike other content-wise similar diagnostic interviews, PRISM-5 is designed to specifically differentiate independent mental disorders from substance-induced mental disorders in heavy substance use populations and also includes a section about gambling disorder. SCID-5-CV, MINI 7.0.2, and other interviews with a wide array of mental disorders have little or no guidance on how to differentiate and no specific, tailored differential questions, probes, and guidance for this task. The same substance use-related limitation seems to be the case in content-wise comparable ICD-11 interviews that are being developed. This diagnostic vulnerability triggers a reflection about bias, information gathering and processing, and competency: How can clinicians compensate for this shortage in several diagnostic interviews, and do reliable differential diagnosis, especially in symptom-compounded, poly-substance use cases? Perceptions about compensating with your intuition, perceived skills, and experience are not the obvious and only answer to that question.

Differential Diagnosis

The instruments mentioned above, and others, need to be integrated into a wide multidisciplinary mapping, including assessing many diagnostic sections, because of the high level of comorbidity and the myriad of relevant factors that might be relevant in each case. This strongly indicates the need for careful differential diagnosis and thorough formulation, where you triangulate the data collected from several sources, ideally done over a longer period (e.g., more than 30 days) when patient-related assessment feasibility varies and the current situation and context imply a possibility to go into more detail. An attitude relevant to such a lengthy approach is that it is better to, when feasible, be too thorough than too random or mostly intuitional and quick. See Box 3.3 with examples on pitfalls and vulnerabilities.

Box 3.3: Pitfalls and Risks in Assessments

- Lack of working alliance and common assessment goal between the patient and clinician.
- Cultural differences between patient and clinician.
- Patient factors (e.g., memory problems, language barriers and defensive mechanisms).
- Symptoms change over time.
- Relying too much on assessing behavior when the patient is unable/has difficulty to express emotions.
- Relying too much on information from others (other than the patient).
- The clinicians' prejudice/resistance to or inclination towards (certain) diagnosis.

(continued)

Box 3.3 (continued)

- Too- or only open or rigid interview style.
- Overconfidence in one's own experienced diagnostic skills and intuition.
- Lack of assessment experience and training, and/or rigid, one sided preconceptions.
- Time pressure that threatens assessment feasibility, or unwillingness to invest enough time in assessments.
- Thinking that "insight" is about the degree to which a patient agrees with the mental health professionals' interpretation.

This is not a matter of overdiagnosis or symptom-only focus, or only be concerned about clear-cut disorder expressions and specific, isolated interventions. It is about being humble about the myriad of possible separate, overlapping, and intertwined factors involved in a person's daily life, to achieve the best possible follow-up. To maintain or achieve such a "best practice" attitude will depend on the amount of personnel, available competency, and economic resources. Furthermore, you can have such an attitude and make the best out of it in your resource-thrifty daily work, with ongoing considerations of what is reasonable or possible to use from available resources in a specific context.

Another important point is to know which substances can induce which symptoms during intoxication (I) and withdrawal (W), as exemplified in Table 3.1 [3, p. 545]. The 1-month boundary related to considering independent mental disorders is communicated for the sake of simplicity, and you have to be differentially diagnostic before that, because the duration of withdrawal symptoms varies greatly. In most cases, 1 month is probably on the long side, whereas for drugs with a very long half-life (e.g., clonazepam), 1 month might be too short. Clinicians are thus supposed to use their clinical judgment when applying this time frame. Further, see examples about withdrawal onset and duration in Table 3.2 [7, p. 484].

Related to communicating about specific mental disorders not influenced by, e.g., substance intoxication and withdrawal, the American Psychiatric Association (2022) changed the term "primary" to "independent" in 2013 when they published DSM-5, while the World Health Organization (2024) has kept the term "primary" in ICD-11. Both words have their limitations when communicating about causality when a person has a history of heavy substance use. "Primary" might make it sound like there is a type of rank, as if it's decided that some mental disorders are more important or severe than others, or occurred first. While "independent" might make it sound like a mental disorder has no causality related to other factors and mental disorders (e.g., substance-induced mental disorders). You need to be aware of a possible fault of looking at substance use as the only causal factor, and underestimating the importance of other risk factors [29]. This is also generally pointed out by the American Psychiatric Association [3, p. 25]: "The use of 'independent mental disorder' should not be construed to mean that the disorder is independent of other potential causal factors…".

Table 3.1 Diagnosis associated with substance class

	Psychotic disorders	Bipolar and related disorders	Depressive disorders	Anxiety disorders
Alcohol	I/W	I/W	I/W	I/W
Cannabis	I			I
Hallucinogenes	I	I	I	I
Opioids			I/W	W
Sedatives, hypnotics, or anxiolytics	I/W	I/W	I/W	W
Stimulants	I	I/W	I/W	I/W

Table 3.2 Examples of the onset and duration of substance withdrawal

Substance	Onset and duration of withdrawal
Alcohol	Onset typically occurs within 6–12 h after last use. Mild or moderate withdrawal typically last for 3–7 days after cessation use
Cannabis	Onset typically occurs at some point between 12 h and 3 days after cessation or reduction of use. Symptom severity typically peaks at 4–7 days and may last for 1–3 weeks after cessation of use. Withdrawal may also be briefer, in some cases lasting only a few days
Opioids	Withdrawal from short-acting opioids such as injected heroin or morphine typically begins within 4–12 h of cessation of use and lasts for 4–10 days Withdrawal from longer-acting opioids such as codeine, oxycodone and similar pharmaceutical agents may not be evident for 2–4 days and may last for 1–2 weeks Withdrawal state from long-acting drugs such as methadone may persist for up to 2 months after cessation of use
Sedatives, hypnotics, anxiolytics	The severity and time course of withdrawal is related to the particular substance taken, its half-life and duration of action, and the amount, frequency and duration of use before cessation or reduction of use. The withdrawal state associated with short-acting drugs typically has its onset within 12–24 h after cessation of use and has a course of up to 14 days Withdrawal onset may be delayed by 3–5 days with longer-acting drugs and may persist for several weeks
Cocaine	Typically occurs within 6–24 h of cessation of use The withdrawal state may last up to 7 days Craving is prominent in the later stages
Stimulants, including amfetamines, methamphetamine and methcathinone	Withdrawal typically occurs within 24 h to 4 days of cessation of use. The severity and duration of the withdrawal state is widely variable based on the type of stimulant taken and the amount, frequency and duration of such use prior to its cessation. In the first phase of stimulant withdrawal, which typically lasts for 7–14 days, low mood, lethargy and hypersomnia predominate. After this phase, irritability and craving are prominent and may persist for 6–8 weeks
MDMA or related drugs, including MDA	Onset of withdrawal typically occurs within 12–24 h after last use. The features vary in type, severity, onset and duration according to the amount, frequency and duration of use prior to cessation of use. The duration of withdrawal may be up to 10 days. Craving may be prominent during the later stages

The Way Forward After an Assessment

Both the assessment as a whole and bits and pieces of the (eventually some temporary) perspectives and conclusions in an assessment can represent crucial turning points in bettering the patients' life quality in both the short and long term. The purpose of an assessment is to take the person's suffering and problem areas seriously, by offering a thorough exploration of the whole life, and getting an overview of the individual's desires and needs in everyday life. In short, the goal is to shape a therapeutic, recovery-oriented path forward. This could mean reducing symptoms or problems, avoiding relapse or further complications, aiming to assist the patient in mastering their own life, and improving overall quality of life.

It is not always easy for all patients, after several years of chaos, instability, losses, persistent stress, and limited opportunities for positive expression and unfolding, to provide an "in the moment on demand" comprehensive answer about what they expect and need, what meaningful activities every day their life could be filled with, or to express in detail what's needed from the health care services. This is a personal process that varies from person to person, hence the importance of discussing plans and goals on several occasions during the assessment and especially in the follow-up afterward. New desires and needs may arise or change, which should be discussed and integrated into the follow-up.

For an assessment to be useful, a case formulation must be developed with the patient, with a thorough description of all aspects that can contribute to the understanding of the problem areas, strengths, and the way forward with goals and plans. The development, adaptation, and updates of the treatment plan must be based on clinical characteristics, as well as the patient's needs related to work, housing, self-care, social network, and education, with a focus on identity, meaning-making, and resilience [30]. The support system also needs to focus on all negative factors that can affect the potential for a meaningful everyday life: loss of meaning, poverty, social isolation, symptoms that reduce functional level [31], mattering [32], and demoralization. Integrated treatment in this context means having a culturally sensitive, multidisciplinary approach, where the services work coordinated, and support each other well across service levels and roles, while acknowledging each parties' competence and responsibility. Last, the people who are involved in the follow-up need to encourage the patient to be an active part in their own recovery [33], where meaningful activity and having access to and being welcome in various safe, supportive, and stable social arenas are also very important.

Summary

- Many people with SUD/MH live with unexplained, compounded, or unclear but obvious suffering for years, with a crisscrossing of medical, existential, social, and psychological burden.

- Getting an alliance and positioning yourself to get to know a person, and getting an overview and insight into a person's life, is generally a comprehensive task.
- Assessments can be time and resource-demanding, where the type and amount of content are affected by service level, context, local preferences, available resources, and assessment competency.
- Identifying and sorting needs, symptoms, problem areas, and strengths, and how this is intertwined and woven into daily life, is an important guide toward better understanding and offering appropriate support, interventions, and treatment. This requires mental health workers to strive for maximizing assessment utility by embracing a plurality of diagnostic and explanatory frameworks, including being competent in differential diagnosis.

Reflection Questions

- Whether you work municipally or in a specialist service: Do you cooperate with the other service levels during the assessment? If no or insufficient: Why not, and how can you or your workplace improve it?
- On what basis do you think your way of doing assessments, including eventually standardized content in your assessments, is a good enough or the best way to do it? Is it mainly based on your personal or collegial entitlement and convictions? Why are you eventually sure it's detailed enough and differential diagnostically reliable?
- Why might it be important to involve caregivers in the assessment, including ongoing and further follow-up, apart from obtaining comparative information?
- How do you go through the information from the assessment with the patient before you formally diagnose?
- How do you handle situations where the patient does not agree with your opinion about probable diagnostic conclusions or feels misunderstood?
- How do you usually deal with descriptions you do not understand or strongly disagree with from a completed assessment? Do you address it with the patient, those who have done the assessment, or other service collaborators?
- How do you work to get—and maintain—a consistent co-understanding with the patient and other parties, about suffering, needs, and strengths—where a fresh assessment has shed new light on the current situation?

Recommended Literature and Online Resources

American Psychiatric Association. *Diagnostic and statistical manual of mental disorders* (5th ed., text rev.). Arlington: American Psychiatric Association; 2022.

Kind A. How Does the Psychiatrist Know? On the Epistemology of Psychiatric Diagnostic Reasoning. Bielefeld: Transcript Publishing; 2024. Online version available for free at transcript-publishing.com

Reed, GM, Ritchie, PLJ, Maercker A, Rebello TJ (Eds.). A psychological approach to diagnosis: Using the ICD-11 as a framework. Washington: American Psychological Association; 2024.

Stein, DJ. Problems of living. Amsterdam: Elsevier Inc.; 2021.

World Health Organization. Clinical descriptions and diagnostic requirements for ICD-11 mental, behavioural and neurodevelopmental disorders. Geneva: World Health Organization; 2024. Available for free at who.int/publications/i/item/9789240077263

References

1. Kessler RC, Nelson CB, McGonagle KA, Edlund MJ, Frank RG, Leaf PJ. The epidemiology of co-occurring addictive and mental disorders: implications for prevention and service utilization. Am Orthopsychiatric Assoc. 1996;66:17–31. https://doi.org/10.1037/h0080151.
2. Regier DA, Farmer ME, Rae DS, Locke BZ, Keith SJ, Judd LL, Goodwin FK. Comorbidity of mental disorders with alcohol and other drug abuse: results from the epidemiologic catchment area (ECA) study. JAMA. 1990;264(19):2511–8. https://doi.org/10.1001/jama.1990.03450190043026.
3. American Psychiatric Association. Diagnostic and statistical manual of mental disorders. 5th ed, text rev. Arlington: American Psychiatric Association; 2022.
4. Reed GM, Ritchie PL-J, Maercker A, Rebello TJ, editors. A psychological approach to diagnosis: using the ICD-11 as a framework. Washington, DC: American Psychological Association; 2024.
5. Krishnamurthy R, Hass GA, Natoli AP, Smith BL, Arbisi PA, Gottfried ED. Professional practice guidelines for personality assessment. J Pers Assess. 2022;104(1):1–16. https://doi.org/10.1080/00223891.2021.1942020.
6. Flinn L, Braham L, das Nair R. How reliable are case formulations? A systematic literature review. Br J Clin Psychol. 2015;54(3):266–90. https://doi.org/10.1111/bjc.12073.
7. World Health Organization. Clinical descriptions and diagnostic requirements for ICD-11 mental, behavioural and neurodevelopmental disorders. Geneva: World Health Organization; 2024. Available at https://www.who.int/publications/i/item/9789240077263.
8. Aftab A, Banicki K, Ruffalo ML, Frances A. Psychiatric diagnosis: a clinical guide to navigating diagnostic pluralism. J Nerv Ment Dis. 2024;212(8):445–54. https://doi.org/10.1097/nmd.0000000000001791.
9. Zimmerman M, Morgan TA, Stanton K. The severity of psychiatric disorders. World Psychiatry. 2018;17:258–75. https://doi.org/10.1002/wps.20569.
10. Frances A. A report card on the utility of psychiatric diagnosis. World Psychiatry. 2016;15(1):32–3. https://doi.org/10.1002/wps.20285.
11. Frances A, Widiger T. Psychiatric diagnosis: lessons from the DSM-IV past and cautions for the DSM-5 future. Annu Rev Clin Psychol. 2012;8:109–30. https://doi.org/10.1146/annurev-clinpsy-032511-143102.
12. Crunelle CL, van den Brink W, Moggi F, Konstenius M, Franck J, Levin FR, van de Glind G, Demetrovics Z, Coetzee C, Luderer M, Schellekens A, ICASA Consensus Group, Matthys F. International consensus statement on screening, diagnosis and treatment of substance use disorder patients with comorbid attention deficit/hyperactivity disorder. Eur Addict Res. 2018;24(1):43–51. https://doi.org/10.1159/000487767.
13. Andreassen OA, Malt UF, Malt EA, Melle I, editors. Lærebok i psykiatri. Basisversjon. Første utgave. [Textbook of psychiatry. Basic version. First edition]. Oslo: Gyldendal; 2020.
14. Norwegian Neuropsychological Association. Veileder i klinisk nevropsykologi – prinsipper for utøvelse av klinisk nevropsykologisk virksomhet (Guidance in clinical neuropsychology – principles for the practice of clinical neuropsychological activities). [Internet]. 2024. Available

at https://psykologforening.fra1.digitaloceanspaces.com/Foreningen/Utvalg-r%C3%A5d-og-interesseforeninger/Norsk-Nevropsykologisk-Forening/Veileder-i-klinisk-nevropsykologi-3-utgave.pdf.

15. Norwegian National Advisory Unit on Concurrent Substance Abuse and Mental Health Disorders. Må ta hensyn til kognitiv svikt hos pasienter med rusmiddelproblemer [Must take cognitive impairment into account in patients with substance use problems] [Internet]. Ottestad: Norwegian National Advisory Unit on Concurrent Substance Abuse and Mental Health Disorders; 2019. https://rop.no/aktuelt/ma-ta-hensyn-til-kognitiv-svikt-hos-pasienter-med-rusmiddelproblemer/. Accessed 13 Feb 2025.
16. Norwegian National Advisory Unit on Concurrent Substance Abuse and Mental Health Disorders. Psykisk utviklingshemming hos rusavhengige blir ikke fanget opp [Intellectual disabilities among people with substance use disorder is not detected] [Internet]. Ottestad: Norwegian National Advisory Unit on Concurrent Substance Abuse and Mental Health Disorders; 2019. https://rop.no/aktuelt/psykisk-utviklingshemming-hos-rusavhengige-blir-ikke-fanget-opp/. Accessed 13th February 2025.
17. Norwegian National Advisory Unit on Concurrent Substance Abuse and Mental Health Disorders. Hvordan utrede rusavhengighet hos personer med utviklingshemming? [How to assess substance use disorder in people with intellectual disabilities?]. [Internet]. Ottestad: Norwegian National Advisory Unit on Concurrent Substance Abuse and Mental Health Disorders. https://rop.no/aktuelt/hvordan-utrede-rusavhengighet-hos-personer-med-utvikling-shemming/. Accessed 13 Feb 2025.
18. Spitzer RL. Psychiatric diagnosis: are clinicians still necessary? Compr Psychiatry. 1983;24(5):399–411. https://doi.org/10.1016/0010-440x(83)90032-9.
19. Maj M, van Os J, De Hert M, Gaebel W, Galderisi S, Green MF, et al. The clinical characterization of the patient with primary psychosis aimed at personalization of management. World Psychiatry. 2021;20:4–33. https://doi.org/10.1002/wps.20809.
20. Gureje O, Lewis-Fernandez R, Hall BJ, Reed GM. Systematic inclusion of culture-related information in ICD-11. World Psychiatry. 2019;18(3):357–8. https://doi.org/10.1002/wps.20676.
21. Gureje O, Lewis-Fernandez R, Hall BJ, Reed GM. Cultural considerations in the classification of mental disorders: why and how in ICD-11. BMC Med. 2020;18(1):25. https://doi.org/10.1186/s12916-020-1493-4.
22. McHugo GJ, Krassenbaum S, Donley S, Corrigan JD, Bogner J, Drake RE. The prevalence of traumatic brain injury among people with co-occurring mental health and substance use disorders. J Head Trauma Rehabil. 2017;32(3):E65–74. https://doi.org/10.1097/htr.0000000000000249.
23. Mestre-Pintó JI, Domingo-Salvany A, Martín-Santos R, Torrens M, PsyCoBarcelona Group. Dual diagnosis screening interview to identify psychiatric comorbidity in substance users: development and validation of a brief instrument. Eur Addict Res. 2014;20(1):41–8. https://doi.org/10.1159/000351519.
24. Bach B, Kerber A, Aluja A, Bastiaens T, Keeley JW, Claes L, Fossati A, Gutierrez F, Oliveira SES, Pires R, Riegel KD, Rolland JP, Roskam I, Sellbom M, Somma A, Spanemberg L, Strus W, Thimm JC, Wright AGC, Zimmermann J. International assessment of DSM-5 and ICD-11 personality disorder traits: toward a common nosology in DSM-5.1. Psychopathology. 2020;53(3–4):179–88. https://doi.org/10.1159/000507589.
25. Priebe S, Golden E, McCabe R, et al. Patient-reported outcome data generated in a clinical intervention in community mental health care – psychometric properties. BMC Psychiatry. 2012;12:113. https://doi.org/10.1186/1471-244x-12-113.
26. Clausen H, Ruud T. The practical and social functioning (PSF) scale: development and measurement properties of an instrument for assessing activity and social participation among people with serious mental illness. BMC Psychiatry. 2024;24:693. https://doi.org/10.1186/s12888-024-06135-x.

27. Bach B, Sellbom M. Instruments and other sources of diagnostic information. In: Bach B, editor. ICD-11 personality disorders: assessment and treatment. Oxford: Oxford University Press; 2025.
28. Hasin D, Shmulewitz D, Stohl M, Greenstein E, Roncone S, Aharonovich E, Wall M. Test-retest reliability of DSM-5 substance disorder measures as assessed with the PRISM-5, a clinician-administered diagnostic interview. Drug Alcohol Depend. 2020;216:108294. https://doi.org/10.1016/j.drugalcdep.2020.108294.
29. Rognli EB, Høye A, Bramness JG. Methamphetamine-induced psychosis and schizophrenia: a call for special attention: response to Zhu et al. Am J Psychiatry. 2024;181(2):168–9. https://doi.org/10.1176/appi.ajp.20230522.
30. Maj M. Beyond diagnosis in psychiatric practice. Ann General Psychiatry. 2020;19:27. https://doi.org/10.1186/s12991-020-00279-2.
31. Braslow JT, Brekke JS, Levenson J. Psychiatry's myopia-reclaiming the social, cultural, and psychological in the psychiatric gaze. JAMA Psychiatry. 2020 Sep 9. https://doi.org/10.1001/jamapsychiatry.2020.2722.
32. Flett GL. An introduction, review, and conceptual analysis of mattering as an essential construct and an essential way of life. J Psychoeduc Assess. 2021;40(1):3–36. https://doi.org/10.1177/07342829211057640.
33. Davidson L, Tondora J. Person-centered care planning as foundational to clinical practice. World Psychiatry. 2022;21:1–2. https://doi.org/10.1002/wps.20922.

Housing and Supported Housing

4

Tore Willy Lie

Abstract

Housing and supported housing are basic, critical assets when helping an individual in their recovery process, and a very important piece in integrated treatment. Having a specific place to stay is just the first step on the path to having a stable and safe place you can call home. Some people with co-occurring substance use disorders and mental disorders (SUD/MH) make those steps on their own, and others do not, where the need for intensity and type of supported housing will vary a lot in each case and between each person. This chapter explores topics like what makes housing challenging, suitable housing, housing first, assessing the need for housing support, how to plan transitions between inpatient units, prison, and the municipality, how to meet someone in their own home, and more.

Keywords

Housing · Housing first · Housing support · Homelessness · Supportive housing · Recovery housing · Emergency accommodation

A permanent home is important for personal identity, and it can tell a lot about the life and values of the person living there, and feeling safe where you live is fundamental for all of us. However, a home does not mean safety for a certain number of people with SUD/MH, as they have experienced high levels of stress in their own home. Lack of social network, employment, or other meaningful activity, where

T. W. Lie (✉)
Department of Health and Nursing Sciences and Section for Mental Health and Rehabilitation, University of Inland Norway, Elverum, Norway
e-mail: tore.lie@inn.no

T. W. Lie, L. Lien (eds.), *Integrated Treatment of Co-occurring Substance Use and Mental Health Disorders*, https://doi.org/10.1007/978-3-032-20049-5_4

some stay most of the time in their own home, can also increase feelings of loneliness [1]. Some also have ongoing high levels of stress due to domestic partner violence, while others may feel high levels of anxiety about being evicted due to non-payment of rent or an unsafe neighborhood. In other cases, some have for various reasons been on the move several times in a short period of time, and have little experience of settling down in one place, including eventually a lack of practical support associated with housing.

A home becomes a home when the person or people who live there are allowed to make their mark on it. It should be possible to invite people to visit and be a place where you can retreat. This is important regardless of whether you have acquired private housing or whether you live in municipal housing, and it is about much more than generally just having somewhere to live [2]. At the same time, predictable, stable housing is generally very important to get the most out of other types of follow-up and treatment, as many factors can directly or indirectly affect each other—and thereby the services need to work on all domains at the same time. Stability and predictability of basic housing needs are also a foundation for achieving other things in life.

Many people with SUD/MH have an unstable housing status, and a certain proportion of those with severe SUD/MH have no or limited positive experience over time of living predictably and well. Losing their home will often influence substance use, mental health, and medical problems, while at the same time, this worsening can make it more challenging for the services to provide cross-sectorial, integrated treatment. Another challenge can be the transition between longer stays in prison or inpatient treatment and their own home, including the effort to find proper housing if the patient doesn't have that or has lost it during the stay. Some also move to a new place right after release or discharge, maybe with little clothes and basic inventory available (e.g., bed, refrigerator, oven, phone subscription, bank card, etc.), might be financially poor, and lack related social and practical support (e.g., transporting and lifting products to their own home and assemble furniture). All these daily living aspects are about lowering relapse risk and are basic prerequisites for a dignified life [2], which the services might lack focus on for different reasons.

Housing Policy

For a good number of municipalities that offer official housing, it is challenging to settle people with SUD/MH, maybe with major internal discussions before various local housing policy decisions are made. This can involve reviewing suitable property, type of neighborhood, choice of housing type, choice of inventory related to the persons' functional level, and whether the housing should be with/without staffing, and how to prioritize and place all who need housing. There is a lot to consider on top of the eventual thoughtful intentions of developing and maintaining dignified housing offers. Supported housing is often a part of the regular staffing budget and competes with other important municipal tasks, while construction can, e.g., take place via various loan schemes and external grants. Lack of knowledge about all this and more among partners tends to skew their expectations about local housing availability and the speed of housing case management, including the timing of when housing needs are communicated externally before inpatient discharge, and more.

There might be a need to change or improve housing approaches by evaluating municipalities' experiences with housing for people with SUD/MH, to provide a better understanding of the factors necessary for better housing and service models. This includes involving the (future) resident to a certain point in design, color, and material choices and evaluating how such involvement can affect their dignity and daily living competence.

When establishing municipal housing for this target group, it is important to have strategies for neighborhood and local community work included in the planning [1]. Municipalities that succeed in housing conditions for people with substance use problems have a clear and long-term strategy for how to solve it, and the strategy must have political anchoring and a feasible action plan [3].

What Is Suitable Housing and Supported Housing?

There is great uncertainty and divided opinions about what is the most suitable housing for this heterogeneous group of people and what is considered to be a satisfactory physical housing standard varies between countries. People with SUD/MH have very different housing and service needs, and it must be assessed individually in each case. Having a housing complex where several people with substance use problems live can be challenging, because residents who manage (or are working on) to limit or avoid the use of substances can be adversely affected by those who are not in the same situation. It can therefore increase the risk of relapse or deterioration.

Therefore, it may be useful to build municipal housing offers that are spread, e.g., two houses for themselves, or building four-family houses where each apartment has its own entrance. When building co-located housing, it is not recommended to have more than six housing units. Service offers with easily available follow-up, and on-site staffing will often require co-location of several homes in the same place. If there are common areas in such housing complexes, it often requires (24-h) staffing for it to work [4]. Common areas in co-located housing offers can increase the level of- or induce conflicts, therefore it is important to consult those who live there. It is advantageous that people who are regularly acting out or with known high risk of it live in separate housing units, and not in the middle of a residential area. Another aspect, considering the usefulness of co-located housing, is that people with severe mental illness with poor interpersonal functioning can have their feelings of loneliness reinforced by living in an independent home [5]. Age composition is also important considering various aspects of group dynamics and neighborhoods with younger adults and the elderly. It is also experienced that it is challenging to settle younger disadvantaged people in the age group 16–23 with substance use problems and social anxiety, who have dropped out of school and have no income [6].

A home with follow-up can provide better functional level and quality of life [4], and can contribute to promoting the persons' independence and self-determination by [7]:

1. Assisting the resident in developing greater awareness of a meaningful and array of choices.
2. Respecting the persons' daily choices.
3. Providing training in the skills the resident needs to function as independently as possible. In housing follow-up, you must recognize the varying needs and levels of function of the resident, and substantiate the goals and desire to strengthen and develop self-determination.

When building new official housing or adjusting established areas, it should ideally not be a long distance to bus or train, grocery store, pharmacy, and more, as many do not have a car, and might have issues with planning, where eventual problems with time and dates will further exacerbate this.

It is also advantageous that there are available 24-h services for those who obviously need that. Another important aspect is that the resident should not lose the housing because they are not complying with certain activities or expectations. Municipalities can also offer differentiated housing with varying degrees of

Table 4.1 Housing based on the resident's treatment stage [8, p. 245]

Housing type	Level of tolerance for substance use	Treatment stage (IDDT)	Primary function of the housing
"Wet" housing	Relatively tolerant	Engagement—consideration	Safety Stable housing (i.e. reduction of problems related to homelessness) Tolerating substance use problems to give opportunity to engage the resident
"Humid" housing	A little tolerance	Consideration—active treatment	Stable housing that has some limits to use substances, make it easier to reduce use Supporting the resident in considering how substance use affects their life Limiting substance use to make it easier to reduce problems and maintain sobriety or type of substance use with significantly less consequences
"Dry" housing	Relatively intolerant	Active treatment—relapse prevention	Help the resident to maintain sobriety or substance use with few if any long term consequences Stable housing that helps the resident to stay away from relations associated with substance use problems Facilitate focus on other life domains, like employment and relationships

tolerance for drug use, depending on which phase the user is in (read about the treatment stages in IDDT in Chap. 2), as shown in Table 4.1.

This type of housing differentiation, and possible moving between housing offers as needed, can appear as a flexible and ideal recovery-oriented approach. With regard to the tenancy law in respective countries, there might be limited juridical room for action for this type of approach, unless a consent to be in a (treatment stage) phase-based housing program is contractually agreed upon with the resident. Regardless, this housing framework is something to strive for within each countries' legal framework.

Emergency Accommodation: Temporary—But Persistent for Some

When considering what is appropriate official housing for people with substance use problems and mental problems, it is important to look a closer at various temporary housing that might be offered by official authorities. Emergency accommodation is often simpler, smaller types of housing, where the intention is that the resident should not live there "longer than necessary", with regard to the further process of obtaining proper housing. It can, e.g., be a kind of barracks, very small standalone (eventually movable) houses, a cabin rented at a campsite, or a hostel. You also have worst-case examples where the official welfare administration has given inhabitants a tent, and defined it as "housing", when there has concurrently been a lack of other housing offers. Most of the temporary housing offers will put some limits on treatment planning and setting goals with the patient and the often organizational separated support system. It is a risk that the patient stays for a long time as a result of renewal of the housing offer, which increases the risk of relapse and worsening the current condition.

Various emergency accommodations have received much criticism through the years for both location, housing type, and standard. Some of them are located in a decentralized—partly hidden from other inhabitants, and sometimes in areas that are not associated with being a residential area. This can appear as a lack of dignity for the resident, and can communicate that the resident is unwanted in society. Whether that is the intention or not, it increases the risk of maintaining and heightening stigma and lack of social inclusion. Such housing placement becomes extra troublesome for those who, e.g., have severe problems with interpersonal functioning, cognitive impairment, financial issues, or physical disability. Further, municipalities might not be legally obliged to offer different types of transport related to daily chores, but such measures can be some of the most important you do for daily dignity, stability, predictability, it makes sure the treatment plan is followed, and it can be worth its weight in gold for maintaining or improving the alliance—especially in the initial phase of the follow-up.

Housing First

This housing concept has received a lot of attention for several years. It is a user-driven method for offering housing and services to homeless people who have a substance use problem and/or mental illness [9]. The user's need for comprehensive and integrated follow-up with varying intensity is central in this model. The principle that you get housing first does not mean that this approach overrides all other interventions that the user needs in order to strengthen the life situation in different areas, such as finance, work, education, mental and physical health. The difference compared to a model where the user without housing must go through various temporary measures to gain access to permanent housing is that Housing First focuses

Box 4.1: Housing First Key Principles

- Housing is a human right
- Choice and control for service users
- Separation of housing and treatment
- Recovery orientation
- Harm reduction
- Active engagement without coercion
- Person-centered planning
- Flexible support for as long as required

on obtaining suitable housing along with relevant services. The most important aspects of this approach are that one has abandoned the idea that a person must first show housing-related daily living ability [1, 9], and allegiance to the key principles in the model, see overview in Box 4.1 [10].

The goal is to ensure a stable living situation, with a lot of emphasis on the user's wishes. Several of the principles in Box 4.1 must be included to achieve good results [11]. It should be no requirement for sobriety, or that one must receive specific types of services to gain access to this type of housing. This model does not come without any challenges, and they are the same as in other regular municipality housing, with, e.g., too few and varied types of residencies, and a lack of interaction and integration between the specialist and municipal services. But, some health care providers have found a solution to this, where they have merged, e.g., a FACT team (read more about FACT in Chap. 12) and Housing First services.

Housing-Related Mapping

Mapping someone's life situation in their own home is consciously and unconsciously influenced by our own ideas of what a good living situation and quality of life are. What is seen as normal or natural by most people in a society is not necessarily the best way to live for everyone. It is important to be aware that you need to distinguish between what are unfortunate living conditions and that some do not have the same preferences as you (see Box 4.2 for mapping tips).

Unfortunate living conditions can, e.g., be accumulation of garbage, a lack of cleaning (that affects hygiene to a questionable degree, affects neighbors, physically affects building material and infrastructure, etc.), and various forms of mess and chaos that make it difficult to stay in the home [1]. In some cases, it might be that the home technically is not in a satisfactory condition, and will, if not taken care of, e.g., lead to very drafty windows, a poor electrical system, roof leaks, mold, rot, lack of heating, lack of insulation, etc. Associated with this is the usefulness of routinely going through a checklist related to possible fire hazards (maybe in cooperation with the local fire station) when allocating municipal housing. Then an increased risk of fire can be discovered, and fire hazard-reducing measures can be initiated.

The purpose of the whole mapping is to create a plan together with the resident for follow-up with regard to the resident's resources, wishes, needs, and problem areas. It must be mapped broadly how the living conditions can be mastered, including screening of mental illness and substance use problems (read about primary care screening of SUD/MH in Chap. 3). It is useful to get information about experiences

Box 4.2: A Selection of Questions That Can Be Useful in Various Situations [12]

- Does the home you have remind you of substance use, traumatic events, or other issues, and can trigger relapse or maintain persistent, heavy substance use?
- Do you think anyone who has substance use problems or sells drugs will visit you? Is it difficult to reject or keep a distance from them? Can it tempt you into a relapse or maintain the current pattern of substance use?
- Do you want to train on rejecting drug offers? Do you need to practice staying sober at your home?
- Do you want to move to a new place?
- Do you have enough mental energy and motivation to get to know new people in the healthcare system?
- Are you too far from family and a sober social network?

Box 4.3: Questions That Should Be Considered, Related to the Mapping [1]

- Does the resident need to set boundaries for or be protected due to the type or severity of his or her mental problems?
- Has the resident had substance use problems from early in life, and thus not followed normal socialization? Is it such a comprehensive problem that it is a question of addiction? What experiences does the user have with being drug-free?
- Does the user have somatic complaints that are unclear? Does he or she have access to a regular doctor who also focuses on other health problems than the substance use problem? What is the resident's experience with managing the use of prescribed medication on their own?
- Does the user have intellectual disabilities that are significant for the living conditions, for a short or persistent time? E.g., problems with receiving messages, memory, carrying out or completing tasks, difficulty planning, and generally lack of an overview of everyday measures that should be followed up on or done?
- Consider the type of follow-up and goals: Is it habilitation or rehabilitation?
- What makes the resident feel insecure, and how does he or she protect themselves?
- Does the user have unresolved cases with the criminal justice system, or problems related to a drug milieu, such as debt or threats of violence?
- What social network does a resident have beyond people involved in the follow-up?
- Who can live in the same housing complex?

the user has from previous housing, what went well or poorly, and what you can learn from those experiences, which are relevant for current or future living conditions and follow-up (see examples in Box 4.3 above). If needs are revealed beyond what the service can offer, it must be discussed with the user, who else can contribute, and whether there is a need for referral to the specialist service.

Cognition

It is important to screen the residents' possible cognitive impairment in order to tailor follow-up according to level of functioning, or else the services might overestimate the level of functioning. Services might also express expectations or "push" the resident to do things on their own that they actually can't manage, which just adds another problem for the resident. Another problem is when the resident forgets to perform daily or weekly chores at home, where the services might conclude that it's about motivation, drug-related, or laziness—while it's really about, e.g., mild intellectual disability (MID) or borderline intellectual functioning (BIF). The cognitive difficulties can be related to memory, concentration, planning, getting started, completing tasks, impulsivity, anger, and more. Some may also cover up the problems and compensate in various ways that initially make it difficult to discover the actual level of functioning. It is important to find a balance between not overestimating or underestimating the resident and challenging one's own subjective assessments continuously.

It is also important to achieve good observations and documentation of this, and you might end up with a specialist service collaboration for a more comprehensive assessment and other follow-up. A thorough differential diagnostic and an overall comprehensive assessment by the specialist service can be important for those who provide supported housing, with regard to understanding and calibrating housing-related measures. Furthermore, the specialist service can benefit from those who work with housing follow-up: They can have a lot of important information from observations, interventions, and interactions over a long time, and have valuable information about what seems to have worked and not worked in the follow-up.

Assess Practical and Social Skills

It is recommended to use the Practical and Social Functioning scale (PSF3) [13], which is an instrument for assessing social and practical skills. It can also be significant in the assessment of the resident's cognitive abilities. PSF3 should preferably be combined with a form that assesses perceived quality of life, like DIALOG [14]. The areas assessed in PSF are: own health, personal hygiene, cooking, own belongings, financial management, use of transport, contact with others, behavior in conversations, work ability, and leisure activities. The wording in the form is designed to be positively formulated based on what the user can do, and it should be scored based on what the user actually does, not what you think he or she can manage. It is scored by the supported housing worker, based on observations and conversations with the user over the past 4 weeks. The form can be used as an indicator of and a rough overview of what is important to follow-up on or work with. It can also be used as a measure of improvement if the assessment is repeated after a certain period [1], e.g., after 6 or 12 months. It is recommended that the assessment is then repeated by the same employee, since the form is based on judgment—which can affect the score across those who fill out.

After the Assessment, What Now?

After initial assessment, there must be further dialogue with the resident about the need for supported housing, what it should entail, expectations clarification, level of ambition, and the goal for services and the resident.

Living in a regular home can motivate the individual to take better care of the housing [6]. Some will argue that a home should be at least 40 m^2 and ideally have regular, western housing functionality and infrastructure [4]. In this context, it is important to be aware that the smallest apartments that can be purchased on the housing market, especially in the largest cities, are down to, e.g., 25 m^2, where housing and outdoor areas lack light due to high-rise surrounding constructions [15]. Therefore, it is difficult to set a universal guideline on minimum size and other contextual requirements for housing that is allocated, beyond the usual standard, with regard to housing functions. Consideration must also be given to the resident's possible care- or visitation rights for their own children [4]. Other practical aspects, from a western point of view, are that it should not be installed too small hot water tanks and lack access to internet. Lack of internet can in certain amount of countries create problems with keeping up with everyday duties and contribute to digital exclusion.

Another point is that it is generally a challenge that housing for people with SUD/MH is characterized by some turnover and high wear and tear (beyond normal use wear and tear), which means that there are special requirements for standard and material choice. With that as a starting point, there is not a contradiction between environmental robustness and the feeling of living well [6].

The Neighborhood

Some neighbors react strongly and negatively when municipality housing complexes are nearby or might be built, where people with substance use problems live. A resident does not have good opportunities to become part of the neighborhood if they are not wanted. Based on experience, ghetto-like housing setups are not appropriate, as they are often characterized by many people who are actively using drugs, with a number of negative consequences. There can be several reasons why neighborhoods react, and they are usually related to prejudices against and attitudes towards people with substance use and mental problems. It might be possible to influence reputation and skepticism by the municipality, e.g., by focusing on landscaping and housing that are maintained, along with the supported housing. A good reason for neighbors to react could be threats or other unpleasant and unpredictable behavior from one or more residents. All of this can create unrest, especially for families with children. Others are worried that their own home will become less attractive in the housing market as a result of the area's reputation, or that they react to, e.g., persistent poor waste management, police being observed regularly in the neighborhood, the lawn never being mowed, or noticeable accumulations of various things in the yard.

If there are conflicts with neighbors, it may be necessary to seek help from a mediation council, the police, or the legal system in various ways. Supported housing workers should assist residents in conflict-ridden situations with neighbors, but they are not responsible for resolving it.

Confidentiality weighs heavily in such situations, where other content and information must be balanced based on the situation. The role of the housing support personnel can be to guide the resident and facilitate dialogue, to contribute to the developing of the resident's d cultural and social skills related to neighborliness. This can be conflict-preventing in the long run. Another important aspect is that neighborliness cannot be reduced to only dealing with the individual resident, it is necessary to include targeted measures at the group and community level [1]. Neighborliness is about finding a balance between people's security and the integration of residents.

How to Meet Someone in Their Own Home?

Doing follow-up in someone's home is different from meeting the person at the service office, an outpatient unit, or a 24-h housing unit. In the service provider's arenas, more of the power relationship lies with the personnel, in terms of deciding if and how long the users should be there. In a home, you must respect the resident's boundaries and not be too insistent on what should be sorted out during the visits. How the visits are over time can affect quality of life, and it is important to have conversations about what can be challenging with resettlement. Here are some important qualities and approaches for housing support personnel [16]:

- Commitment to working with the target group, ability to adapt to the individual's needs.
- Flexible, structured, solution-oriented, self-reliant, creative.
- Able to set boundaries, act predictably, be confident in oneself, and be patient.
- Ability for interdisciplinary collaboration and coordination.
- Able to remain calm, withstand working under stress, and handle challenges.
- Withstand being rejected, withstand the user becoming angry and irritated, do not get in position and still stand in it.
- Actively seek out and highlight the user's positive sides.
- In conversations, be respectful, clear, friendly, predictable, sensitive, and listen.
- Be observant of the use of your own and the user's gaze, body language, and tone of voice.
- Some are extra vulnerable to various forms of rejection. Be aware of how you inform, and have processes around assumed difficult conversations.
- Create safe frames, be patient, flexible, and available—and spend time on achieving a collaborating atmosphere.

Actively Participate in Practical Tasks

Some users have, over several years, experienced many broken relationships and have, for various reasons, little trust in the support system. Therefore, it is important to be patient initially, so that the users get an experience that the housing follow-up workers are trustworthy [16]. To achieve good housing follow-up services, those who follow-up must agree with and reconsider with the user what the purpose of home visits is, and that it is clear what services can be offered. The person living in a home decides who is let in, and the resident's right not to open must be respected [1]. On the other hand, this can be a dilemma: For how long do you wait to take action when you can't get in touch with the resident? It is useful to have a dialogue with the resident about how to handle such situations. Some might want you to, via a formal consent, get an extra key to lock yourself in, or want you to contact caregivers.

The following presents practical tips in connection with home visits. Some of the points are pointedly formulated and will therefore be suitable for reflection and discussion (based on guidance from the Substance Abuse and Mental Health Services Administration, [17]):

- Inform others at your workplace about where you are, approximately how long you will be away, and if you have a coworker with you.
- Call first, send a text message, or leave a note about the time.
- Do not come without having the time confirmed. If you still travel, what consequences can the visit have?
- Think about the purpose of the visit, is this something the resident is obliged to receive?
- Check the daily form before the visit. Ask if a visit is ok, do not take for granted that everyone wants a visit.
- Knock/ring and ask if you can come in. Explain why you are visiting.
- Do not enter without the resident inviting you to do so. Respect the private sphere. Ask if it's okay before you sit down or touch anything in the home.

When you are allowed to come in, the motivation for it may be something completely different than what was the original purpose of the visit. It is then important to understand what you are being invited to, and prioritize it before—or instead—the reason you went there [18]. It is also important to be aware that you are in a private arena where you are to protect the resident's integrity, and thus, the relationship between you can be vulnerable. To create and maintain a relationship, there are three things that are important: Adapt to the resident's needs, avoid taking control during visits, and help the resident articulate uncertainty and things that hinder living and related cooperation. Further, it is useful with a supportive team where disappointments and difficult situations can be addressed, and colleagues can listen and provide input [1].

If the resident has caregivers, they can be an important resource in supported housing. They may have knowledge and experiences that can be important in finding suitable housing and types of supported housing. The effort of caregivers will sometimes be absolutely crucial for stability and dignity for the resident, and a necessary part for the support to be useful. Read more about the role of caregivers in Chap. 13.

Someone's Home, Others' Work Environment

The work environment for those who offer supported housing is an important aspect, and is equally applicable in such services as in other working contexts in general. This with regard to various forms of safety, infection control, and physical conditions. The latter can be, e.g., about access to the home, parking of the car, and outdoor and indoor lighting.

In some cases, it may be necessary to express some needs/wishes to the resident related to the visits, e.g., pets (allergies, aggressive behavior), that syringes and other things that pose an infection risk are collected and handled by the resident themselves, or that the housing is aired before visits. Other aspects can, e.g., be about whether the electrical system is in accordance with regulations. It is important that the personnel report relevant aspects to their leader, with regard to ongoing needs, to consider and, if possible, adjust work environment challenges. Individual decisions can be made in connection with services, where the resident commits to follow certain rules or procedures for the service to be provided. Such conditions must have a clear connection with the content and purpose of the decision, and be according to eventual legislation in the respective country. It can be related to, e.g., hygienic conditions, safety, or other aspects related to the work environment [1].

Violence Risk in Someone's Home

Some people have a low threshold for becoming verbally threatening or physically acting out. It can also occur that some deliberately want to make you feel insecure, either with body language or by, e.g., leaving a weapon visible in their home. It is well documented that it can be very stressful to work with people who have a certain risk of being physically and mentally threatening, aggressive, or violent. In risk assessments, the employees must map out different situations and assess possible consequences and outcomes, collect relevant information, and create preventive routines and safety procedures for each case [1].

As a housing support worker, you must have the ability to de-escalate situations and have good judgment of when you should withdraw [16]. When it comes to special safety measures, it must be assessed whether there is a need for more employees to go together. In safety routines, it must be clearly stated when to ask for assistance from the emergency services, and the employees must know how to facilitate good cooperation with the agency for the best possible outcome for the user and the least possible damage or risk to society. Sometimes housing support personnel also have to acknowledge that there are insolvable dilemmas and situations with danger to others' lives and health, where one cannot help without putting one's own life and health at risk.

It is important that each employee reflects on their own contributions in a difficult situation that has arisen, as a proportion of situations arise as a result of the employee's approach. If there have been episodes involving violence or threats, the manager should ensure that the employee(s) receive debriefing and possibly be shielded from other assignments that day. Employees must always report deviations and/or damage in connection with violence and threats. If there have been serious episodes, the need for further follow-up should be assessed by the manager. It is important to detect insecurity and uncertainty early among the employees, as well as prevent with good preparations and management plans [16]. Taking care of the staff must be prioritized highly. A good working environment prevents regular turnover of employees and ensures stability; it is a safety measure in itself [1]. Read more in Chap. 10 about follow-up when the risk of violence is a problem area.

Record Keeping

In each country, there might not be clear rules related to the documentation of residential follow-up. In most cases with housing follow-up, which is not defined as a health service, there is no requirement for documentation. However, requirements for professionalism and professionally sound work necessitate documentation, and in this way, you can, e.g., be indirectly regulated by acts [1]. Furthermore, good documentation of a resident's functional level over time related to residential management can also be very useful information for the specialist health service in connection with assessment, provided that the resident consents to the distribution of the information. Residential follow-up should be documented [19] because:

- It makes the actual follow-up visible, it gives an overview of the status and current usefulness of interventions, or lack thereof.
- It provides insight into what is actually offered.
- Opportunity for quality assurance and evaluation, and systematically monitor eventual progress in the resident's functional level.

Transition from Institution to Housing

If a hospitalized patient needs help with arranging existing housing or acquiring new housing before discharge, the municipality must be contacted quickly to start looking at possibilities for planning new housing or eventual adjustments related to existing housing [19].

Here are some practical tips related to discharge:

- The people responsible for follow-up/treatment municipality/specialist service, clarify the discharge date with the patient/user, caregivers, and relevant cooperating partners.
- For some patients/users, it may be beneficial to be able to retain the day place/contact with the day unit/institution for an agreed period in the transition phase when moving into their own home.
- A (cross-sectorial) team meeting is held if there is an agreed need for it, and consent has been obtained from the patient/user or on behalf of the patient/user.

The purpose of the meeting is to review and coordinate all aspects related to discharge, and clarify any remaining uncertainty that must be resolved before discharge.
- It is important that the specialist services at discharge have good routines to inform relevant municipal services about treatment interventions that have changed during the stay, which are of immediate importance for the patient at discharge. The epicrisis is not always immediately available to municipal services, and e.g., digital short-form, cross-sectorial messaging systems do not always contain necessary information, which increases the risk of harm and lack of compliance in the follow-up.
- Plan/individual plan for follow-up after discharge is prepared or updated. It is clarified who is responsible for further treatment and follow-up, and who the patient/user and caregivers can turn to with any questions and challenges.

Discharge from Specialist Security Unit

This patient group clearly differs from most other groups of patients in terms of the type of needs and scope of treatment, and thus also how resource-demanding treatment and follow-up will be. There can be challenges related to self-care, aggressive or threatening behavior, a tendency to isolation, as well as reduced interpersonal abilities related to shared decision-making and alliance building. The patients often reject contact with others and often have SUD and co-occurring somatic disorders. Other characteristics are homelessness or problems with maintaining a home, frequent and unplanned admissions, and the consequences of relapse in terms of mental challenges are large, e.g., new psychosis breakthroughs [20].

Lack of legal basis can be a hindrance to intervening where some patients have deteriorated or been exploited. The juridical protection for the individual can be weakened if ways of controlling and regulating are implemented that are in violation of human and other juridical rights. This group is largely dependent on safety, predictability, and trust due to their severe mental illness, and societal protection related to prevention of new episodes of violence, and requires gradual reduction of coercion and security-based interventions while cautiously increasing new stimuli.

Release from Prison

Convicts should be offered needs and resource mapping in the correctional services as early as possible in the execution of the sentence. Through this mapping, among other things, including later mapping, the need to acquire or maintain housing will emerge. This information is used to concretize interventions, in order to try to ensure the inmate a safe and good living situation. This can be done with the help of a treatment plan and group meetings in prison or, eventually, digitally when the prison is technically set up for such possibilities, between present services. The correctional services, along with in-prison health care personnel, should ensure that there is established contact with relevant services well before release [21]. This usually means that it is necessary to establish this contact more than a couple of weeks before release in order to make the transition as smooth and useful as possible, and avoid the high risk of quick relapse. It is important that the support system contributes to basic practical things the first time after release. Here are some tips for prison and staff associated with housing and housing follow-up (partly based on [21]):

- Tasks related to housing should start as soon as possible after imprisonment. Contact the imprisoned individual's hometown to address needs and express the need for binding, mutual cooperation. Proper housing is one of the most important factors that must be in place to offer real opportunities for reintegration, (re) habilitation, and recovery.
- A person who is summoned to serve a sentence should have a clear plan for future rental, storage for private properties, how pets should be taken care of, etc. Those who follow-up the person should start assessing the need for assistance related to this as soon as the date for the sentence start is known. This type of practical focus is a general joint responsibility for all service levels. Much of this is difficult in prisons with high security levels, e.g., access to an ID card, online banking, digital login on official services, personal email, available phone time, and so on.
- Inmates should at discharge, have a copy of the mapping done, including eventual future plans set up, appointments, treatment plan, contact information to specific personnel or services, etc.

Read more about mental health care services related to prison in Chap. 11.

Summary

- Low-threshold housing types may be necessary, but to a limited extent. Temporary housing should only be used in connection with acute situations, and should therefore not extend over a long period of time.
- There is a need for different types of municipal housing for people with SUD/MH, ideally with different housing types that have each threshold for substance use and challenging behavior. Not everyone can live in small houses, not everyone can live with others, and some need 24/7 staffing.
- Treatment-like supportive housing is absolutely necessary for some to stay in their home and create a home.
- Housing and any clarification of what the follow-up in the home should be must be clarified or started process well in advance of discharge from an inpatient ward or release from prison.
- There is no single, universal definition of what constitutes good housing conditions, as it varies from resident to resident and countries in-between. On the

other hand, each country has its references, which set the tone for a physical and technical standard, e.g., certain types of available electronics (washing machine, oven), electrical installation, type and quality of isolation, building materials, etc.
- The core is to have a home that is stable and safe, be able to create a home, and be able to handle daily living in line with the ongoing level of function.

Reflection Questions

- What characterizes a messy home environment? What is your personal limit for poor cleanliness, and can that affect how you interact with the resident and offer housing support?
- What importance can cultural factors have in terms of how individuals or families want to live, and can it affect how you consider someone's needs and level of functioning?
- How would you react if you were directly or indirectly pressured to agree to premises, rules, and interventions you do not want, which are directly/indirectly, with various elements of informal and formal coercion, forced on you in order for you to get a home or to keep it?
- Regardless of what the agreement on follow-up is with the resident, you will sometimes see and hear things that the resident may not have thought about and that are not related to the housing support. How do you relate to that? What dilemmas can arise?
- Think about your own past and present neighborhoods: When do you think that someone in your neighborhood can be a nuisance? What kinds of behavior and events make you feel unsafe or bothered? Do you think the person you offer supported housing might have similar opinions as you?
- Could someone with a substance use disorder or severe mental disorder rent an apartment in your home? If no or unsure: Does your opinion affect your interaction with service users/patients when helping them to obtain housing on the private market?
- Can't residents be left in peace even if they live a life in their own home that primarily harms their own quality of life?

Recommended Literature

- Best practices for recovery housing (2023): library.samhsa.gov/sites/default/files/best-practices-for-recovery-housing-pep23-10-00-002.pdf
- Housing first Europe Hub: housingfirsteurope.eu
- Housing first Institute: pathwayshousingfirst.org

References

1. Aakerholt A, Vea A, Tønnesen BL. Hjelp til å bo. Oppfølging i bolig til personer med rusog psykisk lidelse [Housing support. Housing support for people with substance use disorder and mental illness]. Oslo: Universitetsforlaget; 2016.
2. Norwegian University of Life Sciences. Folk som sliter med rus og psyken trenger et hjem, ikke bare et sted å bo [People struggling with substance use and mental health needs a home, not just a place to live]. Oslo: forskning.no; 2020. Available at https://www.forskning.no/medisinske-metoder-nmbu-norges-miljo-og-biovitenskapelige-universitet-partner/folk-som-sliter-med-rus-og-psyken-trenger-et-hjem-ikke-bare-et-sted-a-bo/1668192.
3. Kommunal landspensjonskasse. Kommunale utleieboliger. Risikoreduksjon [Municipal rental housing. Risk reduction]. Oslo: Kommunal landspensjonskasse; 2014. Available at https://klp.no/virksomhet/hms/skadeforebygging/_/attachment/download/3351da1a-d07f-4746-b00d-62d017621812:5d45c7ad891b8dab0203d1b58565d6f9aa48fb53/KLP_Temahefte_utleie2017_A4_web.pdf.
4. The Norwegian State Housing Bank. Personer med rusmiddelavhengighet og/eller psykiske lidelser [People with substance use disorder and/or mental illness]. Bodø: Husbanken; 2025. Available at https://www.husbanken.no/kommune/lan-og-tilskudd/investeringstilskudd/veileder-omsorgsbygg/ulike-beboeres-bo%2D%2Dog-aktivitetsbehov/personer-med-rus%2D%2Dog-psykiske-helseutfordringer/.
5. The Norwegian Directorate of Health. Kommunens ansvar for varig botilbud [The municipality's responsibility for permanent housing]. In: Nasjonal faglig retningslinje for utredning, behandling og oppfølging av personer med samtidig ruslidelse og psykisk lidelse – ROP-lidelser Sammensatte tjenester – samtidig behandling [National guideline for assessment, treatment and follow-up of people with co-occurring substance use disorder and mental health disorder – dual diagnosis. Compounded services – co-occurring treatment]. Oslo: The Norwegian Directorate of Health; 2012. Available at https://www.helsedirektoratet.no/retningslinjer/samtidig-ruslidelse-og-psykisk-lidelse-rop-lidelser/Utredning,%20behandling%20og%20oppf%C3%B8lging%20av%20personer%20med%20ROP-lidelser%20%E2%80%93%20Nasjonal%20faglig%20retningslinje%20(fullversjon).pdf/_/attachment/inline/c3cf6958-227f-499a-8f0b-0055dca9fc2c:286222117d81c9f269cddbee85a495a47bf9df29/Utredning,%20behandling%20og%20oppf%C3%B8lging%20av%20personer%20med%20ROP-lidelser%20%E2%80%93%20Nasjonal%20faglig%20retningslinje%20(fullversjon).pdf.
6. SINTEF. Boligen er viktig for helsa til psykisk syke [Housing is important for the health of mentally ill people]. Trondheim: SINTEF; 2019. Available at https://sintef.no/siste-nytt/boligen-er-viktig-for-helsa-til-psykisk-syke/.
7. Aakerholt A. ACT-håndbok (2. utg.) [ACT handbok (2nd edt.)]. Hamar: Norwegian National Advisory Unit on Concurrent Substance Abuse and Mental Health Disorders; 2013. Available at https://omsorgsforskning.brage.unit.no/omsorgsforskning-xmlui/handle/11250/2444658.
8. Mueser KT, Noordsy DL, Drake RE, Fox L. Integrert behandling av rusproblemer og psykiske lidelser [Integrated dual disorder treatment]. Oslo: Universitetsforlaget; 2006.
9. Tsemberis S. The pathways model to end homelessness for people with mental health and substance use disorders. Minnesota: Hazelden; 2010.
10. Housing First Europe Hub. What is Housing First? Available at https://housingfirsteurope.eu/what-is-hf/.
11. Norwegian Resource Centre for Community Mental Health. Housing first. Trondheim: Nasjonalt kompetansesenter for psykisk helsearbeid; 2025. Available at https://napha.no/temaside/housing-first.
12. Molde municipality. Håndbok for en rusfri hverdag [Handbook for a drug-free everyday life]. Molde kommune; 2020. Available at https://rusfrihverdag.no/
13. Clausen H, Ruud T. The practical and social functioning (PSF) scale: development and measurement properties of an instrument for assessing activity and social participation among

people with serious mental illness. BMC Psychiatry. 2024;24(1):693. https://doi.org/10.1186/s12888-024-06135-x.
14. Priebe S, McCabe R, Bullenkamp J, Hansson L, Lauber C, Martinez-Leal R, Rössler W, Salize H, Svensson B, Torres-Gonzales F, van den Brink R, Wiersma D, Wright DJ. Structured patient-clinician communication and 1-year outcome in community mental healthcare: cluster randomised controlled trial. Br J Psychiatry. 2007;191:420–6. https://doi.org/10.1192/bjp.bp.107.036939.
15. Martens J-F, Stugu S. Fire boligpolitiske forslag [Four housing policy proposals]. Klassekampen; 2020. Available at https://klassekampen.no/utgave/2020-12-07/fire-boligpolitiske-forslag
16. Welfare Administration, Oslo. Bosetting av personer med sikkerhetsproblematikk i egne boliger [Settlement of people with safety issues in their own homes]. Oslo: Oslo kommune; 2020. Available at https://www.oslo.kommune.no/getfile.php/13389257-1607948331/Tjenester%20og%20tilbud/Politikk%20og%20administrasjon/Bydeler/Bydel%20Grorud/Politikk%20i%20Bydel%20Grorud/Grorud%20bydelsutvalg/M%C3%B8ter/2020-03-19/Sammen%20om%20bolig/Digital%20metodeh%C3%A5ndbok%20-%20Bosetting%20av%20personer%20med%20sikkerhetsproblematikk%20i%20egne%20hjem.pdf.
17. Substance Abuse and Mental Health Services Administration. Permanent supportive housing: training frontline staff, HHS Pub. Id. SMA-10-4509. Rockville: Center for Mental Health Services, Substance Abuse, and Mental Health Services Administration, U.S. Department of Health and Human Services; 2010.
18. Mauseth KW. Å ha et beboerperspektiv på hjemmebesøk [Having a resident perspective on home visits]. In: Brodtkorb, E. og Rugkåsa, M. (eds.). Under tak – mellom vegger. [Under the roof – between walls]. Oslo: Gyldendal; 2007.
19. Linde S, Nordlund I. Innføring i profesjonelt miljøarbeid. Systematikk, kvalitet og dokumentasjon [Introduction to professional environmental work. Systematics, quality and documentation]. Oslo: Universitetsforlaget; 2006.
20. SIFER Utskrivningsklare pasienter i sikkerhetspsykiatrien – en kartlegging av utskrivningsprosessen fra sikkerhetsavdeling til kommune [Discharge-ready patients in security psychiatry – a mapping of the discharge process from secure psychiatric unit to the municipality]. SIFER; 2020. Available at https://sifer.no/wp-content/uploads/2022/02/Utskrivningsklare-pasienter-i-sikkerhetspsykiatrien-en-kartlegging-av-utskrivelsesprosessen-fra-sikkerhet-savdeling-til-kommune-1.pdf.
21. The Norwegian Correctional Service. Bolig. [Housing]. Lillestrøm: Kriminalomsorgen; 2024. Available at https://xn--tilbakefring-2jb.no/bolig/.

Supported Employment: IPS

5

Karl Petter Gjeterud, Therese Bekkevold, Grethe Breirem-Sveen, Mads Kristian Johansen, and Tore Willy Lie

Abstract

Employment can lead to enhanced income, psychosocial benefits, clinical improvements, and decreased use of mental health services. Individuals with SUD/MH have a very high unemployment rate and can face many challenges in obtaining and maintaining employment. Among them are treatment providers who believe employment services are not in their scope of practice, including underestimating the patients' working ability. On the other hand, several services also recognize that supported employment is an important part of recovery for this target group, especially when it is integrated with other services. One of the preferred models is Individual Placement and Support (IPS), which is an evidence-based practice for individuals with severe mental illness. It has emerged as

K. P. Gjeterud
Norwegian Labour and Welfare Administration (Nav), Moss, Norway
e-mail: karl.petter.gjeterud@nav.no

T. Bekkevold
Norwegian Labour and Welfare Administration (Nav), Fredrikstad, Norway
e-mail: therese.bekkevold@nav.no

G. Breirem-Sveen
Fontenehuset Gjøvik, Gjøvik, Norway
e-mail: grethe@fontenehusetgjovik.no

M. K. Johansen (✉)
Norwegian Labour and Welfare Administration (Nav), Bodø, Norway
e-mail: mads.kristian.johansen@nav.no

T. W. Lie
Department of Health and Nursing Sciences and Section for Mental Health and Rehabilitation, University of Inland Norway, Elverum, Norway
e-mail: tore.lie@inn.no

T. W. Lie, L. Lien (eds.), *Integrated Treatment of Co-occurring Substance Use and Mental Health Disorders*, https://doi.org/10.1007/978-3-032-20049-5_5

a robust approach to helping individuals obtain and succeed in competitive employment. This chapter has an introduction to the rationale and principles of IPS, experiences of using the model for individuals with SUD/MH, and a list of examples of other supported employment measures.

Keywords

Individual placement and support · Supported employment · Psychosocial rehabilitation · Work participation · Vocational rehabilitation · Competitive employment · Empowerment-based support model

Participating in competitive work despite SUD/MH problems can be of great importance for the individual. For example, it may provide structure and fill daily free time with meaningful activity and decrease opportunities to use substances among other factors [1]. It can also be important for society, which implies the usefulness of having a cross-political agreement that we should have a society and a working life that includes and provides opportunities for everyone. Through a joint strategy, politicians can connect the labor and welfare administration and health sector to open up opportunities for IPS implementation, which is an integrated treatment service for individuals with moderate to severe mental disorders. It has been tried with new target groups, among them individuals with SUD. Many personnel and participants have expressed positive feedback about the method's efficacy and usefulness, but there is little research on IPS for individuals who have SUD/MH. Currently available analyses indicate an effect of IPS employment for this target group [1, 2]. An RCT shows that IPS participants worked more hours and earned a higher total salary than control group participants [3], and other RCT studies are going on [4, 5].

Description of the Method

IPS was developed especially for individuals with severe mental illness and later expanded to also include moderate mental illness. It is a comprehensive program where several criteria must be met according to a fidelity scale, including that the program is integrated with mental health services [6]. The method is evidence-based [7] and has eight central principles [8]:

1. Focus on competitive employment: Agencies providing IPS services are committed to competitive employment as an attainable goal for individuals with behavioral health conditions seeking employment. Education and specialized training may enhance career paths.
2. Eligibility based on client choice: Individuals are not excluded because of perceived lack of readiness, diagnoses, symptoms, substance use history, psychiatric hospitalizations, homelessness, level of disability, or legal system involvement.

3. Integration of rehabilitation and mental health services: IPS programs are closely integrated with mental health treatment teams.
4. Attention to worker preferences: Services are based on each person's preferences and choices, rather than providers' judgments.
5. Personalized benefits counseling: Employment specialists help individuals obtain personalized, understandable, and accurate information about their Social Security, Medicaid, and other government entitlements.
6. Rapid job search: IPS programs use a rapid job search approach to help job seekers obtain jobs directly, rather than providing lengthy pre-employment assessment, training, and counseling. If further education is part of their plan, IPS specialists assist in these activities as needed.
7. Systematic job development: Employment specialists systematically visit employers, who are selected based on job seeker preferences, to learn about their business needs and hiring preferences.
8. Time-unlimited and individualized Support: Job support is individualized and continues for as long as each worker wants and needs the support.

In IPS, everyone who wants to work is eligible. Participation is determined by the individual's own wish for competitive employment—no one is excluded. This core principle and other key elements contribute to IPS being a robust evidence-based model for supporting people with substance use and mental health problems [9]. It is built on a binding cooperation between the welfare and health care services.

The main goal of IPS is to support individuals to be employed in regular work without unpaid internships or probationary periods. Regular work is defined as work that anyone can apply for in society, which provides regular pay, at least the minimum wage [10]. There is no requirement or expectation that it should be full-time, there can be different percentages of positions from 1 h a week to a full-time position according to the participant's preferences. The goal is to create a permanent and predictable connection to the working world at a level that the participant experiences as reasonable and desired. Often, participants who start in smaller positions can increase as they master and have a desire for this. For some, it may be appropriate to take more education to reach the goal of regular work, in which case they will be able to receive IPS as part of their treatment when they seek education and support during the education period.

IPS Is Integrated with Mental Health Services

In IPS, employment-oriented services are integrated with rehabilitation and mental health services. IPS is a team approach, where a treatment team consists of an employment specialist, therapists, and other employees in mental health and substance use services. In IPS, the employment specialist is part of a multidisciplinary treatment team, in line with health personnel, such as psychiatrists, psychologists, social workers, nurses, and more. In addition, the employment specialist is part of an employment-oriented team together with other employment specialists, where they have a common method supervisor. The method supervisor leads the employment-oriented team and has an important role in promoting the integration of the IPS service and regularly participates in meetings of the multidisciplinary treatment teams.

Some examples of services that can offer IPS as a part of their follow-up concept:

- SUD inpatient and outpatient treatment units. There are also examples of OAT services that have IPS integrated as a part of their service.
- Municipality health services, where they also have cooperation with other housing and municipal services.
- ACT and FACT teams, which are often a formal collaboration between the specialist service and the municipal health service.

IPS in FACT

ACT and FACT are treatment models that are based on formalizing cross-sectional, multidisciplinary collaboration, in the form of an agreement between the specialist service and the municipalities involved. It is desirable that IPS is strengthened in the ACT/FACT teams. The IPS method involves integrating the treatment apparatus into the follow-up toward ordinary work. A success criterion for this to happen is a binding collaboration between the municipal/specialist health service and the Norwegian Labour and Welfare Administration. Employment specialists have now been introduced in several FACT teams, where the approach has been well received, and the implementation has worked well in practice. IPS is applied in the same way in FACT as in other treatment settings. Together, FACT and IPS create a good platform for coordinated support throughout the treatment process. We find it challenging that both IPS and FACT have different fidelity scales, which sometimes conflict with each other's tasks and roles. Read more about ACT and FACT teams in Chap. 12.

Adapted Benefits and Benefit Guidance

Participants in IPS shall receive individually adapted social services and benefits to secure the participant's finances. This may involve financial social assistance for living, housing, health, and dental treatment, as well as financial advice and possibly help in entering into an agreement with a creditor in the event of debt problems. The participant's fear of losing benefits is often a barrier to work participation. The purpose of individually adapted financial advice is for the participant to be secure in their finances in the event of changes in salary, employment rate, and benefit changes, especially in the event of a transition to regular work. Several articles have been written about the connection between mental illness and financial problems, and it seems as if it can go both ways: Mental illness can often lead to financial problems [11], but financial problems also affect mental health [12].

Here is an example that underlines that the need for individually tailored financial advice is not only about the amount, but also about creating predictability and a sense of security: During a conversation with an employment specialist in a FACT team, a participant said, "I decided to quit my job because the financial framework wasn't clear enough. A fixed disability pension gave me more predictability, and that felt more important than earning a little extra."

Starting the Job Search Process

Contact with employers begins shortly after a participant has expressed a desire to work. Rapid job search is about starting the process of developing the participant's career profile and job development plan and does not necessarily require the participant to have applied for a job within the first 30 days. The employment specialist quickly begins systematic job development after the first meeting with the participant to get to know what the potential job market for the individual participant may be. Contact with the job market and knowledge of employers is also used in the conversation with the participant to explore possible job tasks and the work environment at different employers that the participant has expressed an interest in and may suit the participant.

In IPS, long-term mapping work, review of work ability, and use of job training are avoided before trying to find regular work. The participant can choose to look for jobs and contact employers on their own or receive support from the employment specialist to get in touch with potential employers. A first physical meeting with a relevant employer for the participant can then be conducted by the individual themselves, along with the employment specialist, or the employment specialist alone at the individual's request. It is often experienced as motivating when the individual experiences that their desire for work is taken seriously. Some may feel that it is scary. Then the employment specialist uses the contact with the employers to inform themselves and the participant about what the labor market looks like.

Building Relationships with Employers

Through systematic job development, employment specialists build relationships with a network of employers based on the participant's interests and preferences. The employment specialist contacts employers to get to know the business, work tasks, and needs and informs the companies about what the IPS services can offer (close support and follow-up if the participant wishes and follow-up by the employer). Through systematic job development, the employment specialist supports the participant and employer in finding good solutions together and through this creates a good job match. For those who find it a little scary to approach work, the employment specialist works to create good relationships with employers. This is to be close to the participant and arrange not-so-formal meetings to get to know different employers. The process is adapted to the individual's wishes and needs.

Job Support with No Time Limit

The intention of time-limited job support is to ensure that participants receive follow-up after they have found work. Job support is individually tailored based on work tasks, previous experiences, challenges related to SUD/MH, and other issues. Job support should continue for as long as the participant wishes. Then, ideally, follow-up should be transferred to another person in the participant's network (relative, colleague at work, general practitioner, or others) so that the threshold for saying something if it starts to get difficult is as low as possible. It is better that we catch it early and correct it than that they fall back into old habits and thought patterns. Many participants try several jobs during their time in IPS. They change jobs because they want development or other tasks or because it simply does not work. Even if they are dismissed from their position due to, e.g., SUD, the IPS service or treatment is not interrupted. Substance use problems have also often been a problem in previous employment relationships. Each experience related to it is analyzed together with the participant and is considered a learning opportunity.

Respect for the Participant's Preferences

All choices related to the employment-oriented services are made on the basis of the individuals' wishes, resources, and experiences. Employees associated with the IPS service support the individual to make their own decisions about the type of work, job support, openness about background, etc. The individuals' preferences and goals should be considered rather than the situation in the labor market, such as vacancies or needs within certain industries. An important argument for this is that the right job (tasks, working environment, working hours, scope, etc.) to a greater extent ensures continuity and a stronger connection to working life. Especially in the beginning, it is important to minimize risk factors and focus on managing the situation one step at a time.

When it comes to being open about one's own challenges related to substance use and mental health, there are different opinions and experiences, and some may experience that they lose job opportunities by being open about it [13]. In the context of IPS, one explores what the individual thinks about being open about health issues and how they want to share their background with a potential employer. This is a conversation the employment specialist has with the individual and maybe the therapist or caregivers. Ultimately, it is the individual who decides how and what they want to share with employers. Experience has shown that this can change over time. Therefore, this is a process that is repeated as new experiences are gained and used to eventually adjust what is seen as shareable information. The employment specialist contributes with their previous experiences, as well as guidance on what can be said and how, so that the individual can make their own informed choice.

IPS Fidelity Scale

The IPS fidelity scale, also called IPS 25, describes how fidelity reviews are carried out and the intention of the review is described [11]. It consists of 25 criteria that together provide guidance on what characterizes a well-implemented IPS service. Each point is graded from 1 (not implemented) to 5 (fully implemented). The scale is divided into three main areas:

1. Staffing: Includes three criteria that describe how the employment specialist's everyday life is structured. How many participants the employment specialist should follow-up, the phases of the specialists' follow-up, and that they are dedicated to the role and are not working on other tasks.
2. Organization: Includes eight points that describe how the service is organized, how the organization creates the conditions for a good IPS offer for patients, including cooperation with and anchoring in management.
3. Follow-up: This is the most comprehensive part and contains fourteen points that describe how the service is implemented. These points describe how to work together to achieve the goal of a permanent connection to the working world for the participant/patient.

The degree of method fidelity according to the IPS fidelity scale is related to whether participants enter work and remain employed over time. The goal with these reviews is for the organization to gain better ownership and knowledge of the content of the fidelity scale and to ensure operation according to the IPS method.

For newly established IPS services, the recommendation is that they should conduct the first review after 6–9 months. Then, regularly, once or twice per year, depending on how well the IPS has been implemented. Reviews are carried out by one or more individuals with good knowledge of the IPS fidelity scale. The review involves reviewing documents and documentation, conversations with stakeholders, and observations of meetings, etc. This gives both an overall impression and an impression of how the different elements of the method have been implemented. Although each point describes a specific element, it is important for those carrying out the fidelity review to look at how these points are interconnected, to be able to provide good guidance for further work on the implementation of the IPS method. The practice today is self-assessment with support, where well-qualified IPS advisors guide the IPS service throughout the entire process. This way of carrying out assessments provides better opportunities for creating good ownership and knowledge of the content of the fidelity scale. It can also contribute to increased knowledge of the IPS method, the intentions behind the points in the fidelity scale, and good insight into one's own practice. The review provides a basis for the service to work further on the implementation of IPS in their organization. Review of services using a fidelity scale has shown a good effect on the degree of implementation [14].

IPS Practice Experiences

The following are three case examples presented from different perspectives and services in Norway (at Fredrikstad IPS, FACT Gjøvik, and a psychologist's first experiences with IPS) to illustrate IPS in practice.

Fredrikstad IPS

Fredrikstad IPS has two employment specialists in multidisciplinary specialist treatment for SUD and one employment specialist linked to the municipal service. We refer to experiences from this service (with names changed), with the consent of all involved, to highlight what constitutes good IPS practice for people with SUD/MH [15].

This example is about John, who has had substance use problems and ADHD. For several years, he has received follow-up from a mental health worker in the municipality, as well as in the specialist health service, for periods. He has had periods in his life where things have worked better and has several employment relationships behind him. However, he has not been able to completely take the step out of his substance use problem, even though he has attempted treatment several times. When he turned 40, John felt that he had really decided to change. He was then granted long-term treatment and was in SUD treatment at an inpatient unit for about 12 months. John had been referred to IPS several times before by a therapist in the specialist outpatient clinic, but did not get started due to relapse. However, he was aware of the offer. Well before John finished his long-term treatment, the employment specialist was contacted. John had been clear that he needed a job to be able to take the step into a different life with less substance use. Substance use was often the coping strategy in tough, stressful circumstances or when restlessness struck.

The goal was to be working upon discharge, so he would not have to go home and most likely end up in the same situation as many times before. Even though John had been referred to IPS several times, but had not gotten started, his desire for a job was also taken seriously this time.

In the first period, it was essential that the employment specialist Maria establish a good relationship with John. She attended two joint meetings at the treatment site and met John when he was home on leave. The employment specialist expressed that what made them successful in establishing a good relationship was that she was genuinely curious about both John's experiences and qualities, as well as what he wanted to work on.

John was very clear about his own desires and competencies. Where the participant is unsure or unclear about what he/she wants, it is important that the employment specialist takes the time to explore interests and talk to individuals in the network. One employment specialist refers to this as "looking for gold," finding where the motivation lies, or finding employers/tasks that light the "spark in the eye."

This illustrates the principle of following the participant's preferences. John had good confidence in his/her own abilities, but this is not always the case for all participants. It can often be important to challenge the participant to dare to believe in his/her own skills and opportunities for work. Supporters must at times be "bearers of faith, hope and love," as the employment specialist puts it. The job wish that underlies inclusion is fresh, and it often happens that participants give up along the way. It is then important that the supporters show that they believe that the participant has something to do in working life and contribute to reminding the participant of this by highlighting specific characteristics or experiences that show that there is a basis for the belief in a job, or the "job hope."

Initially, there were difficult periods that resulted in John not coming to meetings and appointments, but no one gave up. Eventually, the mental health worker left, and the therapist at the specialist outpatient unit was left alone with the follow-up together with the employment specialist. With such a solution, John did not have to deal with a new person and could continue in a safe environment with the employment specialist and his therapist. This happened in dialogue and was a natural development when the need for follow-up was no longer as great.

In IPS, one is concerned with maintaining established relationships and not changing employment specialists along the way, as some participants suffer from relationship damage. It is then crucial to create security in the relationship and allow the participant not to have to tell his story several times. John expressed early on that he found it tiring to tell his story repeatedly, as he had gone through several measures and offers previously. The employment specialist could then, with John's consent, be updated on what was relevant to her from the mental health worker and the therapist at the specialist outpatient unit. The close interaction between the mental health worker and the therapist in the specialist service in this situation created space for a recovery-oriented practice across sectors, in an appropriate way from the participant's process and progression. In this example, it could also have been relevant to connect with caregivers or other important individuals in the participant's network, who can contribute with other perspectives and experiences. Many caregivers have lost faith that things will get better. Caregivers can also be important to stay in touch with when the individual drops out or does not attend. Contact with caregivers must take place with the individual's consent.

FACT Gjøvik

The Flexible Assertive Community Treatment team, FACT Gjøvik [16], has a total of eleven employees in the team, where four of them do not have case manager responsibilities: a psychologist, a psychiatrist, a music therapist, and an occupational therapist. There is also a user specialist in the team (a trained social worker). Working in a FACT team is different from IPS in other areas. The team is used to thinking multidisciplinary—and as an occupational therapist, you quickly become a natural part of the team. It is experienced as a strength that the FACT teams are structured in such a way that it is easy for the IPS method to become an integrated part of the team.

In the FACT model, work is an important part of the treatment. The occupational therapist can contribute to the treatment process, for example, to gain more insight into executive functions. This can provide important observations of what the participants are able to do and what they struggle with at work.

At FACT Gjøvik, the importance of work being a starting point for the next step in life and a treatment goal for the patient is emphasized. The team conducts the job interview within a week of the appointment or calls the employment specialist during the treatment sessions and consultations. If the patient says that they want a job on Monday, it may not be as relevant on Thursday. In that case, it is important to capture the interest/motivation when it is there. Many patients have an opinion that it will not work based on previous experiences. In that case, it may be a harmless method to pick up the phone and have a short chat with the employment specialist, and approach work gradually.

In IPS, the emphasis is on meeting participants in their local environment or at home to build relationships with the participants in an arena where they feel safe. When individuals do not show up or disappear, the FACT team is effective in catching up with the participants. This strengthens the employment specialist's opportunities to stay in touch with participants who are struggling to meet.

Daily whiteboard meetings according to the FACT method are central to having an overview of the different patients in the portfolio and being able to quickly identify deviations or challenges. The employment specialist participates at least once a week. IPS or work is part of what is followed up on the whiteboard. FACT Gjøvik has developed the treatment plan so that work is highlighted. This helps to focus on work for all patients in the portfolio.

Everyone in the FACT team has experience and education that contribute to the interdisciplinary perspective. For example, when a participant wanted to work with music and singing, the music therapist helped produce a demo that the participant could then use in their search for a suitable job. Or a psychiatrist follows up on medication, which can help create better conditions for job success. The last one is about a person who had challenges getting started on their own. Then the therapist traveled to the person's home in the morning to help with various things, so that the person was ready to leave. Then the employment specialist came and drove the participant to work. Relatively many of the patients in the FACT team have disability insurance. This means that more are satisfied with working in an adapted, non-binding offer (also see the section on other work-oriented measures later in the chapter). The compensation for this does not affect the payment of disability benefits, as the amount is often below the limit for what one can earn as a disabled person, and at the same time, it is completely non-binding, and there is no expectation or requirement that the person will come. For those who want some activity and earn some money, this can be an alternative. This is about financial predictability and security. Several individuals may also be in the assessment phase to receive disability benefits and therefore cannot participate in a work-oriented measure until the case processing is complete, and a decision has been made. It is important to have individually adapted financial guidance, in parallel with other treatment/follow-up and the work-oriented services from the employment specialist. There are FACT teams that have their own supervisor from the Norwegian Labour and Welfare Administration in the team to ensure some financial guidance.

Situations may arise outside the participant's home where immediate contact with a therapist or others in the FACT team is crucial. For example, in the case of a drug-induced psychosis with delusions and conspiracy thoughts in the participant. By making a phone call to the therapist, the employment specialist got the therapist to follow-up. The employment specialist feels that this creates security in the meeting with participants. The therapist is keen to update the employment specialist on the status of participants in the IPS portfolio so that they are well updated.

The Importance of Meeting Someone in Their Arena

An IPS participant trained a lot, and it was difficult to get a meeting, even though we tried to go for a walk, meet at the FACT team's office, or do something else. The employment specialist ended up taking a training session with her, which included mapping. In several training sessions, she told her whole life story. It gradually became clear that work did not fit into her schedule. She was disabled and felt that everyone else's expectations of work were the same. She herself was very happy to have found accommodation, new friends, a good training environment, and money to live on with disability insurance. She did not quite see how work would fit in now, but after several joint training sessions, she was convinced to explore opportunities. She has since participated in projects and is going to start education and eventually return to work. She felt an obligation to have an employment specialist, and felt she was letting the employment specialist down by saying no.

Defining Personal Job Desires

It can be challenging to help participants define their job desires. Many have poor experiences from working life, or little previous experience and little knowledge of what opportunities exist. It is therefore important to work with this in ways other than just based on what they want or have done, interest tests, etc. Here is a good example of how an employment specialist at FACT Gjøvik did it:

The employment specialist began the conversation by focusing on the experiences they have gained so far. For example, many have experience with buying and selling drugs. This can be a useful experience even if they were previously associated with something illegal. The positive aspects are emphasized. This emphasizes the importance of exploring previous experiences and interests to bring out resources and relevant expertise.

Another example is about a participant with a lot of different work experience, who presented a long list of jobs and work tasks that he absolutely did not want. When reviewing previous experiences, the employment specialist asked the person to describe his previous work tasks and why these were no longer relevant. It then emerged that heat workers and sheet metal workers were not relevant due to the risk of injuring eyes and hands due to heat and sparks. This led to a discussion about the Health, Safety, and Environment (HSE) standard today. When asked why the person in question was afraid of injuring eyes and hands, it emerged that playing the guitar and writing/reading notes was a leisure interest that had great value for the participant. This eventually resulted in a job with children at an activity center where the participant was given space to use his interest by singing and playing for the children and having music-based activities with them. This freed up time for the educational staff so that they could focus on other tasks.

The person in the example above eventually says that he made the list so that he would not get a job. He was used to being presented with what he perceived as good opportunities, without it having previously led to anything. He had put up a wall to protect himself, but IPS includes as much as is important to address in the meeting with new or potential participants.

There is often talk of a good job match. This means that work tasks, interests, and skills match each other. Some have tried many different things that have not worked, and have later found permanent jobs where they are going well. The qualities that we have seen as challenging in one job have been a strength in another.

A Psychologist's First Encounter with IPS

This part is about a psychologist's first experience with IPS at a specialist outpatient unit: Philip was 44 years old. Over the past 5 years, he has experienced losing his job, contact with his children, and his social network. He had had an alcohol problem for several years. His alcohol use had contributed to the loss of things that were previously important to him. Nevertheless, he drank a lot. When he came to treatment, he was both tired and ashamed. Tired of drinking and ashamed that it had gone so far. In addition, he was no longer entitled to employment benefits and was placed on unemployment benefits.

He expressed that he was now ready for change. He wanted to have contact with his children and realized that he would then have to reduce his alcohol consumption. He also wanted to start working. The process of applying for a job was difficult for him. He was afraid of rejection and felt ashamed when he thought back to his previous workplace, where he had lost his job due to substance use. The changes happened quickly. He reduced his alcohol consumption considerably, and within a relatively short time, he only drank occasionally on weekdays. He was still drinking on the weekends and could sometimes lose control of his drinking. He had regained contact with his children. He had not yet been able to apply for a job and found this too difficult. In the conversations, we concentrated on managing his alcohol use and did not go into much detail about the process of getting a job.

Philip reflected on his own process and wondered why he had to quit drinking when there was nothing to stand up for. At the same time, we had found an employment specialist associated with the drug and alcohol outpatient clinic. With Philip's consent, the employment specialist was invited to a joint conversation, and we began working together. We worked closely together at first. Shortly after they had established contact, Philip began applying for jobs. The shame and fear of rejection had been reduced. He eventually took complete control of the process. After a few rejections, he got a permanent job after about 6 months. He then decided to quit drinking completely. He saw that drinking on the weekends affected his performance at work. Six months later, he was still not drinking alcohol and working in the same job.

As a therapist, I learned a lot from working with Philip and the IPS employment specialist. I learned that working to get back into work can act as an additional motivation for change. A motivation for change that I often fell short of creating in the therapy room. I got to see other sides of him that I would never have seen if it were solely office-based psychotherapy, and I see the need for co-occurring multidisciplinary support from other personnel in several cases I have worked with since.

Other Work-Oriented Measures

There are several different work-oriented services for individuals with SUD/MH in addition to the IPS services. What they have in common is that they place a high value on activity and work agenda and see this as important for reducing or gaining better control over the substance use problem.

It can be a measure where it is a requirement that you are not under the influence of alcohol or other drugs when you show up. Like work collectives, which are mainly run by the members themselves, with offers of work-oriented rehabilitation. For example, meetings are held where work tasks are distributed according to the needs and wishes of each visitor. The goal for the members is to take over as many tasks as possible, take responsibility, just like in a regular workplace. Further, support for writing a CV, training on interview situations and job searching, and arranging job dinners for employers in the local area, to create an arena where members and employers meet. It can be a type of job support, where ordinary workplaces are used as an arena for job training, where permanent employment is the goal.

Another variant is transitional work, where the institution has agreements with different employers to solve a specific job. The jobs are simple, so anyone can do them. This gives members the opportunity to work, e.g., half a year at a collective wage. Such places can also be a support for many, regardless of whether it is a transitional job or an ordinary job. It can function as a social arena where one meets other individuals in a similar situation.

There are many types of employment measures that may be relevant for individuals with SUD/MH. Availability, adaptation, and types depend on how administration and legislation are set up in each country, and how—and if they are based on an assessment of work ability. The work ability assessment can, e.g., be made by the person in dialogue with the supervisor in the labor and welfare administration. Some of the specific measures are, e.g.:

- Supported employment (SE) is a measure that targets individuals who need support to achieve and maintain employment, providing close and individualized follow-up from a local employment specialist. The program is based on the SE methodology, which is closely related to the Individual Placement and Support (IPS) model and emphasizes rapid job placement and ongoing support in ordinary workplaces.

- A measure aimed at individuals who are unsure of what they can work with, e.g., due to poor health or they have been out of work for a long time.
- "Follow-up" measures for individuals who need support or guidance to find or keep a job. It can be a mentor at work or support from a supervisor.
- Measures that are intended to strengthen work ability and that, through rehabilitation, provide support to overcome health-related and social problems such as work obstacles.
- Measures for individuals with disability insurance who need work in a sheltered enterprise. This is permanent adapted work with work tasks that are adapted to the participant. This can also be individual positions in ordinary enterprises.
- Qualification programs: Can, e.g., be for individuals who want employment, but need extra follow-up to get a job. In Norway, as an example, this is a municipal measure, unlike the above, which are state measures.

It is important to have a variety of offers as different individuals with SUD/MH may have different preferences in terms of both form and content. However, there are currently no employment measures that can show the same results as IPS, where research shows that over twice as many individuals find work with IPS compared to other measures [7, 17].

Summary

- IPS is an evidence-based method, which includes a fidelity scale with characterizations of how the service should be set up.
- Research has shown that it works better than other work-related services, but there is a need for more studies that examine the effect of IPS for individuals with SUD/MH.
- IPS can be established in the municipal health service, specialist health service, and, e.g., ACT/FACT teams.
- IPS is a recovery-oriented practice that is based on a holistic perspective, where, among other things, treatment and work-oriented services are carried out simultaneously and integrated.

Reflection Questions

- Do you generally underestimate individuals with SUD/MH's ability to work? What makes you confident in your judgment about others' work-related functional level? What can you do to change that attitude?
- The biggest challenge with IPS is that it is a cross-sectoral approach that requires close cooperation between the municipal health service, specialist service, and labor and welfare service. How can we ensure cross-sectional cooperation to optimize the potential of IPS?

- How can the different roles contribute to employment, and how can we utilize each other's strengths for the benefit of the patient?
- Why are multidisciplinary dynamics important for IPS?

Recommended Literature and Online Resources

- Handbook for IPS Peer Specialists; 2017.ipsworks.org/wp-content/uploads/2024/01/HANDBOOK-FOR-IPS-PEER-SPECIALISTS-1.10.24.pdf
- Individual Placement and Support (IPS)—A Supported Employment Model. Online resource by Substance Abuse and mental Health services administration (SAMHSA); 2025. library.samhsa.gov/product/individual-placement-and-support-ips-supported-employment-model/pep25-01-002
- IPS Employment Center: ipsworks.org
- IPS training courses: ipsgrow.org.uk/providers/training-courses/
- Supported employment fidelity review manual, fourth edition. A companion guide to the evidence-based IPS Supported Employment Fidelity Scale; 2019. ipsworks.org/index.php/product/fidelity-manual/
- Swanson SJ, Becker DR. IPS Supported Employment: A Practical Guide, 2022 Edition. IPS Employment Center; 2022. ipsworks.org/index.php/product/ips-supported-employment-a-practical-guide-2022-edition/

References

1. Mueser KT, Campbell K, Drake RE. The effectiveness of supported employment in people with dual disorders. J Dual Diagn. 2011;7:90.
2. Hellström L, Pedersen P, Christensen TN, Wallstroem IG, Bojesen AB, Stenager E, et al. Vocational outcomes of the individual placement and support model in subgroups of diagnoses, substance abuse, and forensic conditions: a systematic review and analysis of pooled original data. J Occup Rehabil. 2021;31(4):1–710.
3. Rognli EB, KAA A, Aas EM, Reme SE, Lystad JU, Stavseth MR, Arnevik EA. The effectiveness of Individual Placement and Support on vocational outcomes for patients with substance use disorders: A pragmatic superiority randomized controlled trial of Individual Placement and Support versus enhanced self-help. Addiction. 2025; https://doi.org/10.1111/add.70155.
4. Bejerholm U, Håkansson A, Knutagård M, Hillborg H. Individual Placement and Support for persons with alcohol and drug addiction in a Swedish context (IPS-ADAS): study protocol for a randomised controlled trial. Trials. 2024;25(1):222.
5. Marsden J, Anders P, Shaw C, Amasiatu C, Collate W, Eastwood B, Horgan P, Khetani M, Knight J, Knight S, Melaugh A, Clark H, Stannard J. Superiority and cost-effectiveness of Individual Placement and Support versus standard employment support for people with alcohol and drug dependence: a pragmatic, parallel-group, open-label, multicentre, randomised, controlled, phase 3 trial. EClinicalMedicine. 2024;68:102400.
6. Forsetlund L, Smedslund G, Hval G, Bergsund HB. Individual placement and support for people with moderate to severe mental illnesses or substance abuse disorder: a systematic review; 2023. Available at https://www.fhi.no/en/publ/2023/Individual-placement-and-support-for-people-with-moderate-to-severe-mental-illnesses-substance-abuse-disorder/.

7. Drake RE, Bond GR, Becker DR. Individual placement and support—an evidence-based approach to supported employment. New York: Oxford University Press; 2012.
8. IPS Employment Center. IPS practice and principles. Available at https://ipsworks.org/index.php/documents/ips-practice-and-principles/.
9. Harrison J, Krieger MJ, Johnson HA. Review of individual placement and support employment intervention for persons with substance use disorder. Subst Use Misuse. 2020;55(4):636–43. https://doi.org/10.1080/10826084.2019.1692035. Epub 2019 Nov 29. PMID: 31782349.
10. Becker DR, Swanson SJ, Reese SL, Bond GR, McLeman BM. Supported employment Fidelity review manual; 2019. Available at https://ipsworks.org/wp-content/uploads/2019/12/Final-Fidelity-Manual-Fourth-Edition-112619.pdf.
11. Holte A. Psykisk sykdom øker risiko for uhåndterlig gjeld, som igjen hindrer tilfriskning fra sykdommen – en usystematisk oversikt [Mental illness increases the risk of unmanageable debt, which in turn hinders recovery from the illness – an unsystematic review]. 2020. Available at https://psykologisk.no/2020/06/psykisk-sykdom-oker-risiko-for-uhandterlig-gjeld-som-igjen-hindrer-tilfriskning-fra-sykdommen-en-usystematisk-oversikt/.
12. Holte A. Gjeld øker risikoen for psykiske helseplager – en usystematisk oversikt [Debt increases the risk of mental health problems – an unsystematic overview]. 2020. Available at https://psykologisk.no/2020/06/gjeld-oker-risikoen-for-psykiske-helseplager-en-usystematisk-oversikt/.
13. Faltin T. Hvor høy er prisen for å være åpen om fortida? Fortalte om rusfortida, jobben glapp [How high is the price for being open about your past? Told about past drug use, didn't get the job]. 2021. Available at https://www.rus.no/aktuelt/hvor-hoy-er-prisen-for-a-vare-apen-om-fortida-fortalte-om-rusfortida-jobben-glapp.
14. McHugo GJ, Drake RE, Whitley R, Bond GR, Campbell K, Rapp CA, et al. Fidelity outcomes in the National Implementing Evidence-Based Practices Project. Psychiatr Serv. 2007; https://doi.org/10.1176/ps.2007.58.10.1279.
15. Bekkevold T, Olsen M, Melkic S, Kirkeng M. Experiences from Fredrikstad IPS (Norway) [personal communication, confirmed for use in this chapter]; 2021.
16. Breirem-Sveen G, Stensby I. Experiences from FACT Gjøvik (Norway) [personal communication, confirmed for use in chapter]; 2021.
17. Norwegian Institute of Public Health. Supported Employment for people with disabilities: a systematic review; 2017. Available at https://www.fhi.no/en/publ/2017/supported-employment-for-arbeidssokere-med-bistandsbehov-en-systematisk-ove/.

6 Drugs: Use and Addiction

Jørgen Gustav Bramness

Abstract

As seen in other chapters, there is a profound and frequent relationship between drug use and mental disorders. Many patients with mental disorders have extensive drug use, and many patients with substance use disorders (SUDs) have mental disorders. But it can be difficult to determine the causal pathway. Does it start with a mental disorder or with drug use? Many believe that the temporal relationship is helpful for deciding what to address first, but that may be a too simplistic understanding.

This chapter starts with some numbers. How common is substance use, and how many are addicted? Then we review the different drugs and drug groups. Knowledge about drugs can help us to a deeper understanding of the problems. What are the different drugs, and what are the consequences of their use? Finally, the concept of addiction is explained. Addiction is a commonly used word. We believe we have an intuitive understanding of the concept. But at closer inspection, many are bewildered. Addiction or dependence is difficult to explain.

J. G. Bramness (✉)
UiT The Arctic University of Norway, Tromsø, Norway

Department of Clinical Addiction Research, Oslo University Hospital, Oslo, Norway

Research Centre for Substance Use Disorders and Mental Illness, Hamar, Norway

European Federation for Addiction Societies, Salzburg, Austria
e-mail: joebra@ous-hf.no

T. W. Lie, L. Lien (eds.), *Integrated Treatment of Co-occurring Substance Use and Mental Health Disorders*, https://doi.org/10.1007/978-3-032-20049-5_6

Keywords

Dual disorder · Substance use disorder · Addiction · Dependence · Abuse

The Epidemiology of Substance Use

What is the prevalence of drug use and SUD? This is more difficult to answer than you might think. There are several problems associated with ascertaining the prevalence of drug use and SUD. Firstly: what to measure? Should we count all those who have tried a drug, those who use it regularly, or just those with drug problems? Secondly, we lack good data. You can't just go out on a street and ask people about their drug habits and expect honest replies. You won't meet everybody there, not everyone would want to talk to you and not everyone will reply truthfully. Drug use is perceived as shameful, and it is illegal.

We could try other approaches. For alcohol, we could look at sales figures: stores, duty-free and serving of alcohol. For illegal drugs, we could look at seizures by the police or customs. One can count those who come for treatment for substance abuse, even if much substance use goes untreated. Or you can look at search trends on the internet, as Google Trends may reveal what drugs people use or crave. Some even do wastewater (sewage) analysis. None of these information sources is perfect, but when numbers from different sources line up, we become more confident.

These numbers say that as many as 90% of the population have tried alcohol at some point in their lives, and more than 70% of the adult population have consumed alcohol in the past year. Men drink more often and more than women. Older people drink more often but consume way less than younger people. Those with higher education or high-income drink more than those from lower social strata but still have fewer negative effects related to their alcohol use. The annual sales figures for alcohol in Norway suggest that each Norwegian drinks about seven liters of pure alcohol a year, a slight decrease over the past 10 years and way below the European average, with only Italy with lower registered alcohol use. In Norway, alcohol is mostly consumed as beer or wine. The numbers for how many have harmful use of drugs or alcohol addiction are more difficult to ascertain. Each year, about 20,000 people are treated for alcohol problems in the specialist service. But research indicates that this constitutes only 5–10% of those with alcohol problems. From this, one can assume that at any given time, there are about 2–300,000 people who have alcohol use disorders (AUD) in Norway. This corresponds quite well with the few Norwegian and many foreign epidemiological studies that point to a 12-month prevalence of around 4–6% of the adult population [1]. Lifetime prevalence (the chance of ever having had an AUD) is about double.

For illegal drugs, the numbers are much lower. While most of the adult population has tried alcohol, the majority have never tried illegal drugs. Cannabis is the most used illegal drug. One in four have ever tried cannabis, with around 5% having used it in the past year. Recent cannabis use is most prevalent in the young, and among these, we see a moderate increase in use. More men than women use cannabis. After cannabis, it is stimulants like cocaine, amphetamines, and ecstasy/ MDMA that are the most widespread drugs. Around 2% of the population report having tried this at some point, while well under 1% report use in the past year. Cocaine has shown the sharpest increase during the latter years. For opioids and other drugs, the numbers are low.

Drug Effects

This section will review the most common drugs of abuse. Emphasis will be placed on the impact the various drugs have on mental disease. There are a myriad of different drugs with varying effects. It may be challenging to grasp this, but broadly speaking, drug effects may be divided into three groups according to effect: sedative, stimulating, and hallucinogens (see Fig. 6.1). Most known drugs can be placed in such a figure, but each will also have their peculiarities.

Sedative effects may come from influencing various inhibitory neurotransmitter systems. These systems are widespread within the central nervous system (CNS), and thus almost all brain functions can be inhibited. This may influence vital processes such as breathing, heart rate, blood pressure, and digestion but may also involve learning, memory, motivation, and experience of pleasure.

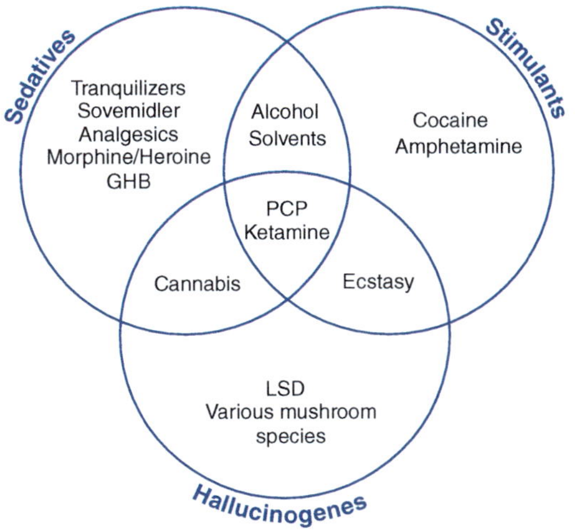

Fig. 6.1 Three overlapping circles compare types of drugs by their effects: sedatives, stimulants, and hallucinogens. The sedatives circle includes tranquilizers, analgesics, morphine or heroine, and GHB. The stimulants circle includes cocaine and amphetamine. The hallucinogens circle includes LSD and various mushroom species. Where sedatives and stimulants overlap are alcohol and solvents. Where sedatives and hallucinogens overlap is cannabis. Where stimulants and hallucinogens overlap is ecstasy. In the center, where all three overlap, are PCP and ketamine. This diagram helps understand how some drugs share effects from more than one category [2]

Stimulating effects result from influencing dopaminergic and, partially even serotonergic and noradrenergic neurons. These neurotransmitter systems are less widespread, but are important for functions such as motivation, the ability to feel pleasure, and closeness. Psychomotor speed, appetite, and sleep and wakefulness patterns will also be affected by central stimulants. So will phenomena such as anxiety, compulsion, and depression.

Hallucinogenic substances will often be able to exert their effect through influence on serotonergic and glutamatergic neurons. As the name suggests, these substances can give altered sensory impressions.

Such a presentation is, of course, simplified. The various neurotransmitter systems will influence each other, so there is not a one-to-one relationship between drug use and single neurotransmitter processes in the CNS. The effects of drugs will also depend on dose, route of administration, and personal vulnerabilities of the individual. Many drugs will have mixed effects that lie between the main effects mentioned. This is attempted to be illustrated in Fig. 6.1 by placing them between the main effects.

Drugs with the Most Widespread Use

Alcohol

Alcohol is our oldest known intoxicating drug and has, except for a short prohibition period, been legally used by humans throughout all written history. Alcohol has many different effects: elevated mood, reduced concentration, impaired short-term memory, decreased learning ability, but also decreased critical sense and increased impulsivity and aggressiveness.

There are large individual differences in how people react to alcohol. These individual differences may be due to age, gender, how used we are to drinking, whether we are on a rising or falling blood alcohol concentration (BAC), the time of day, our physical and mental health, how alert we feel, whether we have eaten, and what expectations we have of the alcohol intoxication. Still, there are some rules of thumb and the effects are related to how high the BAC is, measured in grams per deciliter of blood, or percent (%). At a BAC of 0.05%, our perception and ability for precise reaction will begin to decrease. At 0.1%, most people will experience increased reaction time: decreased balance, movement, coordination, concentration ability, and attention. At 0.15%, you will feel tired and have inhibited psychomotor skills, slurred speech, and memory problems. At 0.2% and above, one gets symptoms of poisoning, lack of control over body functions, and risk of death. The large individual differences can be illustrated by the fact that we have seen deaths below 0.2% BAC, while some have survived 0.5% BAC.

Most people have a tempered relationship with alcohol and use it for pleasure and in moderation. It is perceived as a positive thing, and for most people, the use of alcohol is not associated with a high health risk. But alcohol use, and especially high alcohol use and AUD, is a risk factor for many diseases and disorders to a smaller or larger degree. Some diseases are *caused* by alcohol, i.e., somatic diseases such as alcohol-related diseases in the heart, stomach, liver, pancreas, and the peripheral nervous system. Use of alcohol during pregnancy can harm the fetus and lead to so-called fetal alcohol syndrome. In addition, there are more than 200 other diseases or conditions where alcohol *contributes* negatively but is not the sole cause of the malady [3]. Such conditions include cardiovascular diseases such as high blood pressure, heart attack, and stroke. But alcohol even increases the risk of cancer in many organs and worsens the prognosis. Alcohol suppresses the immune system and makes one more vulnerable to a range of infections.

Similarly, some mental disorders are *caused* by alcohol, i.e., delirium tremens, Korsakoff's psychosis, other alcohol-related psychoses, and Wernicke's encephalopathy. The mental disorders *caused* by alcohol use, of course, include harmful use of alcohol and alcohol dependence (together AUD). But perhaps most importantly, there are the mental disorders where alcohol is a negative *contributing* factor. It is well known to many that alcohol can suppress anxiety. We welcome people with a drink at parties to reduce the little social anxiety we all have. But just as much as alcohol effectively suppresses anxiety, the hangover effect, and especially with heavy use over time, shows us that alcohol worsens anxiety over time. Similar arguments can be made for sleep and depression. There is no doubt that mental illness can be caused by and worsened by alcohol. This applies also to more serious mental illnesses, like bipolar disorder and non-affective psychosis.

It is also important to remember the problems related to alcohol use of a social and societal nature. Under acute intoxication, our ability to make sound judgment decreases, and alcohol use increases the chance of traffic accidents, falls, drownings, violence, especially in relationships, but also of abuse and suicide. Alcohol problems may lead to decreased work participation and an increase in sick leave and problems in the family, especially for children as next-of-kin.

It is a frequently discussed topic whether a little alcohol may have some health benefits [4]. This stems from studies showing that those who abstain from alcohol may have an increased risk of cardiovascular disease. This research has been welcomed by many, and some recommend having a glass for your health. It is possible, but definitely not proven, that this is correct. People usually abstain for a reason, perhaps because they have an increased risk or are already sick (sick abstainers). If you consider total morbidity and mortality (not just cardiovascular diseases), the advantage also disappears. Lastly, the amount that could have possible health benefits is very low, less than one unit per day. Larger amounts increase the risk of all diseases. In real life, alcohol cannot be recommended due to its health benefits.

Cannabis

Cannabis is our second most used drug. It is derived from the plants *cannabis sativa* or *cannabis indica*. Cannabis is traditionally used in two ways. Either as marijuana from dried leaves, apical bud, and flowers from the female plant, or as hashish from the plant resin. Both variants are smoked, marijuana as such, and hashish, most often mixed with tobacco. However, cannabis can be ingested in many ways: drunk as tea, added to food, or used in lotions.

There are over 400 chemical constituants in cannabis, and more than 100 of these are psychoactive cannabinoids of various kinds. The most important is, however, $^{\Delta}$9-tetrahydrocannabinol (THC) [5]. Most effects of cannabis are related to how much THC one consumes. There are a variety of cannabis products and semisynthetic and synthetic cannabinoids, the latter not chemically similar to the cannabinoids of the cannabis plant, but giving many of the same effects.

Acutely, cannabis may alter sensory impressions and behavior. A "high" will involve a feeling of euphoria, happiness, joy, and well-being. The effect will vary from person to person. Some become relaxed, some active. Some find that things become very funny. It has been described that one becomes more aware of colors, patterns, and music. Some describe that one gains deeper insight. This is purely subjective, and measured with more objective studies, intellectual and psychomotor skills are reduced. With the intake of higher doses, some may experience anxiety, panic, paranoia, and psychosis. Short-term memory is greatly reduced, and one can have problems distinguishing dreams from reality.

Cannabis affects bodily coordination and motor skills. The user may have problems coordinating sensory stimuli, but to a lesser extent than seen with alcohol. Unlike what is seen with alcohol, a cannabis intoxicated person will be aware of their impaired abilities and will try to compensate for this. Common signs of cannabis intoxication are dilated pupils, bloodshot eyes, rings around the eyes, and dry mouth. Intoxication may also induce sugar and food cravings.

As for alcohol, most people who consume only a limited amount of cannabis, or only a few times, will experience few problems related to this. It may also be that the problems that follow cannabis use are less than those that follow alcohol use, but few good studies compare the two drugs in an adequate manner. But as for alcohol, some will experience health problems related to the use of cannabis. Acute intake can lead to anxiety reactions, depression, and hallucinations. Since cannabis also affects heart rhythm, in rare cases, arrhythmias have been seen.

Used over time, one can become addicted to cannabis. One experiences tolerance development and withdrawal if one tries to taper off or quit. If one uses cannabis regularly, there are reports that up to 1 in 3 develop addiction [6]. Some may not develop addiction but are left with little other activities and goals in life. Cannabis is linked to fewer somatic diseases than alcohol, but if one smokes cannabis, there is an increased incidence of lung diseases, primarily chronic bronchitis, but some also claim lung cancer and chronic obstructive lung disease. In recent years, there have also been cases of intractable severe nausea. This is probably due to cannabis' anti-nausea properties as a medicine (see below).

Cannabis causes some reduced cognitive function in users, in young people, to an extent that may not completely be reversed by abstinence. Cannabis can double the risk of anxiety and depression. Some maintain cannabis use because they experience anxiety and depression in withdrawal. Anxiety and depression are quite common disorders, so a doubling of risk is significant [7]. There is agreement today that the use of cannabis increases the risk of psychosis/schizophrenia. The more one consumes and the earlier one starts, the greater the chance of developing schizophrenia increases [8]. The general risk of about 1% in the population increases to

2–3% in cannabis users. Cannabis smoking usually precedes the schizophrenia diagnosis, and it can be difficult to argue that the relationship goes the other way: that schizophrenia leads to cannabis smoking. On the other hand, it is often difficult to say when schizophrenia starts. It is also the case that many with an established psychosis/schizophrenia diagnosis use cannabis. Such use of cannabis significantly worsens the prognosis for the disease.

Cannabis can be used as a medicinal drug. Several studies have shown that cannabis can be used as pain medication, as an antiemetic for MS patients, and as palliative care for terminal patients and cancer patients [9]. These results stem from many placebo-controlled, double-blind, randomized studies of good quality. At the same time, we must acknowledge that a good part of the medical use of cannabis is not prescribed by a doctor for established medical indications but is used because it is subjectively felt to be good, without real medical benefit.

Opioids Including Heroin

Opioids were originally extracted from or synthesized from the opium poppy. This was originally opium, from which morphine was eventually produced. Later, heroin was synthesized, and the two substances (morphine and heroin: opiates) and a few other derivatives were for many years the only ones on the market. In recent decades, many morphine-like substances that work in the same way have been synthesized. We call this broader group *opioids*.

Opioids work on opioid receptors in the CNS. These are present in many different variants, and their chemistry and properties are complex. There are endogenous substances (endorphins and enkephalins) that interfere with these receptors. These are important in the regulation of pain and pain perception, making opioids good pain relievers. But they are also involved in such diverse things as mood, sleep/wakefulness, hunger/satiety, regulation of breathing and the eye, memory, and experience of exhilaration/euphoria.

As with other drugs, the effects of opioids depend on the amount taken, the potency of the drug, the route of administration (oral or intravenous), but also personal characteristics, the context in which the drug is taken, and, not least, how accustomed one is to taking opioids. When taking small doses, one can experience acute pain relief, while larger doses result in a marked "high" with euphoria, drowsiness, and disorientation. Effects on the cardiovascular and respiratory systems are also central: decreased heart rate, blood pressure, and breathing. This is associated with a high overdose risk. Since opioids also affect the whole body, the user may experience dry mouth and small pupils. The gastrointestinal tract is also affected, and one can see nausea, vomiting, acid reflux, and constipation. There may also be urine retention.

The tolerance development for opioids is significant, and it is difficult to taper off. This is why one must be careful with using opioids in the treatment of chronic conditions, even though there is significant gain in modern medicine to use opioids in the treatment of acute pain, such as injuries or surgery. Opioids show good effects for cancer patients and in terminal treatment. But used for other pain conditions, and over time, opioid use leads to more problems than it solves. From the 1990s onward, hundreds of thousands of American patients developed an addiction to opioids because many doctors (heavily and unethically influenced by the pharmaceutical industry) prescribed opioids indiscriminately [7]. When they later became more restrictive, many turned to heroin. In 2021, there were more than 100,000 overdose deaths due to the use of opioids in the USA. On the European continent, we have mostly been spared this because doctors here have been more diligent in prescribing.

Except for the extreme tolerance development and overdose risk, opioids themselves (when administered in smaller doses) have relatively few health problems related to their use. The danger comes largely from the accompanying problems. Adulterated substances can cause poisonings, mixing with other drugs increases overdose risk, and use of unclean injection equipment can cause local or systemic infections. Because of the development of tolerance, the risk of habituation and addiction is great. Many find it impossible to taper off. This is the background for opioid agonist therapy (OAT).

OAT was started in the 1960s when it was discovered that the illegal street use of heroin could be replaced with a prescribed long-acting opioid. Methadone treatment was introduced [10]. Instead of being forced to live on the street with crime to finance drugs, and instead of buying drugs of unknown quality and strength, often added harmful substances, and with the risk of overdose, patients were prescribed a long-acting opioid. This meant that one did not need to be weaned off but had a steady supply of opioids throughout the day. This resulted in reduced crime, morbidity, and mortality. Patients could take part in rehabilitation through education and work, and many could live in their own homes. Usually, long-acting opioids such as methadone, buprenorphine, and 24-h morphine are used for substitution, but in principle, any opioid can be used for OAT, even heroin.

Not everyone benefits from OAT, and there has been some resistance to this intervention. Some believe it is problematic that we give drugs to patients and see harm reduction as a second-rate solution. There are dilemmas in OAT, such as the fact that some women become pregnant and give birth to children with withdrawal. But OAT is predominantly a good thing and the best we have to offer patients in a very difficult life situation.

Central Stimulants

Central stimulant drugs include several different drugs, the most important being cocaine and amphetamines. Cocaine is synthesized from the coca plant growing in South America, while amphetamines (amphetamine and methamphetamine) are synthetic drugs. There are numerous other central stimulants, such as ephedrine (cough suppressant), cathinone (the active ingredient in khat), caffeine, and methylphenidate (which is used to treat ADHD). For many drugs, a minor central stimulant effect is one of several effects, e.g., for alcohol and ecstasy.

Central stimulants work by increasing the amount of free dopamine in certain parts of the CNS. The drugs also affect neurotransmitters like noradrenaline and serotonin. This induces a strong and immediate "high." Again, the effects experienced and how affected one is will depend on dose, potency, administration method, and personal factors. The "high" is often described as a strong euphoric experience with increased alertness, increased ability to concentrate, increased energy, and decreased fatigue. Increased psychomotor pace is experienced, as well as increased self-confidence to the point of feeling invincible. Basic needs are often neglected. One can go a long time without food or sleep. This is part of the reason why central stimulants have been used by soldiers in war, but also by students who want to put in the extra hours. However, critical sense and learning ability also decrease with the use of central stimulants, and it is doubtful whether one can achieve better grades by such intake.

Both amphetamine and methamphetamine are sold in Northern Europe as white powders, while methamphetamine in parts of the world is produced and sold as the more potent and purer crystalline methamphetamine ("ice"). The powder form is mostly snorted or injected, while crystalline amphetamines can be smoked. Injection as a method of administration is more common in Northern Europe.

Even if the intake of small doses of central stimulants is not harmful to health (e.g., a cup of coffee or treatment of ADHD), the use of higher doses and stronger stimulants will pose significant health risks. The physical side effects are largely due to stimulant effects on the cardiovascular system, with increased heart rate, high blood pressure, and risk of both cardiac events and cerebral stroke. The mental adverse effects will, to some extent, overlap with the desired effects of the drugs, but then in an exaggerated form. Anxiety, irritability, aggression, violence, and paranoia may follow. Paranoid traits and eventually fully developed psychosis can occur with high doses and/or long-term use. Probably, a component of personal vulnerability and sleep deprivation will play a role in the risk of psychosis.

Stimulant drugs have been used for medicinal purposes as weight loss drugs or by shift workers who need to stay awake for prolonged times. The most widespread use today is for the treatment of hyperactivity disorders (ADHD) in children and adolescents (to some extent also in adults) and for the treatment of narcolepsy.

Benzodiazepines

Benzodiazepines are centrally acting sedative drugs used to treat anxiety, sleep problems, and epilepsy. If used correctly, i.e., short-term use, they are safe and effective drugs that pose few health risks. If used inappropriately, i.e., too long or in too high doses, they may cause significant problems.

Benzodiazepines exert their effect by stimulating the $GABA_A$-receptor complex in the CNS. GABA is the most widespread inhibitory neurotransmitter. That is why benzodiazepines work so broadly. In addition to their sleep-inducing, anxiety-reducing, and antiepileptic effects, they will reduce psychomotor performance, cognitive abilities, and respiration.

Some patients may fall into the unfortunate long-term use of benzodiazepines. First, there are intravenous drug users injecting opioids or stimulant drugs. They use benzodiazepines both to enhance the high and to soften the "landing." Amphetamine users will take benzodiazepines for sleep after a period of use, probably a sensible action, while heroin users who mix benzodiazepines with heroin to enhance the high are engaging in a dangerous practice with a significant risk of overdose.

Secondly, we have ill-considered use among those with anxiety disorders, where benzodiazepines may alleviate this in the short term. But one develops tolerance for the effects of benzodiazepines (as with opioids) quite quickly. Some will increase the dose and possibly supplement with other sedative drugs such as opioids and alcohol. This can become very difficult. Thirdly, we have the so-called quasi-therapeutic long-term use [11]. Here, the patient uses benzodiazepines or non-benzodiazepine sleeping agents over a long period of time but does not increase the dose or mix with other drugs. Sometimes the patient uses the drugs intermittently, i.e., not every day. It may be discussed how problematic or harmful this is, but it is clearly outside the recommendations given for the use of benzodiazepines. On the other hand, one should perhaps not condemn all use that is perceived as useful by the patient.

Other Drugs

There are numerous chemical substances that can be used recreationally or as drugs of abuse, and new ones constantly surface. The drugs reviewed above are the ones with the highest prevalence of use. This is followed by a less detailed review of some other drugs. This list is not the least comprehensive.

Designer Drugs/Party Drugs

As various chemical substances were made illicit, some chemists began to play with new variants of the molecular structure of known drugs and "design" new variants. Designer drugs were born. Variants of stimulant drugs, based on amphetamines, are commonly referred to as ecstasy, while variants of cathinone, due to their packaging, have been termed "bath salts". They have effects similar to amphetamines and cocaine, but there is also a stronger serotonergic action. Such effects include entactogenic effects (intense joy and love, closeness, understanding, and connection to others, and mental clarity). We sometimes see depression post use, and there have been reported deaths due to overheating (serotonergic syndrome).

Another group is synthetic cannabinoids. These are potent substances that stimulate cannabis receptors in the brain, thus mimicking the effects of THC, but far more potently. Due to their mode of distribution, often sprayed on different green herbs, they are collectively referred to as "spice". We also have synthetic opioids, which are potent variants of opioids, such as fentanyl and carfentanil, where just a few micrograms can constitute an overdose. We also see synthetic benzodiazepines. Because these substances are new and have partly unknown effects, they are often collectively referred to as "new psychoactive substances" (NPS).

LSD and Other Hallucinogens

LSD (abbreviation for lysergic acid diethylamide) is a powerful psychedelic substance. LSD is tasteless and odorless, and small amounts of LSD cause strong changes in consciousness with different experiences of emotions, senses, memories, and consciousness.

LSD may produce hallucinations with moving geometric patterns, trails of objects, and vivid colors. LSD was, for a period, used therapeutically to give patients consciousness-expanding experiences and possibly better contact with their subconscious. This has been criticized afterward, but new research is underway to see if LSD may have potential as a medical treatment for other conditions. It is unresolved whether LSD and other hallucinogens may have negative long-term consequences, such as "flashbacks."

There are a number of other substances that have been used and are used on similar indications. These include phencyclidine (PCP), mescaline (peyote), psilocybin (magic mushrooms), and ketamine. There is some research around the use of these as therapeutic agents, and some breakthroughs have taken place.

GHB

Gamma-hydroxybutyrate (GHB) is produced from readily available raw materials and with recipes found on the Internet. Optimally synthesized, GHB is odorless and tasteless, and it is a potent central depressant. Due to its steep dose-response curve, it is difficult to dose right. While one dose can be perceived as too small, only a little more can be just right, but also too much. There are two distinct phases in the effect. First comes sedation and then intoxication and euphoria. It frequently causes amnesia. Some claim that GHB can cause increased aggression, but it is unclear whether this is due to a disinhibiting effect that can also be seen with the use of alcohol, benzodiazepines, and other depressants, or if it is a specific effect of GHB.

Solvents

Solvent use may involve a wide range of gases, aerosols, or thinners that are inhaled and absorbed through the lungs. Most substances are ingredients in household or industrial chemical solvents not intended for human use. This applies to organic solvents (found in quick-drying glue and nail polish remover), fuel (gasoline and kerosene), and propellants such as freon and hydrofluorocarbons used as aerosols in hair sprays and sprayable baking fat. The typical solvent user tends to be an individual who has little or no access to alcohol or illegal drugs, such as children, teenagers, inmates, or institutionalized or otherwise marginalized people. Most serious is solvent use in children and teenagers. The effects of solvents range from alcohol-like intoxication and intense euphoria to hallucinations, depending on the type of substance and the dosing. Some solvent users come to harm due to the toxic effects of the solvent or gas, while others are injured by other chemicals in the products. As with other intoxicating substances, users can be injured during intoxication, for example, by driving under the influence. In some cases, users have died from hypoxia, pneumonia, heart failure, or aspiration of vomit.

Harmful Use and Addiction

There are many ways to use drugs. Even if we often hear about the problems related to drug use, and even if we as health workers most often care specifically about these problematic sides, we must not forget that most people use drugs without it being a problem, neither acutely nor in the long term. In a heated debate, this can be easy to overlook. But some have problems with the drugs and use them in a way that involves increased risk of negative health consequences or becoming dependent.

Harmful Substance Use

In the international classification system ICD-10, there are specifically two diagnoses concerned with high drug consumption. These are harmful use (ICD-10 code F1x.1; where the x is replaced depending on which drug we are looking at) or dependence (F1x.2). In some countries, a new version of ICD has been implemented; ICD-11. Here, harmful use is given the code 6A4x.1 and dependence 6A4x.2 [12]. In both ICD-10 and ICD-11, harmful use of a drug involves use in a way that causes health damage. This can be either physical or mental. In ICD-10, the diagnosis is not given if the use of "only" gives negative social consequences or if one is subject to criticism. This is revised in ICD-11, where such consequences also qualify for the diagnosis. The diagnosis may not be set based on adverse events like hangover or withdrawal. Tolerance and withdrawal symptoms can be part of the phenomenon of harmful use, but do not need to be.

The term "misuse" was previously used. However, the term is perceived as too normative and stigmatizing and should not be used, even though it is widespread in everyday language. Some still use "abuse," and it may be difficult to get rid of all stigmatizing everyday language, but "harmful use" is way preferable.

Dependence Syndrome

Dependence syndrome or addiction is characterized by several physiological, behavioral, and cognitive phenomena. In ICD-10, a diagnosis can be set when three or more of the following criteria have occurred simultaneously during the past year:

1. A strong desire, or feeling of compulsion, to take the drug.
2. Problems controlling the intake of the drug: starting, ending, and amount consumed.
3. Withdrawal symptoms occur if the use of the drug is reduced or ceased.
4. Tolerance develops so that larger doses are needed to achieve the same effect as before.
5. Increasing indifference to other pleasures and interests. More and more time is spent on obtaining the drug, using it, or recovering from its use.
6. The use of the drug continues despite clear signs of harm. The user must be (or could be expected to be) aware of these consequences.

In ICD-11, the number of criteria is reduced to three, collapsing criteria 1 and 2, 3 and 4, and 5 and 6. For each of the three new criteria, you only need to fulfill one or the other. For the diagnosis to be set, you need to fulfill at least two criteria during the last year. In sum, this means that the diagnostic cut-off level has been lowered, and several investigations reveal that it will be easier to get a diagnosis of dependence with the ICD-11 than it was with the ICD-10.

Regardless of the diagnostic system, dependence involves an obsessive relationship to the drug. The addiction can be to one drug or to a group of drugs. The use of the drug can be ongoing or just involve a strong urge to take the drug. The urge is often strongest if one tries to refrain from use. Tolerance occurs for many phenomena that do not involve addiction and is not enough to make the diagnosis.

The diagnostic system thus provides a definition of addiction. Below, we will try to look more closely at how we can *understand* addiction.

What Is Addiction?

Only a minority of those who try or use a drug become addicted to it. But some do. Addiction is a complex and incompletely understood phenomenon. There are good theories, supported to a varying degree by research, but we do not have a definitive understanding. Thus, to grasp the phenomenon, we must look at it from different angles. We must have a bio-psycho-social perspective, where both the individual's genes and biology, the individual's experiences and upbringing, in their environment and in society, and the properties of the drugs play a role. The different models of addiction draw their knowledge from such diverse disciplines as philosophy, sociology, epidemiology, teaching, economics, psychology, biology, and medicine. All these fields may contribute and can explain some aspects of the phenomenon. Here, we will try to outline some of the models.

Previously, addiction was mainly understood as a personal and moral problem. The addict was a morally inferior person. This was supported by religious teachings. Several religions impose taboos on substance use. This may lead to stigmatization and exclusion. But we must still not forget that these simple moral rules against drug use have helped many. If one is not exposed to drugs, one cannot become addicted to them. However, we should as much as possible put aside this moral dimension in dealing with and understanding addiction, as people who are addicted do not need additional stigma and shame.

In this chapter, we will discuss other understandings of addiction. The list of explanations is not comprehensive. We have made some selections. The choices are partly made based on this book's theme of mental health. However, it is important to remember that if you encounter other explanatory models, these may also have merit. This does not mean that all models are equally good for understanding the phenomenon. In the following paragraphs, some models for understanding addiction will be presented.

Total Consumption Model

The total consumption model is not an explanation for addiction, but places addiction in an epidemiological context. The model points to how drug use in the

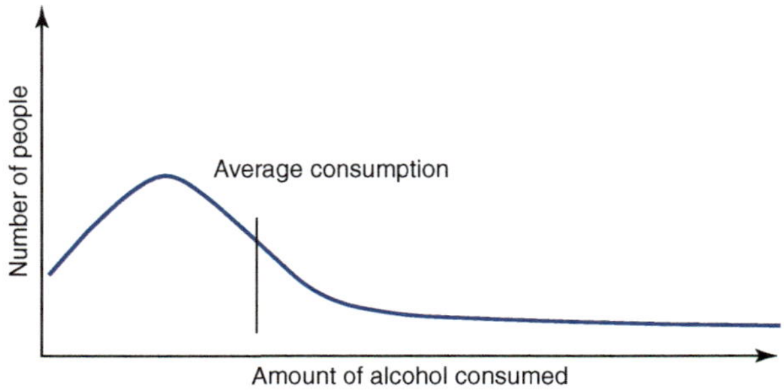

Fig. 6.2 A schematic representation of the total consumption model shows a one-parametric distribution where there is a gradual passage from those who use very little and those who use a lot of alcohol. This model probably applies to all drugs. At the individual level, there is not a one-to-one correlation between the amount of the drug one uses and whether one is addicted. Some will be able to drink a lot, while others less before they get such a diagnosis. But at the societal level, the extent of addiction will be closely related to the amount of the drug that is used. The more of a drug that is used in a population, the more people will get an addiction diagnosis [13]

population is distributed. It is very different how many drugs each individual person consumes. Some are completely abstinent, many consume a little, some more, and a very few a lot or extremely much (see Fig. 6.2).

Those with addiction will be among those who consume a lot, on the far-right side of the graph, even though quantity in itself does not determine addiction (see the criteria for dependence syndrome above).

If we take alcohol as an example, we see that those who drink a lot are not in a distinct group compared to those who drink less. There are not two groups: one with and one without addiction. The amount of alcohol consumed is distributed along a continuum. There is a gradual transition between abstinence and those who drink a little, "normally," a lot, or are addicted. One group does not differ very much from the group that is closest. But Fig. 6.2 also shows that alcohol use is extremely skewed. While most drink a little, a few will drink extremely much. Those who drink a lot will account for a disproportionately large part of the consumption. Many of these will be addicted to alcohol [14]. This model will also apply to other drugs.

This is no trivial observation. Let's imagine that alcohol use did not distribute like this, but, e.g., in two groups: normal use and problem use. The first peak would represent the distribution of those who had a "normal" relationship with alcohol, while the other peak would represent those with addiction. If we were in such a situation to do something about alcohol problems, the best thing would be to treat the addiction. Measures against the entire population would not be necessary (or desirable, then normal consumers could enjoy their alcohol in peace).

But it's not like this. The figure and reality show a so-called one-parametric model for the distribution of alcohol consumption. As with many health-related phenomena, the world cannot be divided into "the normal" and "the abnormal." Other examples are drug abuse, obesity issues, or hypertension. Some would say that such an epidemiological model cannot give us an understanding of what addiction is, but such a one-parameter model tells us that it is not "us" who do not have problems with alcohol and "them" who are alcohol dependent. There is no clear divide. If you consume enough alcohol, anyone can have problems. In a society with high alcohol consumption, more people become dependent. The opposite is perhaps easier to understand: If we do not have access to alcohol, no one becomes addicted.

The total consumption model has formed the basis for many countries' alcohol policies. To prevent overconsumption, there are sales restrictions, age limits, serving time regulations, and high taxation of alcohol. These measures are, however, met with increasing resistance, resulting in extended serving times, reduced taxes, and increased quotas for tax-free. This has led to increased problems with alcohol—and more alcohol-dependent people. The model is also applicable in several areas. In most countries, most other drugs are illegal to use. The illegal status of narcotics worldwide is an attempt to introduce a preventive measure. One can discuss whether it is a good measure, but the underlying thinking is the same. It is also such things that come into play when we want to reduce screen or smartphone time for young people, or when gambling is only allowed in some places.

Addiction as Mislearning and Choice

People drink or take drugs because it makes them feel good and provides favorable, or prevents bad, experiences. It is less in people's minds that drugs can cause harm or be dangerous. A "high" can provide relief from anxiety or other problems. It can provide positive social experiences through belonging and community. The progress from trying a drug, via regular use, to harmful use and addiction can have an element of what we must call operant conditioning (learning through the consequences of the action). We continue to do it because we get positive reinforcement or a reward for doing it. At the same time, trying to quit drugs gives bad experiences, and you learn that you "needs" the drug. This is negative reinforcement. Different people will probably experience such positive and negative reinforcements differently.

But using drugs, even when addicted, will involve making *the choice* to take the drug. No one is forcing the addicted person to indulge in drug use. When someone *chooses* to spend so much time, money, and effort on drug intake, others may think the choice is stupid, but what do we know about other people's preferences? It may be that the balance between goods (positive aspects of drug use) and disadvantages (negative aspects of drug use) speaks in favor of drug use for this person in this situation.

However, such an explanation may be problematic. Even the person who is addicted may claim that he or she wants a change. They seem to have two goals that contrast with one another: the long-term goal of change and abstinence and the short-term satisfaction of drug use. This dilemma may seem irrational, but it is not necessarily so. Our preferences—what we want to do—are unstable phenomena. Even if we have a long-term goal of doing one thing, something else may come up that makes us change plans. This is common for all people. If a person has as their ultimate goal a sober life, the preference for pleasure from intoxication or freedom from anxiety will become greater as the temptation draws closer. When you then have two behaviors (not taking or taking drugs) that are in conflict, one can say that the person is acting rationally, even though it may be destructive.

Such a way of thinking is not only valid in the field of drugs. Many choose to act out in various destructive ways, despite this behavior being associated with pain and shame. The point is that it often feels different in the moment than it does in the long run. And such unstable preferences are more common and more pronounced in those who are addicted, and in relation to their addiction.

Neurobiological Understanding of Addiction

Previously, people talked about the physical dependence on drugs (tolerance and withdrawal) as *the real addiction*, while the rest was *just psychology*. Newer understanding points out that drug addiction must be understood as both a physical and psychological phenomenon. The psychological part of addiction can be the hardest to treat. Modern neurobiology shows us some of the neurobiochemical correlates to the psychological part of addiction.

The development of drug addiction involves a process that starts with trying and controlled, social use of a drug to uncontrolled or almost compulsive use (Fig. 6.3).

The process has its neurobiological correlates in the CNS, especially in the brain's reward and motivation pathways. Here we find the mesolimbic dopaminergic pathways that go from areas in the extended medulla, encompassing domaminergic projection from the Ventral Tegmental Area (VTA) to the Nucleus Accumbens (NAc) (Fig. 6.4). Areas in the prefrontal cortex (PFC), hippocampus (HC), and amygdala are also involved. These parts of the brain are naturally involved in what we perceive as naturally meaningful and are activated by the prospect of satisfying

What should we call it?	Experimentation	Use	Risky use	Harmful use	Addiction
Frequency of use	En gang	Noen ganger	Mange ganger	Svaert ofte	«Alltid»
How are we supposed to understand it?	Normal situation	Recreation		Danger signal	"Disease"
Relevant questions	What are the motivations for trying?		What factors increase the frequency of use?		What can increase or decrease control?

Fig. 6.3 The table explains different stages of substance use, from experimentation to addiction, using five columns. Each stage is described by what it should be called, the frequency of use, how to understand it, and relevant questions to consider. Experimentation is a normal situation with use happening once, raising the question of motivations for trying. Use is recreational, occurring a few times, focusing on factors that increase frequency. Risky use is a danger signal with many uses, questioning what can change control. Harmful use happens often and is seen as a disease, while addiction is described as "always," implying constant use and loss of control. The table helps clarify how to identify and think about different levels of substance use

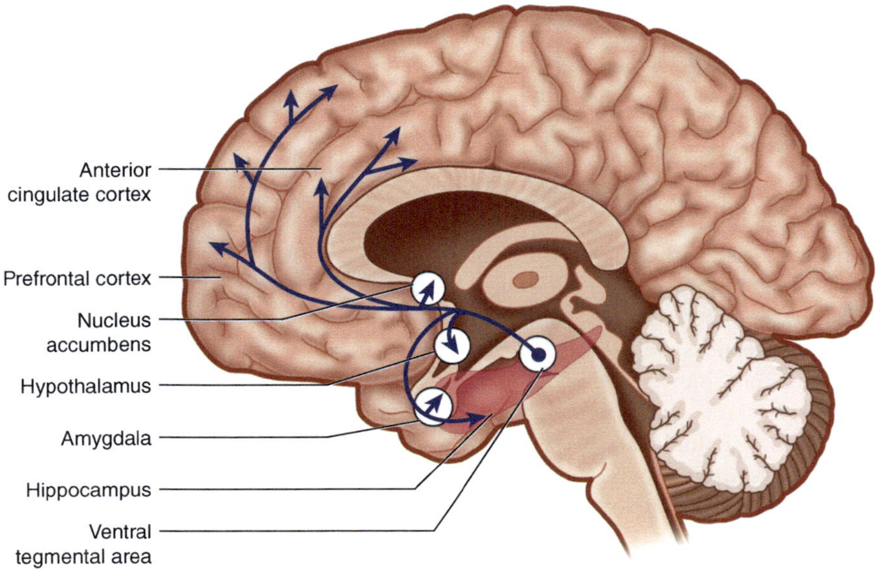

Fig. 6.4 The brain diagram highlights key areas involved in emotional and reward processing, including the anterior cingulate cortex, prefrontal cortex (PFC), nucleus accumbens (NAc), hypothalamus, amygdala, hippocampus (HC), and ventral tegmental area (VTA). Blue arrows show the flow of signals from the ventral tegmental area to these regions, illustrating how they connect and interact. This helps explain how the brain regulates emotions, motivation, and decision-making by linking these important parts

innate needs. It's about what we are motivated to do. It involves meeting basic survival needs such as eating when hungry, drinking when thirsty, comforting and calming our children, or procreating when the opportunity arises. These things are prioritized when needed, and this prioritization is aided by the mesolimbic dopaminergic motivation and reward system.

Neurobiological research has shown that all addictive drugs, indeed, almost all behavior that has an addiction component, work through this system. Addiction is a kind of "hi-jacking" of these mesolimbic dopaminergic pathways. The drug takes over the role of the most significant. Clinically, we see that drug use can continue despite many negative consequences. Drug use takes precedence over food, drink, care, and love for the person being addicted. The neurotransmitter is dopamine. The release of dopamine into the NAc makes us think something is important and is a signal that this is what we should prioritize.

With the use of addictive drugs, the release of dopamine in the NAc is much stronger than when satisfying natural needs. The stronger stimuli will surpass what nature itself can offer in terms of stimulation or meaning. Different drugs work in different places in the system. While central stimulants like amphetamine or cocaine work directly in the synapses in the NAc by increasing available dopamine, alcohol, opiates, or cannabis work "upstream" for the VTA and stimulate increased release

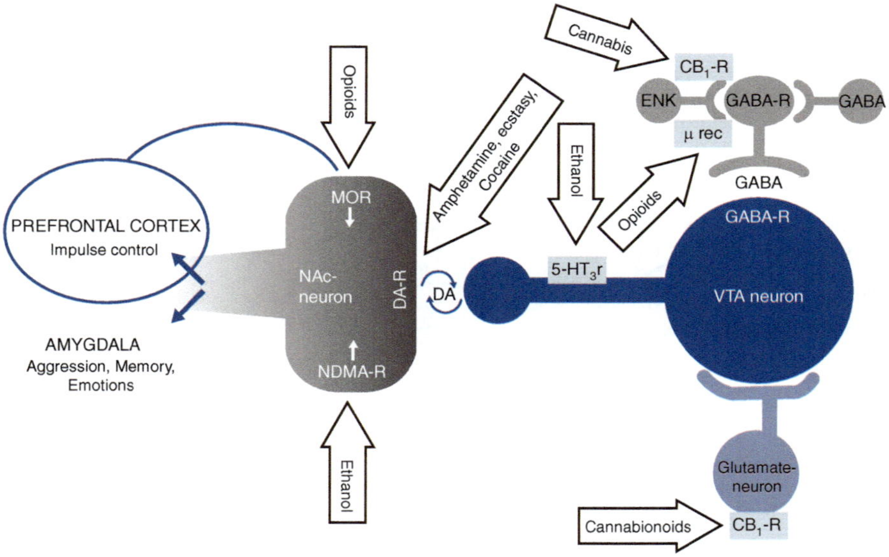

Fig. 6.5 Simplified representation of two neurons in the mesolimbic dopaminergic pathways that extend from the Ventral Tegmental Area (VTA) to the Nucleus Accumbens (NAc). The main neurotransmitter is dopamine (DA) [2]

of dopamine in the NAc through a series of stimulating processes (or inhibition of inhibitory processes) producing the same result (Fig. 6.5).

This knowledge about the mesolimbic dopaminergic pathways may help explain some things about the increased use of and vulnerability to drugs in people with severe mental illness (see below), and why treatment with antipsychotics and blocking of dopamine D2 receptors can lead to an increased propensity for drug use in psychiatric patients. Patients on antipsychotics may experience drugs to "treat" the anhedonic adverse effects that D2 blockade can give.

The picture is, however, more complex. For example, there are also opioid receptors in the NAc. Opioid antagonists like naltrexone can reduce the craving for other drugs, especially alcohol. This is because neurotransmitters other than dopamine also work in this system, and if you block endogenous opioids, you will also remove some of the reinforcing effects of the drugs of abuse.

During the development of addiction, two parallel-running, but different and partly opposite phenomena are experienced [6, 15]. The first phenomenon has to do with how well a drug is perceived; the euphoria it gives, what we call "liking". The second phenomenon is how much you want the drug, what significance the role it plays, and what we call "wanting." The two phenomena are related. It's hard to imagine that you would want a drug if you didn't have positive experiences with it. However, they are two separate phenomena that develop differently throughout an addiction career. While "liking" will decrease with repeated use (tolerance develops), "wanting" will increase (sensitization develops) (Fig. 6.6).

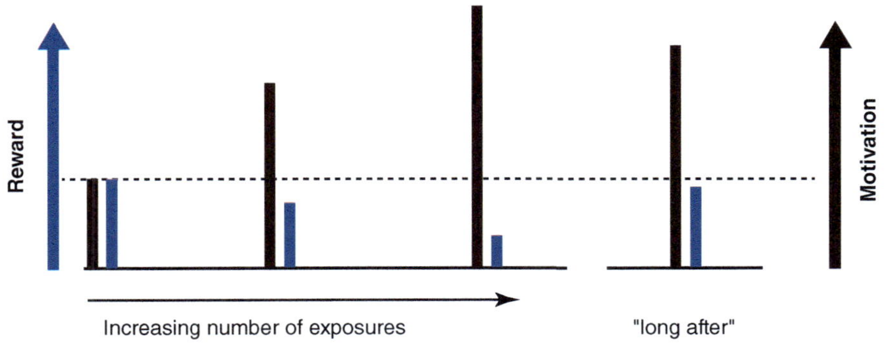

Fig. 6.6 If we set the reward effect (blue column) and the significance/motivation to take a drug (black column) to "1" at first exposure, we see that one develops tolerance for the reward effects over time, while the significance of motivation increases. Motivation is a kind of learning effect that will not return to "normal" even after longer periods of abstinence [16]

The positive yield decreases when you develop tolerance for the drug effects. But the significance of the drug in the addicted person's life increases, even after the drug has stopped giving positive effects. Many addicted persons use drugs almost compulsively despite the fact that it is no longer experienced as positive, sometimes not even freedom from withdrawal. The drug takes up a large space in life, even though it is mostly experienced as negative, even by the person themselves. Studies have shown that even after a long period of abstinence and an almost normalization of the drug effect ("liking"), the significance of the drug and craving ("wanting") may never return to normal. This can explain why relapses occur even after a long period of abstinence. This fits well with an understanding of drug addiction as a disease. The craving for the drug ("craving") can be triggered by many stimuli.

This neurobiological understanding of addiction has given us several insights. It has pointed out the similarity between all the different substances and other addiction-like behaviors. It has given us an understanding of how factors such as neglect and other risk factors increase the likelihood of developing addiction problems. Several experiments show that the mesolimbic dopaminergic pathways are easier to activate if one has such traumas in their past. This model of understanding has explained to us why addiction lasts longer than the pharmacological effect or after-effect that various substances have. And not least, they have given us a deeper understanding of how the various substances work alone or together, and how this understanding can be used in the fight against addiction.

But there are also many things that are not explained by this theory. We have knowledge about vulnerability factors, but we lack a lot of knowledge about why some people can use the same substance in the same amount over a long time but still do not become addicted. We know too little about what predicts the transition from sporadic use to harmful use and then to addiction. We know even less about how one can go the other way, from addiction to getting out of addiction. The theory has given little on the treatment side.

Finally, it must be said that the above presentation of the neurobiological knowledge about addiction is greatly simplified. This is, of course, complex, but it is possible to take away some knowledge without understanding everything.

Co-occurring Substance Disorder and Mental Disorder

SUD have a clear overrepresentation among people with mental illness. And people with mental illnesses often abuse substances and have a higher prevalence of SUD. Even if we exclude nicotine addiction, up to half of all people with psychotic disorders have SUDs. The same will be found in bipolar disorder, especially in the manic phase. Likewise, a large proportion of those seeking treatment for their substance addiction will have many mental health issues.

Distinguishing SUDs from mental illness can be a challenge. Partly, the acute symptoms of substance use or withdrawal resemble various psychiatric disorders. For example, it is so difficult to distinguish an amphetamine-induced psychosis from a schizophreniform psychosis that it has been suggested to use amphetamine-induced psychosis as a model for schizophrenia.

One can question the direction of causality. Are mental problems the cause of SUDs, or is it the other way around (see Fig. 6.7). In the following, these possible explanations are presented. Maybe understanding the relationship between SUD and mental health disorders may reveal important information on addiction.

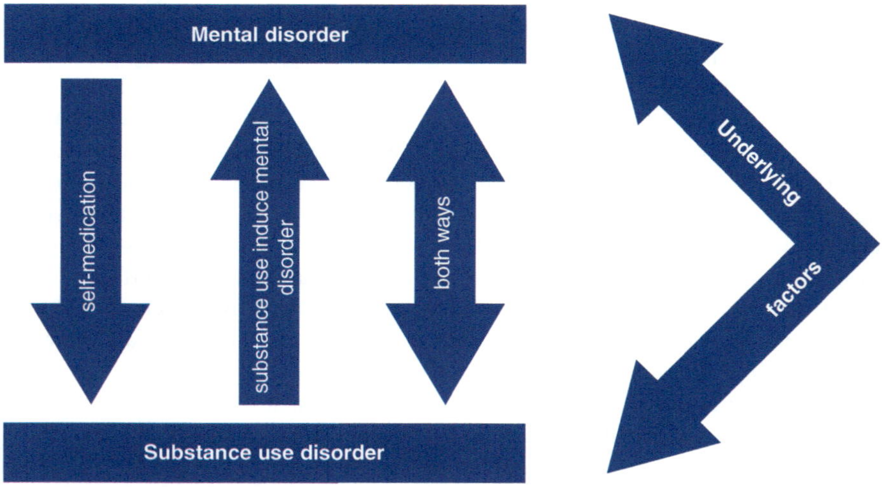

Fig. 6.7 A flow chart shows the relationship between mental disorder and substance use disorder with arrows indicating self-medication, substance use to cope with disorder, and both ways. A separate large arrow labeled "Underlying factors" points diagonally upward, suggesting these factors influence both disorders. The chart highlights how mental disorder and substance use disorder can affect each other and share common causes

Self-Medication

The self-medication theory suggests that substances alleviate symptoms of mental disorders. Drugs of abuse may also counteract some of the negative effects of medications used for the treatment of mental disorders. But even though individuals find it good to engage in substance use and experience it as a kind of self-medication, we often see that substance use exacerbates the mental disorder. Sometimes the self-medication theory makes quite good sense. For example, central stimulants such as amphetamine can be used by people with ADHD because it is perceived as self-treatment. People who have problems with sleep may use cannabis to relax. People with schizophrenia may use substances to counteract the anhedonia that can be caused by high doses of certain (usually first-generation) antipsychotics. Other times, it may seem more random or chaotic and not be easy to understand why exactly that substance is used by exactly that person. Generally, we see that the more serious the mental illness is, the more chaotic the substance use is.

Substances May Cause Mental Illness

Furthermore, substance use can lead to mental disorders. For example, substance use can trigger acute psychosis. Substance-induced psychosis is again a major risk factor for later receiving a schizophrenia diagnosis [17]. Long-term alcohol use can cause depression and anxiety disorders. If one stops a high and long-term use of alcohol, it can lead to an acute, life-threatening psychotic condition (delirium tremens). For all conditions, however, it will depend both on substance use and on personal vulnerability playing a role in the outcome.

The theories of self-medication and substance use as a cause of mental illness are not opposed to one another. Often, both exist simultaneously and lead to a vicious circle. Mental illness exacerbates the substance disorder, and vice versa. As seen in the section on neurobiology, taking control over substance use and being addicted has a lot to do with the function and use of the prefrontal cortex. We know that many people with mental illness have reduced capacity in their prefrontal cortex.

Substance use often predates mental problems. Also, the younger you are when initiating substance use, the greater the risk that it will lead to mental health problems. It is far more dangerous to start drinking alcohol or smoking cannabis when you are 13 than when you are 21 years of age. A young, developing brain probably takes more damage from substance use than a more fully matured one. However, the fact that SUDs precede mental health problems is not a final proof that the substance use is *the cause* of mental health problems, as many may use substances to alleviate symptoms long before the diagnosis is set. Nevertheless, we warn against the use of substances at a young age to prevent mental illness.

Underlying Factors

There are also underlying risk factors that may cause both substance abuse, SUDs, and mental disorders. These can be factors such as social isolation, poverty, lack of structured daily life, and traumatic life events such as sexual abuse and violence. Also, biological factors, perhaps primarily genetics, are important. Many SUDs and mental disorders have a large genetic component, and often, the same genetics explain both disorders.

Summary

- We do not know the exact prevalence of SUDs, but it probably includes 5–10% of the population at any time.
- There are many different substances. For simplicity, we can divide the substances according to their main effects: sedatives, stimulants, and hallucinogens. Some substances have mixed effects.
- Alcohol is our most common and thereby our most problematic substance.
- Harmful use and addiction syndrome are specific diagnoses with distinct diagnostic criteria.
- Addiction is a phenomenon that is not finally understood, but the many explanations can contribute to insight.
- The total consumption model tells us that there is a strong correlation between the prevalence of substance use and the problems related to use, also how many become addicted.
- There are elements of choice both into, within, and out of addiction.
- Neurobiological understanding provides an explanation for why substance use occupies a larger and larger place in people's lives, while it does not feel as good.
- There is a clear overrepresentation of mental disorders in people who have problems with substances and vice versa. This can have many explanations: psychological factors, self-medication, and the fact that substance use can cause mental disorders.

Reflection Questions

- Alcohol is a legal, albeit regulated substance, while all other substances are classified as narcotics and illegal. How do you think this division is considering the negative effects that follow their use?
- Many patients with mental health problems struggle with substance use. Why is this the case? Have you learned anything in this chapter that can shed light on this?
- Both cannabis, opioids, and benzodiazepines can be used as medicines. Yet they are on the narcotics list. Do you find it problematic that we use things as medicines when they can also be used as substances?
- Many use substances without getting problems because of it. How can we understand this when there is so much talk about the dangers of substance use?

Recommended Literature and Online Resources

- Addiction (Oxford Psychiatry Library) second Edition (Oxford University Press, 2018)
- Drugs without the hot air: Making sense of legal and illegal drugs (UIT Cambridge Ltd., 2021)
- U.S. Department of Health and Human Services section about Mental Health & Substance Use Disorder, offer information on drug use and abuse and mental illness: hhs.gov/programs/prevention-and-wellness/mental-health-substance-use-disorder/index.html
- NIDA (National Institute on Drug Abuse) is a premier research institute that provides scientific insights into drug use and addiction, drug facts (from A to Z), but also information prevention, treatment, harm reduction, and stigma: nida.nih.gov
- Oxford handbook of addiction medicine, Third edition (Oxford University Press, 2024)
- SAMHSA (Substance Abuse and Mental Health Services Administration) is a leading U.S. government agency offering extensive resources on substance use disorders and mental health conditions: samhsa.gov
- Textbook of addiction treatment. International perspectives (Springer Nature, 2021)

References

1. Bramness JG. Rusmiddellidelser i Norge [Substance use disorders in Norway]. Oslo: Norwegian Institute of Public Health; 2022. Available at https://www.fhi.no/he/fr/folkehelserapporten/psykisk-helse/rusmiddellidelser/.
2. Mørland J, Waal H. Rus og avhengighet [substance use and addiction]. Oslo: Universitetsforlaget; 2016.
3. Rocco A, Compare D, Angrisani D, Sanduzzi Zamparelli M, Nardone G. Alcoholic disease: liver and beyond. World J Gastroenterol. 2014;20(40):14652–9.
4. Chiva-Blanch G, Badimon L. Benefits and risks of moderate alcohol consumption on cardiovascular disease: current findings and controversies. Nutrients. 2019;12(1):108.
5. Vindenes V, Strand DH, Kristoffersen L, Boix F, Mørland J. Has the intake of THC by cannabis users changed over the last decade? Evidence of increased exposure by analysis of blood THC concentrations in impaired drivers. Forensic Sci Int. 2013;226(1–3):197–201.
6. Leung J, Chan GCK, Hides L, Hall WD. What is the prevalence and risk of cannabis use disorders among people who use cannabis? A systematic review and meta-analysis. Addict Behav. 2020;109:106479.
7. Rognli EB, Bramness JG, von Soest T. Cannabis use in early adulthood is prospectively associated with prescriptions of antipsychotics, mood stabilizers, and antidepressants. Acta Psychiatr Scand. 2020;141(2):149–56.
8. Andréasson S, Allebeck P, Engström A, Rydberg U. Cannabis and schizophrenia. A longitudinal study of Swedish conscripts. Lancet. 1987;2(8574):1483–6.
9. Bramness JG. Medical cannabis. Tidsskr Nor Laegeforen. 2015;135(3):252–3.

10. Dole VP, Nyswander M. Study of methadone as an adjunct in rehabilitation of heroin addicts. IMJ Ill Med J. 1966;130(4):487–9.
11. Griffiths RR, Weerts EM. Benzodiazepine self-administration in humans and laboratory animals – implications for problems of long-term use and abuse. Psychopharmacology. 1997;134:1–37.
12. World Health Organization. Clinical descriptions and diagnostic requirements for ICD-11 mental, behavioural and neurodevelopmental disorders (CDDR). Geneva: World Health Organization; 2024. Available at https://www.who.int/publications/i/item/9789240077263.
13. Rossow I, Baklien B. Alkoholpolitikk og folkehelse [Alcohol policy and public health]. https://www.forebygging.no/Artikler/2022/alkoholpolitikk-ogfolkehelse/.
14. Room R, Livingston M. The distribution of customary behavior in a population: the Total consumption model and alcohol policy. Sociol Perspect. 2017;60(1):10–22.
15. Berridge KC, Robinson TE. Liking, wanting, and the incentive-sensitization theory of addiction. Am Psychol. 2016;71(8):670–9.
16. Bramness JG, Aasland O. Rus og nevrobiologi [Substance use and neurobiology]. Tidsskr Nor legeforen. 2002;122:2311–2.
17. Bramness JG, Rognli EB. Psychosis induced by amphetamines. Curr Opin Psychiatry. 2016;29(4):236–41.

Somatic Illness and Lifestyle Habits

7

Anne Høye and Lars Lien

Abstract

Over the past few years, the reduced lifespan and high incidence of somatic illnesses among patients with mental health and substance use problems, compared to the general population, have received increasing attention. The disparity in morbidity and mortality is particularly pronounced for people with co-occurring substance use disorder and mental health disorders. In this chapter, we will explore various causes of these differences, including lifestyle habits, education levels, economic marginalization, and deficiencies in healthcare services, both within mental and somatic healthcare.

Keywords

Somatic diseases · Mortality · Stigma · Prevention · Lifestyle

A. Høye (✉)
Department of Clinical Medicine, UiT The Arctic University of Norway, Tromsø, Norway

Division of Mental Health and Substance Abuse, University Hospital of North Norway, Tromsø, Norway

Center for Clinical Documentation and Evaluation (SKDE), Tromsø, Norway
e-mail: anne.hoye@unn.no

L. Lien
Department of Health and Nursing Sciences and Section for Mental Health and Rehabilitation, University of Inland Norway, Elverum, Norway

Research Centre for Substance Use Disorders and Mental Illness, Innlandet Hospital Trust, Hamar, Norway
e-mail: lars.lien@inn.no

T. W. Lie, L. Lien (eds.), *Integrated Treatment of Co-occurring Substance Use and Mental Health Disorders*, https://doi.org/10.1007/978-3-032-20049-5_7

From clinical practice, we have numerous examples illustrating how the connection between mental disorders, somatic health, and substance use is often overlooked. For instance, consider the 25-year-old woman subjected to compulsory inpatient treatment for a year, during which she is allowed only 10-min daily exercise periods outside the hospital for extended durations. Over the course of the year, she gained 64 kilograms, increasing her risk of diabetes and cardiovascular disease while also contributing to a poor self-image. Another example is the 39-year-old woman with a history of substance use problems since early adolescence. She develops increasingly psychotic behavior but is unable to "utilize" available treatment options and, as a result, receives no follow-up care. Over time, due to recurring infections, she develops severe heart failure.

Another challenge in healthcare services is that symptoms of serious somatic illness can be misinterpreted as a worsening of mental illness. For example, a 58-year-old man with severe mental illness becomes increasingly tired, apathetic, and confused. These symptoms are attributed to noncompliance with his medication. Eventually, he develops epileptic seizures, which are later diagnosed as being caused by a brain tumor. Conversely, the situation can also occur in reverse. A 42-year-old man, recently divorced, experiences acute breathing problems, dizziness, a rapid pulse, and chest tightness. He is transported by ambulance to the emergency room and undergoes cardiological monitoring eight times over 6 months, with no signs of somatic illness detected. His general practitioner ultimately diagnoses him with a possible panic disorder, and he begins treatment at a mental health center after subsequently developing a substance use problem.

Furthermore, offering treatment for somatic illnesses is not always straightforward. For instance, a 44-year-old man, first admitted when he was 25 years old, has had seven long-term hospital admissions. He is diagnosed with schizophrenia and has been prescribed various medications over the years. Currently, he takes a high dose of antipsychotic medication regularly. He lives alone and manages reasonably well with follow-up care. However, he smokes, is overweight, drinks a lot of alcohol, and occasionally uses cannabis. During a home visit, he reports experiencing chest and arm pain without an apparent cause and becomes short of breath from walking to and from the mailbox. He feels tired and depressed and expresses a desire to stop taking his medication. He is completely resistant to undergoing a somatic examination, and it is difficult to motivate him to engage in any form of physical activity or quit smoking.

Possible Causes for Increased Morbidity and Mortality

These patient stories lie behind the research results we present in this chapter. Patients with severe mental and substance use disorders live approximately 15–20 years less than the general population [1–5]. Mortality increases if the patient has multiple mental disorders, with the highest mortality observed when substance use disorder is one of the diagnoses [6]. Lifespan is most significantly reduced for men, and the difference in mortality compared to the rest of the population is greatest in the youngest age groups. Diseases among people with severe substance use disorder are not only related to drug use but may also be linked to an accelerated aging process [7].

Mortality in the general population varies with factors such as gender, age, and education/income, and it makes little sense to examine mortality independently of the general population. In other words, mortality must be assessed based on what is expected for the same age group and gender in the population during the same time period. For patients with SUD/MH, several studies show that mortality in some groups can be many times higher than in the corresponding gender and age group in the general population [8–12].

For people with severe SUD, overdoses and accidents related to illegal drugs and violence represent the most severe consequences of substance use. Opioid users are ten times more likely to die than others in the same age group, with 50% of these deaths caused by overdoses from various illegal drugs. The remaining 50% is attributed to somatic illnesses often related to illegal drug use, including liver disease, severe infections (particularly those related to injections and the use of dirty needles), HIV/AIDS, cardiovascular diseases, and lung diseases. The sharing of equipment for injecting drug use (IDU) is a significant and growing contributor to the disease burden and a major factor in the transmission of blood-borne viruses throughout the world. Despite significant advances in the treatment of hepatitis C, cirrhosis, and liver cancer, substantial challenges persist for these patients.

For people with severe mental disorders, the primary cause of life years lost is somatic diseases, particularly respiratory and cardiovascular diseases [2, 3]. While suicide is significantly elevated as a cause of death among those with severe mental disorders compared to the general population, the number of suicides or overdose deaths remains relatively low compared to deaths from natural causes. As a result, suicides and overdose deaths have a smaller impact on the overall statistics regarding life years lost. A similar trend applies to deaths related to severe eating disorders, where mortality rates are very high compared to the general population but occur in relatively few cases.

So, what do we know about the causes of these lost life years? Lifestyle factors such as smoking, unhealthy diets, and reduced physical activity are significant contributors [13–16]. Additional factors associated with an increased risk of somatic diseases in people with mental disorders and/or SUD include genetic vulnerability, experienced trauma, and chronic stress. The use of antipsychotic medications is also known to increase the risk of conditions such as cardiometabolic syndrome, although it does not increase mortality. Moreover, evidence suggests that patients with SUD/MH are less likely to be screened or examined and often receive inadequate treatment for established diseases compared to others [17–19]. The reasons for this are complex and multifaceted, including a reduced ability to recognize symptoms, manage personal health, and seek medical help. Contributing factors also include insufficient follow-up from caregivers, general stigma toward persons with mental illness, and systemic failures within the health care system. Let us begin by examining lifestyle factors.

Lifestyle Habits

We know that patients with SUD/MH have a high consumption of alcohol and tobacco, in addition to illegal drugs [20, 21]. Among those with mental illness and substance use problems, up to eight out of ten are daily smokers [22, 23]. Smoking is one of the most important risk factors for cardiovascular disease and death. Additionally, smoking is associated with lung cancer and other lung diseases, such as chronic obstructive pulmonary disease (COPD). Studies show that diseases related to smoking contribute to about half of the deaths among patients with severe mental disorders [24]. Therefore, addressing nicotine addiction is a measure that could make a substantial difference and significantly reduce morbidity and mortality in this group.

Low levels of physical activity and a more sedentary lifestyle contribute to the increased morbidity [25–27]. However, physical activity is not only important for reducing morbidity and mortality; it also plays a crucial role in several other aspects of health. Physical activity acts as a "magic" treatment without side effects and appears to help prevent and treat symptoms of mental disorders such as anxiety, depression, and SUD. It can reduce the need for medication and enhance self-confidence and self-image [28]. In a Norwegian paper [29], fourteen patients who had previously had SUD/MH were asked to describe their path to recovery. For all fourteen, physical activity was an important contributor, though each had their own ways of engaging in it. Other studies point to challenges and barriers for encouraging tailored physical activity [30]. Therefore, it is essential in treatment to identify individually adapted ways to stay active that can be maintained throughout the year.

Generally, patients with mental and substance use problems often have poorer diets compared to the rest of the population [16, 31, 32]. This is particularly related to a preference for easily digestible carbohydrates. Several studies have found that individuals who experience trauma tend to shift their diets to become more carbohydrate-rich. There are several reasons for this, one being that carbohydrates may facilitate easier access to serotonin, one of the neurotransmitters in the brain that regulates mood. Another possible explanation is that carbohydrates provide quick emotional regulation. Additionally, many individuals with mental challenges and substance use problems often face financial difficulties and have less energy to prepare healthy meals. As a result, they tend to choose food that is cheap and easy to make [33].

Trauma, Stress, and Genetics

The relationship between physical symptoms and emotional expression is complex. Many people with severe substance use problems and mental illnesses have experienced trauma during childhood, upbringing, and later in life. Such traumatic experiences can "settle in the body," causing a range of physical symptoms and ailments, such as pain, fatigue, and nausea. Similarly, significant bodily symptoms may be suppressed or misinterpreted, leading individuals to delay seeking healthcare services. Research has shown that children who experience severe trauma, such as physical abuse or maltreatment early in life, exhibit earlier biological signs of aging compared to those who have not experienced trauma [34]. This can contribute to an increased risk of somatic disease. Additionally, prolonged chronic stress activates the hypothalamic–pituitary–adrenal (HPA) axis, which can contribute to the development of depression and other mental disorders [35, 36]. Various degrees of such "toxic stress" can lead to a chronic increased release of stress hormones such as cortisol, corticotropin-releasing factor (CRF), and adrenocorticotropic hormone (ACTH), impairing the "feedback" mechanism that regulates stress hormones like cortisol to normal levels. Chronically elevated cortisol levels can damage important brain areas, such as the hippocampus, which is essential for learning and memory. Recent genetic studies also show a correlation between the risk of mental disorders and cardiovascular disease. However, the relationship between genetic and environmental risk remains complex [37].

Antipsychotic Medications

Side effects associated with antipsychotic medications have been attributed to the excess mortality among patients with severe mental illness. However, several studies suggest that, over time, individuals with severe mental illness who are not on antipsychotic medication experience higher mortality compared to those who are [38–40]. A meta-analysis of data from more than 2.5 million patients with schizophrenia [39] indicates that first-generation antipsychotics are linked to increased cardiovascular mortality in new cases, whereas second-generation antipsychotics and clozapine are associated with lower cardio-cerebrovascular mortality in existing cases. That said, high doses of antipsychotics have been shown to increase mortality from heart and vascular diseases more than low and moderate doses [41]. There is little doubt that second-generation antipsychotics are associated with numerous metabolic side effects [42, 43], but further research is needed to better understand the relationship between increased disease risk, the use of antipsychotic medications, and mortality, as well as how these risks vary depending on individual factors.

The Contribution and Responsibility of the Healthcare Services

Insufficient access to, or reduced availability of, healthcare services has been highlighted as a potential cause of increased morbidity and mortality. Studies show that patients with severe mental disorders face greater challenges in accessing primary healthcare [44] and receive poorer quality somatic specialist health services compared to the general population [17]. For instance, patients with schizophrenia access somatic health services to a lesser extent, even when compared to patients with other mental disorders [45]. A Norwegian study indicates the underdiagnosis of cardiovascular disease in patients with schizophrenia prior to their deaths from such conditions, compared to others who die from cardiovascular disease [18].

Another Norwegian study shows that patients with schizophrenia are less likely to undergo diagnostic procedures and receive treatment for cardiovascular disease in specialist health services [19]. For patients with bipolar disorder, the same trend applies to treatment, though the proportion undergoing diagnostic procedures is comparable to that of the rest of the population. Additionally, a survey involving approximately two million individuals from the UK, USA, Canada, and Australia found that patients with mental and substance-related disorders were prescribed significantly fewer medications across twelve drug categories compared to those without these conditions. This included beta-blockers, statins, insulin, anti-inflammatory drugs, HAART medications for HIV, and anticoagulants [46].

One significant issue is the insufficient follow-up and adaptation within somatic health services and, to some extent, primary health services. The examples presented earlier in this chapter underscore a lack of awareness regarding somatic diseases among doctors and other professionals working in mental health care, SUD treatment, and municipal health and care services. Somatic symptoms and diseases have often been deprioritized or even neglected, with a lack of systematic follow-up and motivation to prevent somatic diseases. As illustrated by the case histories, somatic symptoms have frequently been exacerbated in patients through factors such as weight gain, altered lipid profiles, and the development of diabetes. Furthermore, the lack of activity-based offerings during treatment has contributed to reduced physical activity and increased smoking, often as a response to boredom. There is also a notable absence of nutritional interventions aimed at reducing the consumption of easily digestible carbohydrates, which could otherwise help mitigate these health risks.

How Can We Reduce Excess Morbidity and Mortality?

Clear leadership and the establishment of concrete requirements by political authorities across the healthcare system are among the most critical strategies to address the significantly shorter lifespan of individuals with mental illness and substance-related disorders compared to the general population. Despite increased treatment resources in mental health care and addiction treatment, there is little evidence to suggest that these disparities have diminished [8].

However, there are encouraging developments at both the political level and within health administration in several countries, focusing on the increased risk of somatic diseases and premature death. For example, in Norway, the introduction of a new SUD/MH patient care pathway in 2019 emphasized the issue of excess mortality among individuals receiving treatment in specialist health services. The long-term goal of this initiative is to reduce the mortality gap between these patients and the general population. In addition to the general and diagnosis-specific patient care pathways, a dedicated care pathway for somatic health and lifestyle was introduced. This patient care pathway includes specific measures for the follow-up of somatic diseases and lifestyle changes [47]. However, a significant challenge with this patient care pathway is the lack of integration with specific time frames or reimbursement coding, which has resulted in limited awareness and utilization among healthcare workers.

Another important tool for reducing the gap in life expectancy is the World Health Organization's (WHO) NCD strategy (NCD = noncommunicable diseases) which runs until 2030 and places greater emphasis on the connection between mental and physical health, as reflected in the latest Norwegian public health report [48]. A key priority moving forward will be to focus on specific at-risk groups. It is well understood that good intentions from political authorities are insufficient; the implementation of measures and changes in practice requires dedicated resources and sustained, targeted efforts over time.

Therefore, it is essential for leaders at all levels within the healthcare system to share a collective responsibility for reducing illness and deaths among patients with mental disorders and substance use disorders. A structure is needed to identify risk areas for increased somatic morbidity within each part of the service and to address these issues as concretely as possible. Key questions to consider include: How can somatic diseases be identified? Who holds specific responsibility for follow-up? How can collaboration with general practitioners and somatic healthcare departments be improved? It should also be determined when and how lifestyle interventions can be introduced, and, most critically, who will be responsible for their implementation.

A starting point is to screen and identify common somatic health problems, particularly those related to cardiovascular, respiratory, and gastrointestinal symptoms, as these are prevalent among patients with SUD/MH. It is especially important for this group to be called in for a health check at least once a year, which should include blood tests, blood pressure measurement, and auscultation of the heart and lungs. There is no reason why intervention thresholds should differ from those applied to the general population when treating conditions such as hypertension or high cholesterol levels. On the contrary, more proactive measures should be taken at an earlier stage and at a younger age, as mortality rates have been shown to be highest in younger age groups. These health checks should also ensure that patients in this group undergo screenings and interventions similar to those provided to the general population, such as gynecological examinations with cell samples, mammography, and vaccinations.

As with all effective treatments, the interventions we choose must be clearly described. We must outline the goals of the intervention, the responsibilities involved, and plans for follow-up and long-term objectives. Often, there is a need for tailored measures for each individual patient, with clearly defined responsibilities. This approach may require additional resources throughout the treatment chain, such as ensuring that medications are collected and taken as prescribed, and that their effects and side effects are monitored and recorded.

Closely monitoring the patient when initiating treatment with antipsychotics is essential. This includes obtaining a comprehensive family medical history to assess the familial risk of cardiovascular disease. Measurements of weight, lipid profile, blood pressure, and blood glucose should be conducted prior to starting treatment and monitored regularly thereafter. For example, early weight gain (more than 3 kilograms within the first 3 weeks) often predicts significant long-term weight gain, which can be challenging to track if baseline weight is not recorded before treatment begins. Patients should be treated with the lowest effective dose, and polypharmacy should be avoided whenever possible. Consult the HETI: NSW (Australian) Positive Cardiometabolic Health Algorithm, which has been updated in 2023 (see iphys.org.au) and regionally adapted to several countries, including Norway (see pmc.ncbi.nlm.nih.gov/articles/PMC11863842/).

Changing Lifestyle Habits—Is It Possible?

We know that changing lifestyle habits is difficult for everyone. It is rarely a lack of knowledge but often a lack of motivation that prevents us from improving our diet or starting to exercise after the holidays. Transforming unhealthy habits into good, health-promoting ones requires a high level of discipline and willingness to change—something that can be particularly difficult for those facing major mental health challenges. Furthermore, making such changes often demands mental and financial resources, which may not always be available. For this reason, structural measures are often the most effective approach for patients with mental disorders and substance use disorders, as managing lifestyle changes individually can be particularly challenging for them. These structured measures might include financial and practical support for healthy cooking, free and tailored exercise programs, or access to nature and leisure areas, both at home and during hospital stays.

The most important aspect of supporting patients with co-occurring mental health and substance use disorders is to address lifestyle changes as naturally as discussing substance use or mental symptoms. Often, interventions—such as structured smoking cessation programs—need to be offered multiple times before the patient becomes motivated to make a change. As with all effective addiction treatments, motivational interviewing is a valuable tool for facilitating change. At the same time, those of us working in healthcare must not underestimate the impact of our own attitudes. It is often within this group that resistance to prioritizing lifestyle changes and physical health can be most challenging to overcome. Recognizing the importance of these factors is essential for fostering meaningful change.

Nevertheless, as highlighted in the report from the Lancet Psychiatry Physical Health Commission in 2019 [15], mental health services should prioritize evidence-based lifestyle interventions to promote systemic health benefits for individuals living with mental illness. The increasing acknowledgment of the importance of lifestyle interventions in mental health care—reflected in national and international guidelines and endorsed by prominent organizations like the World Psychiatric Association—certainly presents a timely opportunity for transformative change.

Smoking Cessation

Smoking not only contributes to increased mortality but also significantly reduces health-related quality of life [23]. Those who manage to quit smoking often experience relatively quick improvements in circulation and higher oxygen saturation in the lungs, and they soon feel that they are in better physical shape. Moreover, several studies suggest that addressing nicotine addiction alongside other addictions improves the likelihood of success in overcoming those other addictions. This highlights the importance of diagnosing patients who smoke with nicotine addiction and taking action on it [49].

We have strong opportunities to support patients with substance use and mental disorders in quitting smoking. While some patients express that they are motivated and want help to quit, it can be particularly challenging to motivate staff within psychiatry and substance use treatment [22]. Harm-reduction strategies can also be considered, such as encouraging reduced smoking or suggesting alternatives like snus or e-cigarettes. Although many municipalities offer smoking cessation groups, these groups are often not well-suited for people with severe mental health challenges. To bridge this gap, tailored smoking cessation groups should be offered in both specialized and primary healthcare services. Ideally, these groups would include experience-sharing from individuals in similar situations who have successfully managed to quit smoking, offering relatable and inspiring examples for participants.

Improved Physical Fitness and Increased Oxygen Uptake

Physical activity is often described as a source of joy, fulfillment, and positive experiences of mastery. It influences mood, boosts energy, reduces stress, improves body image, alleviates anxiety and depression, eases withdrawal symptoms, enhances self-esteem and confidence, and improves sleep quality. When performed in group settings, it also strengthens social functioning [50]. It is about seeking the opportunities to integrate activity into your daily life: shoveling snow, taking the stairs, and walking to the store. Several studies show that reducing sedentary behavior is just as impactful in preventing somatic disease as increasing physical activity itself, emphasizing the importance of all forms of movement. Even though not all activities need to have a therapeutic focus, healthcare services often play a crucial role in motivating and facilitating these activities.

Several studies highlight that physical activity has beneficial effects not only on physical health but also on mental health, suggesting it should be considered a complementary treatment, alongside other interventions [51, 52]. Relevant measures to promote physical activity may include organized activity groups at set times, free gym memberships, access to personal trainers, regular exercise opportunities, individualized follow-up even during hospitalization, and financial or practical support for purchasing equipment. The mental health benefits are most pronounced when exercise includes both aerobic components and muscle strength training, is performed regularly (at least three times per week), and includes personal follow-up and guidance from someone with expertise [53]. Therefore, all patients in both municipal and specialist health services should have access to tailored physical activity programs, ideally with oxygen uptake measurements to monitor progress. Achieving this requires resources and long-term planning across all levels of the healthcare system.

Diet

General dietary advice for improving long-term physical health is well-established and incorporated into the guidelines for preventing somatic diseases in individuals with severe mental illnesses (see, e.g., iphys.org.au). However, many patients require support in preparing and consuming healthier, more regular meals. Simply encouraging people to improve their diet is often insufficient, as research unfortunately shows that individual counseling has a limited impact [54]. For the most severely ill patients with concurrent disorders, systematic measures may be necessary, such as providing free meals at home or with others, assisted cooking programs, or reducing the cost of healthy, nutritious food. Additionally, emerging evidence from nutritional psychiatry underscores the vital role of diet in mental health across the lifespan. Meta-analyses reveal strong links between diet quality and mental health, even after adjusting for confounders. Mechanisms like the gut–brain axis, largely studied in animals, may explain these associations. Despite its potential, translating this research into practice faces challenges across individual, clinical, and societal levels.

Dental Health

Many patients with SUD/MH face challenges with poor dental health, including an elevated risk of periodontitis and cavities. These issues often stem from factors such as high sugar intake, inadequate oral hygiene, and medications that directly or indirectly affect teeth, such as through changes in saliva secretion [55]. Dental health is a critical component of physical health, as poor dental health can increase the risk of various diseases such as cardiovascular disease, diabetes, cancer, and respiratory illnesses. Poor dental status can also impair chewing function, promoting a diet rich in easily digestible carbohydrates, and can also affect speech. These issues, combined with visibly poor teeth, may harm self-image and limit social functioning.

There are significant barriers to accessing dental treatment, one of which is the fear of dental treatment (odontophobia). This fear can create a vicious cycle where anxiety and fear lead to avoidance of dental care, worsening dental health, and result in guilt, shame, feelings of inferiority, and further postponement of treatment. Another contributing factor for poor dental health in this group is that we rarely ask about or examine their dental status. The Norwegian Patient Care Pathway "Somatic

Health and Lifestyle Habits" includes a dedicated chapter on dental status, recommending the use of the following introductory questions [47]:

- Do you have pain or other problems in your mouth?
- How long has it been since your last visit to a dentist/dental hygienist?
- If it has been more than 2 years: What is the reason you haven't visited a dentist/dental hygienist for a long time?

If anxiety is identified as the reason, it should be documented in the referral to the dentist or dental hygienist.

For patients with significant dental anxiety, it is important to establish strong collaboration between the dentist and the physician at the institution or general practitioner. This collaboration can help assess premedication to ensure the patient is better prepared and supported during treatment.

Summary

- It cannot be emphasized strongly enough that physical health and lifestyle habits have a significant impact on patients with concurrent mental disorders and substance use disorders, and focusing on this is not exclusive to medical personnel, especially nurses and doctors—it applies to all professional groups.
- We must contribute to a collective effort so that people with mental illness and harmful substance use experience fewer symptoms, reduced disease risk, and receive adequate treatment and follow-up for somatic illness as well. These are conditions for which we have extensive knowledge regarding prevention and treatment in the general population, and we have a responsibility to ensure that patients with mental illness and harmful substance use also benefit from this knowledge.

Ultimately, this will hopefully contribute to significantly reducing the gap in life expectancy.

Reflection Questions

- How can the unit you work at facilitate that somatic follow-up becomes as important as other approaches to patients?
- What structural measures can you implement to help patients on their way to a healthier lifestyle?
- Many of the patients still smoke. What can you contribute to reducing smoking in this group?

Recommended Literature and Online Resources

- Lifestyle Psychiatry (American Psychiatric Association Publishing, 2019).
- Positive Cardiometabolic Health Resource: iphys.org.au

References

1. Nordentoft M, Wahlbeck K, Hallgren J, Westman J, Osby U, Alinaghizadeh H, et al. Excess mortality, causes of death and life expectancy in 270,770 patients with recent onset of mental disorders in Denmark, Finland and Sweden. PLoS One. 2013;8(1):e55176.
2. Walker ER, McGee RE, Druss BG. Mortality in mental disorders and global disease burden implications: a systematic review and meta-analysis. JAMA Psychiatry. 2015;72(4):334–41.
3. Plana-Ripoll O, Pedersen CB, Agerbo E, Holtz Y, Erlangsen A, Canudas-Romo V, et al. A comprehensive analysis of mortality-related health metrics associated with mental disorders: a nationwide, register-based cohort study. Lancet. 2019;394(10211):1827–35.
4. Plana-Ripoll O, Weye N, Momen NC, Christensen MK, Iburg KM, Laursen TM, et al. Changes over time in the differential mortality gap in individuals with mental disorders. JAMA Psychiatry. 2020;77(6):648–50.
5. Laursen TM, Plana-Ripoll O, Andersen PK, McGrath JJ, Tønder A, Nordentoft M, et al. Cause specific life years lost among persons diagnosed with schizophrenia: is it getting better or worse? Schizophr Res. 2019;206:284–90.
6. Plana-Ripoll O, Musliner KL, Dalsgaard S, Momen NC, Weye N, Christensen MK, et al. Nature and prevalence of combinations of mental disorders and their association with excess mortality in a population-based cohort study. World Psychiatry. 2020;19(3):339–49.
7. Luo A, Jung J, Longley M, Rosoff DB, Charlet K, Muench C, et al. Epigenetic aging is accelerated in alcohol use disorder and regulated by genetic variation in APOL2. Neuropsychopharmacology. 2020;45(2):327–36.
8. James SL, Castle CD, Dingels ZV, Fox JT, Hamilton EB, Liu Z, et al. Global injury morbidity and mortality from 1990 to 2017: results from the global burden of Disease Study 2017. Inj Prev. 2020;26(Supp 1):i96–i114.
9. Peacock A, Tran LT, Larney S, Stockings E, Santo T Jr, Jones H, et al. All-cause and cause-specific mortality among people with regular or problematic cocaine use: a systematic review and metaanalysis. Addiction. 2021;116(4):725–42.
10. Degenhardt L, Bucello C, Mathers B, Briegleb C, Ali H, Hickman M, et al. Mortality among regular or dependent users of heroin and other opioids: a systematic review and meta-analysis of cohort studies. Addiction. 2011;106(1):32–51.
11. Stockings E, Tran LT, Santo T Jr, Peacock A, Larney S, Santomauro D, et al. Mortality among people with regular or problematic use of amphetamines: a systematic review and meta-analysis. Addiction. 2019;114(10):1738–50.
12. Heiberg IH, Jacobsen BK, Nesvåg R, Bramness JG, Reichborn-Kjennerud T, Næss O, et al. Total and cause-specific standardized mortality ratios in patients with schizophrenia and/or substance use disorder. PLoS One. 2018;13(8):e0202028.
13. Momen NC, Plana-Ripoll O, Agerbo E, Benros ME, Børglum AD, Christensen MK, et al. Association between mental disorders and subsequent medical conditions. N Engl J Med. 2020;382(18):1721–31.
14. Ayerbe L, Forgnone I, Foguet-Boreu Q, Gonzalez E, Addo J, Ayis S. Disparities in the management of cardiovascular risk factors in patients with psychiatric disorders: a systematic review and meta-analysis. Psychol Med. 2018;48(16):2693–701.

15. Firth J, Siddiqi N, Koyanagi A, Siskind D, Rosenbaum S, Galletly C, et al. The Lancet Psychiatry Commission: a blueprint for protecting physical health in people with mental illness. Lancet Psychiatry. 2019;6(8):675–712.
16. Vancampfort D, Firth J, Correll CU, Solmi M, Siskind D, De Hert M, et al. The impact of pharmacological and non-pharmacological interventions to improve physical health outcomes in people with schizophrenia: a meta-review of meta-analyses of randomized controlled trials. World Psychiatry. 2019;18(1):53–66.
17. Solmi M, Fiedorowicz J, Poddighe L, Delogu M, Miola A, Høye A, et al. Disparities in screening and treatment of cardiovascular diseases in patients with mental disorders across the world: systematic review and meta-analysis of 47 observational studies. Am J Psychiatry. 2021;178:appiajp202121010031.
18. Heiberg IH, Jacobsen BK, Balteskard L, Bramness JG, Næss O, Ystrøm E, et al. Undiagnosed cardiovascular disease prior to cardiovascular death in individuals with severe mental illness. Acta Psychiatr Scand. 2019;139(6):558–71.
19. Heiberg IH, Nesvåg R, Balteskard L, Bramness JG, Hultman CM, Næss O, et al. Diagnostic tests and treatment procedures performed prior to cardiovascular death in individuals with severe mental illness. Acta Psychiatr Scand. 2020;141:439.
20. Dickerson F, Schroeder J, Katsafanas E, Khushalani S, Origoni AE, Savage C, et al. Cigarette smoking by patients with serious mental illness, 1999–2016: an increasing disparity. Psychiatr Serv. 2018;69(2):147–53.
21. Das-Munshi J, Semrau M, Barbui C, Chowdhary N, Gronholm PC, Kolappa K, et al. Gaps and challenges: WHO treatment recommendations for tobacco cessation and management of substance use disorders in people with severe mental illness. BMC Psychiatry. 2020;20(1):237.
22. Lien L. Smoking, mental health and addiction: a review of the literature. J Addict Prev Med. 2016;1(1):1–4.
23. Lien L, Bolstad I, Bramness JG. Smoking among inpatients in treatment for substance use disorders: prevalence and effect on mental health and quality of life. BMC Psychiatry. 2021;21:244.
24. Callaghan RC, Veldhuizen S, Jeysingh T, Orlan C, Graham C, Kakouris G, et al. Patterns of tobacco-related mortality among individuals diagnosed with schizophrenia, bipolar disorder, or depression. J Psychiatr Res. 2014;48(1):102–10.
25. Stubbs B, Vancampfort D, Hallgren M, Firth J, Veronese N, Solmi M, et al. EPA guidance on physical activity as a treatment for severe mental illness: a meta-review of the evidence and Position Statement from the European Psychiatric Association (EPA), supported by the International Organization of Physical Therapists in Mental Health (IOPTMH). Eur Psychiatry. 2018;54:124–44.
26. Stubbs B, Vancampfort D, Smith L, Rosenbaum S, Schuch F, Firth J. Physical activity and mental health. Lancet Psychiatry. 2018;5(11):873.
27. Vancampfort D, Firth J, Schuch FB, Rosenbaum S, Mugisha J, Hallgren M, et al. Sedentary behavior and physical activity levels in people with schizophrenia, bipolar disorder and major depressive disorder: a global systematic review and meta-analysis. World Psychiatry. 2017;16(3):308–15.
28. Svensson M, Brundin L, Erhardt S, Hållmarker U, James S, Deierborg T. Physical activity is associated with lower long-term incidence of anxiety in a population-based, large-scale study. Frontiers in Psychiatry. 2021;12:714014.
29. Landheim A, Lode Wiig F, Brendbekken M, Brodahl M, Biong S. Et bedre liv. Historier, erfaringer og forskning om recovery ved rusmiddelmisbruk og psykiske helseproblemer. [A Better Life. Stories, experiences and research on recovery from substance use disorder and mental health problems]. Oslo: Gyldendal Akademisk; 2016.
30. McCartan CJ, Yap J, Best P, Breedvelt J, Breslin G, Firth J, et al. Factors that influence participation in physical activity for people with bipolar disorder: a synthesis of qualitative evidence. Cochrane Database Syst Rev. 2024;6(6):CD013557.
31. McCreadie RG, Scottish Schizophrenia Lifestyle Group. Diet, smoking and cardiovascular risk in people with schizophrenia: descriptive study. Br J Psychiatry. 2003;183:534–9.

32. Strassnig M, Brar JS, Ganguli R. Nutritional assessment of patients with schizophrenia: a preliminary study. Schizophr Bull. 2003;29(2):393–7.
33. Roer GE, Solbakken HH, Abebe DS, Aaseth JO, Bolstad I, Lien L. Inpatients experiences about the impact of traumatic stress on eating behaviors: an exploratory focus group study. J Eat Disord. 2021;9(1):119.
34. Colich NL, Rosen ML, Williams ES, McLaughlin KA. Biological aging in childhood and adolescence following experiences of threat and deprivation: a systematic review and meta-analysis. Psychol Bull. 2020; https://doi.org/10.1037/bul0000270.
35. Suvarna B, Suvarna A, Phillips R, Juster RP, McDermott B, Sarnyai Z. Health risk behaviours and allostatic load: a systematic review. Neurosci Biobehav Rev. 2020;108:694–711.
36. De Hert M, Detraux J, Vancampfort D. The intriguing relationship between coronary heart disease and mental disorders. Dialogues Clin Neurosci. 2018;20(1):31–40.
37. Andreassen OA, Thompson WK, Schork AJ, Ripke S, Mattingsdal M, Kelsoe JR, et al. Improved detection of common variants associated with schizophrenia and bipolar disorder using pleiotropy-informed conditional false discovery rate. PLoS Genet. 2013;9(4):e1003455.
38. Correll CU, Solmi M, Croatto G, Schneider LK, Rohani-Montez C, Fairley J, et al. Mortality in people with schizophrenia: a systematic review and meta-analysis of relative risk and aggravating or attenuating factors. World Psychiatry. 2022;21(2):248–71.
39. Solmi M, Croatto G, Gupta A, Fabiano N, Wong S, Fornaro M, et al. Effects of antipsychotic treatment on cardio-cerebrovascular related mortality in schizophrenia: a subanalysis of a systematic review and meta-analysis with meta-regression of moderators. Eur Neuropsychopharmacol. 2024;88:6–20.
40. Vermeulen J, van Rooijen G, Doedens P, Numminen E, van Tricht M, de Haan L. Antipsychotic medication and long-term mortality risk in patients with schizophrenia; a systematic review and meta-analysis. Psychol Med. 2017;47(13):2217–28.
41. Torniainen M, Mittendrofer-Rutz E, Tanskanen A, Björkenstam C, Suvisaari J, Alexanderson K, Tiihonen J. Antipsychotic treatment and mortality in schizophrenia. Schizophr Bull. 2015;41(3):656–63.
42. Correll CU, Detraux J, De lepeleire JD, De Hert M. Effects of antipsychotics, antidepressants and mood stabilizers on risk for physical diseases in people with schizophrenia, depression and bipolar disorder. World Psychiatry. 2015;14(2):119–36.
43. Abosi O, Lopes S, Schmitz S, Fiedorowicz J. Cardiometabolic effects of psychotropic medications. Horm Mol Biol Clin Investig. 2018;36(1) https://doi.org/10.1515/hmbci-2017-0065.
44. Bradford DW, Kim MM, Braxton LE, Marx CE, Butterfield M, Elbogen EB. Access to medical care among persons with psychotic and major affective disorders. Psychiatr Serv. 2008;59(8):847–52.
45. Roberts L, Roalfe A, Wilson S, Lester H. Physical health care of patients with schizophrenia in primary care: a comparative study. Fam Pract. 2007;24(1):34–40.
46. Mitchell AJ, Lord O, Malone D. Differences in the prescribing of medication for physical disorders in individuals with v. without mental illness: meta-analysis. Br J Psychiatry. 2012;201(6):435–43.
47. Norwegian Directorate of Health. Somatic care and lifestyle habits in mental illness and/or substance use. Oslo: Helsedirektoratet; 2018. (rev. 2022). Available at https://www.helsedirektoratet.no/nasjonale-forlop/somatisk-helse-og-levevaner-ved-psykiske-lidelser-og-eller-rusmiddelproblemer.
48. Norwegian Ministry of Health and Care Services (HOD). Meld. St. 19 (2018–2019) Folkehelsemeldinga. Gode liv i eit trygt samfunn [Public Health Report – Good lives in a safe society]. Oslo: Helse-og omsorgsdepartementet; 2019. Available at https://www.regjeringen.no/no/dokumenter/meld.-st.-19-20182019/id2639770/.
49. Peckham E, Brabyn S, Cook L, Tew G, Gilbody S. Smoking cessation in severe mental ill health: what works? An updated systematic review and meta-analysis. BMC Psychiatry. 2017;17(1):252.
50. Martinsen EW. Kropp og sinn. Fysisk aktivitet, psykisk helse, kognitive terapi [Body and mind. Physical activity, mental health, cognitive therapy]. Bergen: Fagbokforlaget; 2018.

51. Firth J, Cotter J, Elliott R, French P, Yung AR. A systematic review and meta-analysis of exercise interventions in schizophrenia patients. Psychol Med. 2015;45(7):1343–61.
52. Ashdown-Franks G, Firth J, Carney R, Carvalho AF, Hallgren M, Koyanagi A, et al. Exercise as medicine for mental and substance use disorders: a meta-review of the benefits for neuropsychiatric and cognitive outcomes. Sports Med. 2020;50(1):151–70.
53. Vancampfort D, Rosenbaum S, Schuch F, Ward PB, Richards J, Mugisha J, et al. Cardiorespiratory fitness in severe mental illness: a systematic review and meta-analysis. Sports Med. 2017;47(2):343–52.
54. Jakobsen AS, Speyer H, Nørgaard HCB, Karlsen M, Birk M, Hjorthøj C, et al. Effect of lifestyle coaching versus care coordination versus treatment as usual in people with severe mental illness and overweight: two-years follow-up of the randomized CHANGE trial. PLoS One. 2017;12(10):e0185881.
55. Vanberg K, Husby I, Stykket L, Young A, Willumsen T. Dental health among a selection of injecting heroin users in Oslo. Nor Tannlegeforen Tid. 2016;126:528–34.

Every Patient Has Their Own Doctor

8

Torgeir Gilje Lid

Abstract

In many Western countries, the inhabitants have the right to be registered with a primary care physician, often called a *general practitioner* (GP). Other terms are family physician or primary care physician, but in this chapter, we use the term GP. The GP is an essential resource in primary healthcare and is the first point of contact for almost all health problems, as well as being responsible for long-term follow-up. This involves diagnostic procedures, treatment, and follow-up of the patient, from the banal to very severe conditions, regardless of diagnosis. The GP is responsible for patients regardless of whether medical, physical, or mental health problems or addiction and thus has a shared responsibility for all health problems in all age groups for all, except when the patient is staying in a healthcare institution.

For many patients, the GP is the healthcare professional they have the longest relationship with, and some have had the same GP since childhood. At best, the GP is a bearer of continuity and an important coordinator, as well as a support for the patient. But the GP may also not be involved at all in the treatment and follow-up of a patient. Most often, the reality is somewhere between these extremes.

What characterizes a good patient–doctor relationship with a GP for people with SUD/MH? Specifically, what is required for people with SUD/MH to get the best possible benefit from their GP? This chapter will describe several aspects related to these questions.

T. Gilje Lid (✉)
Center for Alcohol and Drug Research, Stavanger University Hospital, Stavanger, Norway

Department of Public Health, Faculty of Health Sciences, University of Stavanger, Stavanger, Norway
e-mail: torgeir.gilje.lid@sus.no

T. W. Lie, L. Lien (eds.), *Integrated Treatment of Co-occurring Substance Use and Mental Health Disorders*, https://doi.org/10.1007/978-3-032-20049-5_8

Keywords

General practitioner · General practice · Primary health care · Dual diagnosis · Substance use disorder · Primary care physician

The Core Values of General Practice: Norway as an Example

In addition to legal regulations, the GPs' activities are influenced by professional standards, professional culture and traditions. General practice has always been different from all other specialties. Where the other specialties in many ways have divided body and soul between them and developed a clear division of labor, the GP has an overall responsibility. The municipality has an overall responsibility for their inhabitants; it is in the municipality that people live their lives. The GP also has an overall responsibility, both in a life cycle and in an illness trajectory. It is often said that with the GP, the patients are the same, but the diseases come and go, while for the consultant in a hospital, the diseases are the same, while the patients come and go.

Around the turn of the millennium, the Nordic College for General Practitioners developed seven theses for general medicine (see Box 8.1 below) [1]. They are ideals to strive for, and not a realistic description of all days at work for the GP. But the theses provide clear guidelines for the GP's treatment and follow-up of vulnerable groups and are particularly relevant for SUD/MH patients.

The doctor–patient relationship is a core value in general practice, and it is especially important for vulnerable patients. It is also essential to focus on doing what is most important, that which has the greatest significance for the patient's health. And those who have the greatest needs should also get the most treatment. But perhaps the GP needs input from other partners both to see what is most important and to understand the patient's needs. What is most important for the patient must be clarified in collaboration, and the patient's own views should have decisive significance, but both the GP, next of kin, and other helpers can have important input.

Box 8.1 Core Values and Principles of Nordic General Practice/Family Medicine, Short Version [2]. Short Version from the Article, [2]

1. We promote continuity of doctor–patient relationships as a central organizing principle.
2. We provide timely diagnosis and avoid unnecessary tests and overtreatment. Disease prevention and health promotion are integrated into our daily activities.
3. We prioritize those whose needs for healthcare are greatest.
4. We practice person-centered medicine, emphasizing dialogue, context, and the best evidence available.
5. We remain committed to education, research, and quality development.
6. We recognize that social strain, deprivation, and traumatic experiences increase people's susceptibility to disease, and we speak out on relevant issues.
7. We collaborate across professions and disciplines while also taking care not to blur the lines of responsibility.

The seven theses highlight the basic values and principles for the GP's work. But in reality, different doctors will have different understandings of their own role, and the same doctor will have different roles toward different patients. A doctor works for the good of the patient but must follow professional and legal standards for medical practice, sometimes not complying with the patient's wishes. A doctor should not give treatment that is not medically justified, even if the patient strongly desires it. One example can be a SUD/MH patient who wants a prescription for a benzodiazepine, but the doctor will not give it. Another example can be a patient who gets such a prescription from the GP, but where the doctor in secondary healthcare services believes that it is not medically justified.

Professional guidelines and clinical evidence, the doctor's clinical judgment, and the patient's wishes provide a framework for what is right to do in individual situations. But different doctors can have different professional judgments and different knowledge about the specific patient. Even though medical knowledge is becoming increasingly advanced, it is often difficult to transfer knowledge at the group level (from research) to useful strategies in a given situation for a specific patient. But medicine as a practical skill is about *using the best available knowledge in the best possible way* for the individual patient. But it also means that in a specific situation, there are often few clear answers, so the doctor's attitudes, both to the clinical problem and to the patient group, may influence what the doctor believes is medically justified.

Two SUD/MH Practice Examples

Here are two case stories that underline several aspects of the GP's role for people with SUD/MH.

Emma—A Case Story

Emma was a SUD/MH patient who died at home after many years with failing follow-up and treatment. She was sectioned to psychiatric wards 20–30 times, but the admissions were always converted to voluntary admission, and she signed herself out. She did not follow-up on treatment herself, and it was very difficult for both primary and secondary care to maintain contact with her. She never visited her GP.

Emma's GP was interviewed by the local newspaper, and the introduction states: "Emma's GP acknowledges that she did not do enough for Emma." Emma's GP criticized that she was not invited to the collaborative meetings but also acknowledged that she herself should have done more to investigate whether Emma was receiving treatment and support as intended. Emma, herself, never sought her GP and never asked for help from her. Furthermore, Emma's GP expressed in the interview that in the future she will be more proactive and try to establish whether patients like Emma are receiving sufficient treatment and support.

Emma's GP illustrates how difficult the role of the GP can be. She was not invited to join the group meetings, and Emma never sought her GP to ask for help. Emma's GP, therefore, had very little opportunity to help her. In such situations, the GP can be an important collaborator in planning and implementing strategies to help the patient but has very few opportunities to do anything significant on their own.

Olivia—A Case Story

Olivia was receiving opioid agonist therapy (OAT) and died after acute medical illness. She usually received her OAT-medication at her GP's clinic but did not show up due to acute illness. Her GP was criticized for not having followed up on the missing appointments. The OAT clinic saw that she was falling ill and urged her to see her GP, but no one helped her to get there.

Olivia's GP did not want to be interviewed, but in a text message to the newspaper's journalist, he expressed that he did not know that Olivia had missed her appointments, as the dispensing of OAT-medications is done by the support staff, not the doctor himself. He further pointed out that "the office cannot, let alone should, track down all patients who do not show up for their appointment every day."

Legally, it is the GP who is the responsible party, not the doctor's office. A doctor's office with several doctors and support staff is a way to organize the clinic, but it is the GP who is responsible, medically and legally. This means that the GP is responsible for everything that happens at the doctor's office, and largely also for what does not happen, but should have happened. Olivia's GP lacks a recognition of this responsibility and a recognition that Olivia was a patient with more complex needs. But just as important in Olivia's case was that others in the healthcare service around her saw that she was ill and recommended her to go to the doctor, without informing the doctor about this and without taking responsibility for accompanying her to the doctor.

Patients' and Caregivers' Experiences

For SUD/MH patients, some of the challenges are reduced ability and willingness to seek necessary help. But public reports provide information about SUD/MH patients' and relatives' views, indicating that both patients and next of kin experience the GP as an important part of the primary health and social care. It is important to point out here that the choice of GP for oneself is a personal choice, unlike other individuals helping or treating the patient. It is important to ensure the patient's freedom of choice while developing good, practical solutions for collaboration.

Relatives of SUD/MH patients often find themselves in a particularly difficult situation, and the evaluation of the FACT: teams in Norway showed that some have experienced fighting for their family member for years without getting help, and without feeling acknowledged. At the same time, relatives can also be part of the problem for the patient, and it can be challenging for the GP and other healthcare personnel to balance the patient's needs and the relatives' needs.

The Importance of the Relationship

As Box 8.1 pointed out, the first point in the seven theses for general practice is "*We promote continuity of doctor-patient relationships as a central organizing principle.*" The patient enters into a personal relationship with the GP, also in a legal sense, and trust and respect both ways are necessary prerequisites for a good relationship. When this works well, the GP gets to know the patient, and his or her life and history, better. This can contribute to better health and a better quality of life for the patient. The GP can be an important bearer of continuity for the patient in long and complex trajectories. The GP's responsibility does not include deciding everything that should happen to the patient, but it means contributing to tenable comprehensive treatment and follow-up.

In interdisciplinary teams, the GP is often the one who has the longest relationship with the patient and can therefore be an important support and guide for the patient. Sometimes it helps the patient to discuss the agenda with the GP in advance of such meetings, especially if there are difficult and challenging topics. Other times, it may be helpful for the patient to evaluate the meeting with the GP afterward, to understand what happened and why. Such a support role can also be held by others in the interdisciplinary team whom the patient trusts.

But if the relationship is so important, what about those who do not have a GP, or where the relationship with the GP does not work? And what if the patient primarily wants to use the GP to get benzodiazepines or other addictive drugs? A central prerequisite for a good relationship is dialogue. Where there is already a relationship that works, it is important to talk to the patient about what he or she needs in terms of healthcare, and to talk with the GP about how he or she can contribute as best as possible. If the GP is missing or the relationship is not working, it is probably wise to talk to the patient about his or her needs first and offer, e.g., to go along with the patient to the GP. Sometimes the patient may need help to find a new GP.

Who Is the SUD/MH Patient?

Childhood and Upbringing

It is an established truth that experiences also affect the body. Medicine has gradually developed a better understanding of how adverse experiences in childhood and adulthood increase the risk of serious illness. It is well documented that there is a correlation between the extent of adverse experiences as a child and illness and premature death in adults [3]. This applies, for example, to cardiovascular disease, cancer, and chronic obstructive pulmonary disease (COPD), even if we adjust for lifestyle factors such as smoking. This means that increased morbidity and mortality due to unfavorable lifestyle factors add to increased morbidity and mortality due to adverse experiences in childhood and adolescence.

Getz and colleagues' article "Human biology—saturated with experience" [4] describes new knowledge about how allostatic overload (strong and/or persistent threats to a person's existence and integrity) over time can cause exhaustion of the body's flexibility and adaptation. This can cause significant biological effects, which partly explain the increased morbidity and mortality [3]. Serious adverse experiences, especially in childhood, can contribute to increased morbidity and mortality as an adult.

Life Experiences as an Adult

With this knowledge in mind, it is easier to understand that traumatization as an adult can also lead to increased morbidity and mortality. Many SUD/MH patients live under constant stress with high risk of serious illness and death, negative sanctions from their surroundings, and with high risk of violence and traumatization. Many have had adverse experiences both as children and as adults and live with significant risks of new adverse experiences.

SUD/MH patients can also have many negative experiences with the healthcare system. Repeated rejections, direct conflict about payment and prescriptions, and the experience of not being believed or taken seriously when one needs help are examples of such experiences. Signs of serious illness can easily be misinterpreted by a doctor or others and attributed to substance use or withdrawal symptoms or attributed to mental illness (also see the section on "Acute Serious Illness" later in this chapter).

The Significance of Life Experiences for Self-Care, Help-Seeking, and Participation

We who live ordinary lives take many things for granted. And when we take something for granted, it escapes our ability to reflect and our critical sense. The point of learning and development is not just to acquire new knowledge but also to gain better insight into one's own knowledge and attitudes, and not least, increased insights into what we take for granted and therefore do not reflect on. Most of those who work in the healthcare system have had a reasonably safe upbringing and make reasonably sensible life choices as adults. In addition, most of us seek help in sensible ways when we are ill or worried about illness, and we expect to be taken seriously when we seek help.

Things we take for granted

- That the immediate world is reasonably safe and predictable
- That we make reasonably sensible choices
- That we seek help when we need it
- That we are taken seriously when we seek help

But for many of the SUD/MH patients, this is not the case. They often have childhood experiences that not only increase the risk of disease but also cause a lack of trust that the world can be predictable and safe. They have made many choices as teenagers and adults that have made life difficult for both them and their loved ones. In addition, they have sought help for common diseases to a small extent, and when they seek help, they may have experienced rejection and disbelief. All this means that SUD/MH patients must maneuver in a world that is very different from the way we see the world. Their world often requires different action patterns than we expect. This is important to understand to be able to provide help. We therefore need an awareness of what we often take for granted, and we must try to understand the world as it appears to the other.

And here we are approaching a justification for why these paragraphs are written here, in the chapter about the role of the GP. Sometimes the GP has seen all this and can contribute to others around the patient seeing it too. Other times, the GP has not seen this, but others who know the patient can contribute to the GP seeing and understanding the patient better. But it is very important *not to take for granted that others see what oneself sees*. If the patient is urged to go to the GP, in the hope that the GP will then address the medical issues, it may be that the patient goes to the GP primarily to get a prescription for valium. And it may be that the GP sees a patient who has previously tried to deceive him or her, has missed appointments or owes money, and who now once again comes to get a new prescription. After the consultation with the GP, perhaps all parties have reinforced their experience that this is futile. If one talks to the patient in advance about what the GP can contribute and provides good information to the GP about the goal of the appointment, and preferably also accompanies the patient, then it is more likely that all parties can experience the encounter as beneficial.

It is common to refer to Søren Kierkegaard's words that if one is to help someone, one must start where the other is. The Danish theologian Knud Ejler Løgstrup goes a step further in the book The Ethical Demand in 1956 [5]:

The ethical demand says that you should take care of the other: "One should with all one's imagination and judgment do one's utmost to understand what is good for the other, and act accordingly."

Lifestyle Habits

SUD/MH patients have hardly benefitted from the major changes in health habits that the rest of the population in Norway has undergone over the last few decades. In the 1960s, the proportion of daily smokers was around 60 percent, and at the end of the 1990s, it was 30–40 percent. In 2020, only 9 percent of the adult population were daily smokers [6]. The proportion of daily smokers among SUD/MH patients is 9–10 times higher. The diet of the general population is also significantly better today, with a higher proportion of fruit and vegetables and unsaturated fat than in previous generations. The proportion that is physically active is also higher. Equally important is that for most people, living conditions have significantly improved from the 1960s to today. This means that both living conditions and health habits have significantly improved for the general population. In addition, preventive treatment, such as lifestyle advice and early identification and treatment for diabetes and cardiovascular diseases, has become available through the GPs for most people.

SUD/MH patients are also concerned with better health, even if it may not always be at the forefront of their consciousness. But it is important to explore with the patient what they think about health, what they themselves consider important, and how they envision their health in the years to come. This can contribute to a sensible process around health and be a good basis for collaboration with the GP. The goal is to contribute to greater awareness of the patients' health and to measures that can improve health. Read more about somatic illness and lifestyle habits in Chap. 7.

Acute Serious Illness

There is an increased risk of serious physical conditions for a SUD/MH patient compared to the general population, and despite this, it is more likely that a SUD/MH patient will be rejected or misinterpreted when seriously ill. We may say that *those who are at greatest risk of serious illness also have the greatest risk of being rejected when they are seriously ill.* The stories about Emma and Olivia earlier in the chapter are examples of this. With a deterioration in health status or new symptoms in a SUD/MH patient, both the doctor and other healthcare personnel must be aware of the possibility of a serious medical condition. All institutions or other parties working with SUD/MH patients need practical routines for managing several different medical situations (see Box 8.2):

Box 8.2 Three Different Medical Situations

1. Medical emergencies
2. Other medical situations with some degree of urgency
3. Follow-up of severe chronic conditions

These routines will vary, depending on national and local resources and routines, but for all three types of situations, collaboration with other resources is vital.

Most importantly, everyone involved in the follow-up of SUD/MH patients should be aware of the increased risk of acute serious illness, and aware of the increased risk of perceiving serious symptoms of illness as signs of intoxication, withdrawal symptoms, or mental illness.

SUD/MH Patients in Outpatient Treatment

For patients in outpatient treatment, e.g., in opioid agonist therapy (OAT), in assertive community treatment (ACT/FACT-team, read about such teams in Chap. 12), or in a psychiatric outpatient clinic, the GP is often responsible for the medical treatment. The specialist healthcare services' outpatient clinic has a responsibility for ensuring that the patient receives proper medical care and, if necessary, to collaborate to make this happen. This means that the outpatient clinic cannot take for granted that medical follow-up is provided by, for instance, the GP. Some people with SUD/MH do not have a working relationship with a GP (they have moved, the GP has quit, they do not know who the GP is, etc.), or they do not want to see their GP (they owe money, they have threatened the GP to get classified drugs, etc.).

For patients in outpatient follow-up (including ACT/FACT-teams), it is important that the outpatient unit or the team (1) has knowledge about which medical health problems are most frequent in their patient group, (2) has a strategy to establish whether and how a specific patient is followed up medically, and (3) aims to collaborate in establishing proper medical care for a patient if this is lacking. SUD/MH patients often have complex health problems, and to receive good and comprehensive treatment, a collaboration with all relevant parties is needed.

Dilemmas and Challenges

Working with SUD/MH patients, one encounters many dilemmas. The patient's goals and needs, the health and social care personnel's goals, and the GP's understanding of the situation can sometimes seem incompatible. The use of addictive drugs is often part of the patient's complex problems, but sometimes it can also be a necessary piece in the puzzle. Here, the GP can sometimes be perceived as prescribing too liberally, and at other times the GP may be seen as too restrictive.

Child protective services are responsible for assessing the welfare of children and to act accordingly. Some individuals with complex drug and mental health problems are responsible for children. Most often, child protective services are already involved, but all parties responsible for following up SUD/MH patients are obliged to assess potential risks for children and to communicate concerns to the child protection services.

For all SUD/MH patients who are parents, whether they have regular contact with or care for children or neither, it is important to make room for talking about being a parent, about challenges they experience, dreams for the future and about grief and loss. For many without regular contact with their children, the hope of being involved in the children's lives in the future can contribute to a recovery process.

Driver's License

Both the GP and the secondary healthcare services are obliged to clarify whether a SUD/MH patient has a driver's license, and if so, assess whether health requirements for driver's license are met. SUD/MH patients can both legally (prescription drugs) and illegally (bought from others) use drugs or substances that are incompatible with the health requirements in the driver's license regulations. Here, regulations regarding levels of use and who is responsible vary greatly between countries. The patient's overall health condition, including mental disorders, can also be incompatible with the health requirements for a driver's license. But sometimes working to meet the health requirements in the future may be an important part of a rehabilitation process. Regulations for driver's licenses vary internationally, and institutions and clinicians responsible for follow-up of SUD/MH patients should be familiar with the regulations and collaborate with other parties as required in national regulations.

Prescriptions

Medications are an important part of a doctor's toolbox. Most often, medication is one of several possible tools. But for some SUD/MH patients, the GP is perhaps primarily a potential prescriber of classified drugs like opioid painkillers (e.g., codeine, tramadol, oxycodone, and morphine), stimulants (e.g., amphetamines), or benzodiazepines and related drugs (e.g., diazepam and zopiclone).

Many SUD/MH patients are familiar with several of these drugs. The drugs have a significant risk of developing tolerance, which means that with prolonged use, increasingly larger doses are needed to achieve the same effect. They also have a so-called rebound effect, which means that prolonged use causes the symptoms alleviated by the drugs to rebound when the drug use is reduced or stopped. The patient will often interpret this as worsening of the underlying condition (e.g., pain, anxiety, and sleep problems). While the rebound effect is expected and temporary, for the user, it may confirm that one really needs the drug. See also Chap. 6 on drugs and addiction.

GPs sometimes get a reputation as "strict" or "lenient" with medications. Most often, the doctor will have sound professional reasons for his clinical practice, whether perceived as "strict" or "lenient." However, while many "strict" doctors are competent and experienced and want to provide the best possible treatment for the patients without increasing the patient's problems by prescribing addictive drugs, other "strict" doctors may have little interest in patients with complex drug and mental health problems and want to avoid these patients by being strict. Some "lenient" doctors may have a strong desire to help the patients as best as possible and experience strict rules for prescription as negative for the patients, while other "lenient" doctors may be disillusioned and want the least possible discomfort and conflict for themselves.

A dialogue with the doctor can often enable a mutual understanding of a sensible strategy for the individual patient. Sometimes, addictive drugs may have a place. Occasionally, the patient's situation is so difficult and complex that a well-planned course of medication may be an adequate measure. If so, it is important to establish a time frame until reassessment, and what kind of support and follow-up the patient needs in the course of treatment. This can reduce much of the discomfort for both patient and doctor, without "giving up" the patient. It is important to discuss the strategies in the multidisciplinary team to facilitate collaboration.

Sectoral Collaboration

The dismantling of institutions and scarcity of services for these patient groups have led to increased strain on GPs. In addition, both GPs and hospital doctors may feel that the other party has a different understanding of when it is appropriate to admit a patient to specialist health care. It is a major challenge when both parties in a collaboration feel that the other party has a different perception of reality than oneself. Lack of professional support from hospital doctors also puts the GPs in a difficult position toward collaborators in the primary healthcare services and can contribute to GPs hesitating to get involved in complex cases.

Blame Game or Shared Responsibility?

SUD/MH patients often have a difficult life story and extensive and complex problems. They often experience little support in their own network and have limited resources to improve their health and their situation. The GP is an important part of the ecosystem of healthcare services, but dependent upon collaboration with other services, for the benefit of the patient. Such collaboration enables realistic plans and management of acute health problems and crises.

If the collaboration does not work or is lacking, it can easily become a blame game where, e.g., both the hospital and the GP hesitate to take responsibility, and others who are supposed to help the patient experience a lack of support, advice, and assistance from healthcare. A lack of necessary collaboration can be very harmful to the patient and life-threatening. For people with SUD/MH and others with long-term and complex needs, it is important to strive for an interdisciplinary approach, where all parties recognize that they are important, are aware of their responsibility, and ready to contribute in the best possible way when needed.

How can GPs do a good job for people with SUD/MH? These patients often need more time with the doctor, which is difficult to arrange if the doctor often experiences that the patient does not show up anyway. If the patient is accompanied to the doctor, it will be easier to allocate the necessary time. If the patient still does not show up, the time slot can be used for a brief interdisciplinary meeting to plan further measures for the benefit of the patient.

Summary

- Regardless of how motivated and interested the GP is in this group of patients, they will need assistance and help from many different services. The GP has an important role in cross-sectoral follow-up, as one of several parties who can contribute with knowledge and interventions.
- The interdisciplinary team around the patient should be large enough to make sure that those who have a specific role toward the patient are included, and small enough so that the collaboration can be effective.
- In a good and respectful collaboration, it may be possible over time to implement both preventive measures, necessary treatment and follow-up, and good strategies for emergency help when needed.

Reflection Questions

- What can the primary care physician do for SUD/MH patients who do not ask for help themselves or do not show up for appointments?
- What can you and your colleagues in the health and care services do to help SUD/MH patients who do not take the initiative themselves, get the necessary health care?
- What do SUD/MH patients themselves need to develop better health habits?
- How can you and your colleagues in the health and care services contribute to better health habits for SUD/MH patients?

References

1. Sigurdsson JA, Beich A, Stavdal A. A Saga-in-progress: challenges and milestones on our way toward the Nordic Core values and principles of family medicine/general practice. Front Med (Lausanne). 2021;8:681612.
2. Nordic Federation of General Practice (NFGP). Core values and principles of Nordic general practice/family medicine. Scand J Prim Health Care. 2020 Dec;38(4):367–8.
3. Felitti VJ, Anda RF, Nordenberg D, Williamson DF, Spitz AM, Edwards V, et al. Relationship of childhood abuse and household dysfunction to many of the leading causes of death in adults. The Adverse Childhood Experiences (ACE) Study. Am J Prev Med. 1998;14(4):245–58.
4. Getz L, Luise Kirkengen A, Ulvestad E. Menneskets biologi—mettet med erfaring [Human biology—saturated with experience]. Journal of the Norwegian Medical Association. 2011;131(7):683.
5. Løgstrup KE. Den etiske fordring [The ethical requirement]. Copenhagen: Gyldendal; 1957.
6. Norwegian Institute of Public Health. Utbredelse av røyking i Norge [Prevalence of smoking in Norway]. In: Norwegian Institute of Public Health, editor. Oslo: Norwegian Institute of Public Health; 2021.

Coercion in Mental Health and Substance Use Disorder Treatment

9

Julie Granlund Hanssen, Marianne Silsand, and Erlend Bugge

Abstract

This chapter examines coercion in mental health and substance use treatment, focusing on its legal, cultural, and experiential dimensions. Beginning with international human rights frameworks, it outlines the obligations states hold when restricting individual freedom and how these principles are reflected in national legislation. The discussion then turns to formal coercion, such as involuntary hospitalization and forced treatment, highlighting significant cross-national variation in legal criteria and practices. Informal coercion, subtle pressures including persuasion, inducements, and threats, is explored as a widespread yet underregulated phenomenon, deeply shaped by cultural and institutional contexts. The chapter further emphasizes the concept of perceived coercion, drawing attention to patients' subjective experiences of pressure, which may persist even in voluntary treatment. Taken together, these perspectives illustrate how coercion is a complex and multifaceted phenomenon, raising important ethical, clinical, and cultural questions that continue to challenge mental health and substance use services worldwide.

J. Granlund Hanssen (✉) · M. Silsand
Regional Centre for Research and Education in Forensic Psychiatry and Psychology (SIFER), University Hospital of North Norway, Tromsø, Norway

Centre of Expertise on Voluntariness and Coercion, Tromsø, Norway
e-mail: julie.hanssen@unn.no; marianne.elise.myrli.silsand@unn.no

E. Bugge
Regional Centre for Research and Education in Forensic Psychiatry and Psychology (SIFER), University Hospital of North Norway, Tromsø, Norway

Centre of Expertise on Voluntariness and Coercion, Tromsø, Norway

UiT The Arctic University of Norway, Tromsø, Norway
e-mail: erlend.bugge@unn.no

T. W. Lie, L. Lien (eds.), *Integrated Treatment of Co-occurring Substance Use and Mental Health Disorders*, https://doi.org/10.1007/978-3-032-20049-5_9

Keywords

Coercion · Mental health care · Substance use disorder treatment · Human rights · Patient autonomy · Involuntary treatment

In the following chapter, we will examine coercion in mental health and substance use disorders (SUDs). To understand the concept of "coercion," it is central to look at the international human rights that we are required to follow. This chapter also explains how countries around the world regulate and use coercion. These rights form the basis for how countries are expected to treat people who receive health care, including those who are treated for mental illness or drug problems.

The first part of the chapter presents how international human rights describe the use of coercion, and what obligations countries have when they use coercive measures. The next part looks at how different countries use formal coercion, which refers to measures that are based on laws or regulations, such as involuntary admission or forced treatment.

We will then describe informal coercion. This refers to forms of pressure that are not written into laws, but that still influence how people act and what choices they make in treatment. Finally, we look at how people themselves experience coercion. This includes situations where people feel pressured, even if the health care staff believe they are acting helpfully or supportively.

Although many of the examples in this chapter are taken from mental health care, the use of coercion also occurs in treatment services for people with drug problems. Coercion is something that can happen in both fields, and we will highlight that throughout the text.

International Human Rights

The Concept of Human Rights

The basic function of human rights is to safeguard human rights and ensure equal rights for all [1]. However, certain groups experience infringement on, or even loss of, their freedoms. Individuals confined to psychiatric care or SUD treatment may be among these groups. To understand coercion in such institutions, it is essential to look at the overarching principles and regulations in international law. Therefore, the natural starting point would be an overview of international human rights.

The concept of "international human rights" can be understood in various ways depending on academic, cultural, political, and philosophical perspectives. For this reason, a common definition of the term is challenging. Nevertheless, it can be stated that human rights are rights inherent to all individuals by virtue of being human. These rights are irrespective of gender, age, sexual orientation, nationality, religion, and place of residence [1]. This means that the rights are non-derogatory and that they are universal.

A closer examination of the relationship between the state and its individuals reveals that human rights function as a set of rules concerning how the state is obligated to treat individuals and groups. "Rights" can be understood as granting individuals an advantageous position or strengthening their standing in relation to an opposing party. In this context, human rights provide individuals with a stronger position relative to the state [2]. When it comes to coercion in SUD/MH treatment, this means that human rights afford patients a stronger position in relation to the institution.

Human rights represent moral principles and are regulated through legal frameworks. The purpose of human rights is firmly based on protecting the individual from discrimination, abuse, and misuse of power by the state, institutions, or other individuals [3].

To gain a better understanding of international human rights, it is necessary to be familiar with certain key terms. Table 9.1 provides an overview of selected concepts that are frequently used in international human rights. These terms are used in various ways in international instruments, and their precise meaning depends on both the legal context and the intentions of the parties involved.

Universal Declaration of Human Rights

Different continents and regions have varying regulations concerning human rights. Since the aim here is to provide an overview of international human rights, this discussion is based on the United Nations' (UN) *Universal Declaration of Human Rights* (UDHR) of 1948.

Table 9.1 Overview of a selection of key concepts in international human rights

Concept	Definition
Declaration	Various international instruments. Declarations are not always legally binding. The term «declaration» is often deliberately chosen to indicate that the parties do not intend to create binding obligations but merely want to declare certain aspirations [4]. Declarations can also be treaties in the generic sense, intended to be binding at international law. Therefore, it is necessary to establish in each individual case whether the parties intended to create binding obligations. Ascertaining the intention of the parties can be a difficult task [4].

(continued)

Table 9.1 (continued)

Concept	Definition
Convention	Can have both a generic and a specific meaning [4]. Generic meaning: Embraces all international agreements, in the same way as the generic term *"treaty"* does. Therefore, the generic term «convention» is synonymous with the generic term «treaty» [4]. Specific meaning: «Convention» is generally used for formal multilateral treaties with a broad number of parties. They are normally open to participation by the international community as a whole or by a large range of states. Usually, these documents negotiated under the auspices of an international organization are entitled conventions [4].
Treaty	An international agreement concluded between States in written form and governed by international law, whether embodied in a single instrument or in two or more related instruments, and whatever its particular designation [5]. For a treaty to have effect for a state, it is necessary that the state accepts the treaty, for example, through ratification or incorporation [6].
Protocol	The term is used for agreements less formal than those entitled "treaty" or "convention" [4].

Several historical events have contributed to the development of what we today refer to as *international human rights*. The evolution of human rights has taken place over several centuries, with the notion of fundamental rights and freedoms tracing back to ancient Babylon, Greece, and Rome [7]. The development of modern human rights has been shaped and refined through a series of key historical documents, including the *Magna Carta* (England, 1215), the *United States Declaration of Independence* (1776), and the *French Declaration of the Rights of Man and of the Citizen* (1789).

Despite the origins of human rights dating back several centuries, it was only after World War II that they attained universal status [8]. This universal recognition is due to the efforts of the United Nations and other intergovernmental organizations that have placed human rights at the forefront of the international political agenda and facilitated the development of international human rights laws [2].

As a direct consequence of World War II and the atrocities committed against individuals and minority groups, a broad consensus emerged regarding the importance of international human rights. This consensus led to the establishment of the UN and the adoption of the *UDHR* in 1948 [3].

Table 9.2 How human rights can be categorized [2]

Category	Rights
Civil rights safeguards	Life, liberty, and the security of a person Integrity Legal protection Private life and family life Freedom of opinion and expression Freedom of thought, conscience, and religion Right to form and to join trade unions Right to freedom of movement and residence
Political rights safeguards	Right to take part in the government of his country, directly or through freely chosen representatives Right to vote
Economic rights safeguards	Right to work Right to form and to join trade unions Strike Right to a standard of living adequate
Social rights safeguards	Right to security in the event of unemployment, sickness, disability, widowhood, old age, or other lack of livelihood in circumstances beyond his control
Cultural rights safeguards	Education Right freely to participate in the cultural life of the community, to enjoy the arts, and to share in scientific advancement and its benefits Participation in cultural life and enjoyment of scientific progress and copyright protections Right to the protection of the moral and material interests resulting from any scientific, literary, or artistic production of which he is the author

Today, 193 countries worldwide are members of the UN and have a moral and political duty to uphold the principles set forth in the UDHR. However, since the UDHR is a declaration rather than a treaty, it is not legally binding for member states [9].

There is a broad spectrum of international human rights. To create a clearer overview, it can be useful to divide them into categories. Table 9.2 illustrates one such way of classifying these rights.

Convention on the Rights of Persons with Disabilities

As previously discussed, the UDHR is a foundational and universal convention. The United Nations has developed conventions that build upon the principles of the UDHR, but which are more specific and, in some cases, legally binding. Examples of such conventions are the International Covenant on Civil and Political Rights (ICCPR), the International Covenant on Economic, Social and Cultural Rights (ICESCR), the Convention against Torture (CAT), and the Convention on the Rights of Persons with Disabilities (CRPD).

We will take a closer look at the CRPD. The United Nations General Assembly adopted the CRPD in 2006, and the convention entered into force in 2008 [10]. As of March 6, 2025 [11], 191 countries have ratified the convention [12]. It is noteworthy that the USA, Lebanon, and Tajikistan are among the countries that have not committed to the CRPD [11].

The CRPD deals with the rights of people with disabilities. The term "disabilities" refers to "those who have long-term physical, mental, intellectual or sensory impairments which in interaction with various barriers may hinder their full and effective participation in society on an equal basis with others" ([13], article 1, second paragraph). The definition "disabilities" is not exhaustive. This means that where broader definitions of "disabilities" exist in national legislation, such cases will also fall within the scope of the Convention. For instance, individuals with temporary impairments or those who previously have had a disability are also covered by the CRPD [14].

Mental illness is not necessarily associated with disability. However, a clear distinction is not required since the CRPD states principles which should be valid for all human beings, disabled or not [15]. Based on this, individuals subjected to coercion will have their rights protected in accordance with the CRPD.

Approximately 16% of the world's population lives with some form of disability [16]. People with disabilities remain among the most marginalized groups worldwide. Even though international human rights have led to positive changes in several societies, people with disabilities have not benefited to the same extent [14].

CRPD marks a paradigm shift in attitudes and approaches to persons with disabilities [10]. The convention endorses a so-called social model that recognizes disability as the result of "the interaction between persons with impairments and attitudinal and environmental barriers" (14 preamble (e)). Based on this, the purpose of CRPD is to "promote, protect and ensure the full and equal enjoyment of all human rights and fundamental freedoms by all persons with disabilities, and to promote respect for their inherent dignity" ([13], article 1, first paragraph). CRPD ensures that persons with disabilities have the same rights and opportunities as everyone else. The convention covers the many areas where people with disabilities have been discriminated against, including access to justice, participation in political and public life, education, employment, freedom from torture, exploitation, violence, and freedom of movement [14].

In addition, the UN General Assembly has adopted an Optional Protocol to the CRPD [11]. The Optional Protocol entered into force on the same date as the CRPD, on 3 May 2008 [10]. According to the Optional Protocol, individuals or groups whose rights under the convention have not been fulfilled may bring their case before the UN. However, this is subject to the requirement that all domestic remedies must first have been exhausted [11]. A total of 106 countries have ratified the Optional Protocol [12].

Despite the fact that the CRPD strengthens the rights of people with disabilities, its effectiveness is equally dependent on the states' ability to implement and enforce measures that ensure compliance with the convention. The CRPD is the first treaty to include specific requirements for national implementation and monitoring of rights [10]. This is precisely to ensure effective enforcement. The implementation of the convention is a responsibility that lies with the government, while the protection, promotion and monitoring require the leadership of national entities [10].

Since this chapter is intended to provide an overview of international human rights, we will not go into detail regarding how states are to fulfill their obligations toward the Convention. If you wish to learn more about this topic, information can be found in the publication "From Exclusion to Equality: Realizing the Rights of Persons with Disabilities," issued by the Office of the United Nations High Commissioner for Human Rights (OHCHR) in collaboration with the United Nations Department of Economic and Social Affairs (DESA) and the Inter-Parliamentary Union (IPU).

Human Rights in Different Regions of the World

In addition to both the UDHR and the CRPD, are there human rights frameworks that have been developed within and for specific continents and regions? However, providing a comprehensive overview can be challenging due to significant variations in social, cultural, political, and economic conditions across these regions. Such factors influence how human rights function—not only in terms of how they are formulated in legal frameworks, but also in how they are implemented in practice. This, in turn, affects the actual rights individuals are able to claim. This is mentioned only briefly, as a more detailed discussion of the various legal frameworks would be too extensive for the scope of this context.

In the context of mental health care and SUD treatment, one frequently encounters individuals who, as previously noted, have been deprived of their freedom. This group is, therefore, particularly vulnerable to violations of the prohibition against torture or cruel, inhuman, or degrading treatment or punishment ([3], article 5) ([14], article 15). This prohibition becomes especially relevant in situations involving measures such as involuntary hospitalization, the use of coercive means, and forced medication.

Since freedom is a fundamental human right, strict requirements must be met before an institution may lawfully restrict an individual's freedom ([3] article 3). According to article 8 of the European Convention on Human Rights (ECHR), any interference must have a legal basis and must also be proportionate [17].

The requirements of legal basis and proportionality are also reflected in UN instruments, such as the Convention on the Rights of Persons with Disabilities (CRPD). However, the practical implications of these standards for the individual remain unclear and raise a number of complex legal and ethical questions. This uncertainty is partly due to cultural and political differences across countries. Based on these challenges and given that the purpose of providing an overview of human rights is to offer an understanding of the topics discussed later in the chapter, these terms will not be further addressed.

Furthermore, we will examine how coercion is grounded in and implemented through national legal frameworks across different regions and countries.

Coercive Practices

Comparing data across countries on coercive practices in SUD/MH is a somewhat precarious undertaking due to several methodological issues. For instance, legal frameworks and definitions of coercion vary between countries, reflecting cultural and social norms. Additionally, the absence of standardized measurement tools for coercive practices, along with variations in data collection methods and quality, further complicates direct cross-national comparisons. A basic understanding of these methodological issues is a necessary caveat when comparing data on coercion from different countries.

Formal Coercion: Legislation and Legal Definitions

Formal coercion typically refers to involuntary hospitalization, forced treatment, and the use of coercive measures in mental health care (e.g., mechanical restraints, seclusion, etc.), sanctioned by mental health laws and court rulings. However, the legal definitions of voluntariness and coercion differ across jurisdictions, influencing both the classification of coercive practices and the criteria for their implementation. One example is the concept of "danger to self or others" as a criterion for admission to a mental health facility. For instance, in New York State, involuntary hospitalization under the Mental Hygiene Law requires that an individual with mental illness poses a "*substantial threat of harm to self or others*" [18]. This criterion includes risks such as suicide, serious bodily harm, or behavior that induces reasonable fear of serious physical harm in others. By contrast, the Norwegian Supreme Court has ruled that the aggressive behavior of a psychotic parent may fulfil the risk criterion under the Mental Health Act, as such behavior can be considered harmful to the mental health of his/her children [19]. The Swedish mental health legislation offers yet another perspective, as imminent danger is not a prerequisite for involuntary hospitalization. Rather, the legal framework emphasizes the necessity of treatment as the primary justification for admission [20]. The definition of physical restraint is another example, as some countries define physical restraint explicitly as coercion, while others do not, and its practice spans from the use of chains and cage to straps and seclusion [21–23].

Notwithstanding the numerous differences in national legislations and established practices, there is the challenge of semantics. Terms that, in everyday conversation, are translated and used effortlessly between users of different languages may have critically different connotations and practical consequences when applied in a judicial context. Accordingly, when assessing apparently similar legal terms for comparative purposes, the outcome could be imprecise or even misleading. The challenge is even greater when trying to compare practices and legislation on SUD treatment; worldwide, the judicial perspective is highly heterogeneous and ranges from medical to criminal, often with a mixture of both, and sometimes with religion as the point of reference. For example, in the Philippines, Saudi Arabia, and China, drug possession and use are subjected to criminal punishment and coercive treatment [24–26]. By contrast, Portugal, and to a large extent Switzerland, have decriminalized the use of drugs and emphasized voluntariness and harm reduction policies, such as outreach programs and opioid agonist therapy [27, 28]. Though there are some signs of an international trend toward voluntariness [29], supported by studies that indicate that voluntariness is more effective than coercion [30–32], most countries still have laws approving some form of compulsory SUD treatment [33].

The differences between national legislations are suggested to contribute to differences in rates of coercion. For example, a study involving 15 European countries found that nations permitting involuntary hospitalization solely on the basis of treatment need exhibited higher admission rates than those requiring justification based on risk [34]. However, a later study including 22 European countries found no such connections [35]. The researchers did, however, find that higher rates of involuntary hospitalization were associated with how much money a country spends on health care, the number of hospital beds, the level of purchasing power of its citizens, a lower level of poverty, and a higher proportion of foreign-born individuals in the population. These findings suggest that a country's wealth and organization of mental health care play an important role in determining compulsory admission rates.

Data Collection and Quality

Research has shown that there is great variability in characteristics and fidelity of data collection, both within and between countries. Some countries have centralized mental health care reporting systems that enable consistent data collection on a national level, e.g., Norway and Germany, while others rely on regional or local reporting, e.g., Canada and South Korea. Adding to the complexity is *how* data on similar practices are reported, as one study on the use of mechanical restraints in Pacific rim countries demonstrates [36]. The countries included in the study all had national databases on the use of mechanical restraints, but the temporality and the specificity of the reporting differed. Accordingly, the researchers had to find a common denominator that could be extracted from the different national databases, thus ending up with the *average number of restraint events per day per one million people*. The reason for choosing *per day* as the registration interval was simply that one of the countries in the study only provided per-day data. Still, in many cases, a common data denominator cannot be found or calculated, or there is a paucity of data altogether, as illustrated by the WHO Mental Health Atlas. The only coercive measure reported in the atlas is the number of involuntary admissions, and even this is lacking for many big countries: the USA, Brazil, and China being notable examples [37]. Certainly, regional studies could offer insights into the use of coercive practices at the national level. However, caution should be exercised when assessing the representativeness of such studies, given that local variations could be significant, even in smaller countries with a relatively homogeneous population [38].

If national data on coercion in psychiatry is difficult to obtain or to translate into workable statistics, information about coercion in the treatment of substance dependency is even harder to extract. Globally, reporting is patchy at best, and most countries do not offer national statistics on coercive measures.

In summary, there is a huge variety as to the extent of data on involuntary hospitalization and coercive approaches available on a national level. For those countries providing information, the reporting methods also differ in terms of terminology, aims, scale, sampling, and research quality, making generalizations difficult. Notwithstanding these limitations, contrasting data from various countries and regions could offer valuable lessons.

Cultural Factors

Attitudes toward mental health and coercion differ by culture, shaping how involuntary treatment is defined, legally regulated, implemented, and reported. Although it's impossible to quantify cultural influences, it is generally assumed that an attitude toward SUD and mental health disorders characterized by acceptance and non-stigmatization leads to less coercion, as seen in Portugal after drug decriminalization in 2001. However, the actual evidence for this is limited, and though several Western countries have amended their legislation to accommodate demands for protection of patient autonomy, reported rates of coercion are still high [39]. On the other hand, it could be hypothesized that this is a reporting bias, i.e., that the countries at the top of the statistic also have a stronger focus on openness and data fidelity. Put differently, stigmatization may lead to underreporting and misclassification of coercive practices.

Cultural attitudes toward individualism and collectivism may also shape coercion practices. Western societies, especially the USA and Western Europe, typically favor individual autonomy and minimal coercion in mental health care. Legal frameworks and informed consent policies are designed to protect patient rights and restrict involuntary interventions. However, the debate continues about finding the right balance between collectivistic paternalism and individual autonomy, particularly for patients who are unable to provide consent. By contrast, Eastern approaches to mental health care tend to be more collectivistic, prioritizing family and societal welfare over individual autonomy. In several Asian countries, where family authority is a prominent cultural feature, coercive treatments seem to be more acceptable as means to maintain societal and familial harmony. However, these practices have raised concerns about power imbalances and violations of individual rights [40].

Comparing Data

Keeping the aforementioned caveats in mind, what does research say about coercion practices across countries? Data on formal coercion in SUD treatment are still scarce. In mental health care, however, reported coercion rates vary widely. For instance, European data on compulsory hospitalization rates span from 3% in Portugal to 30% in Sweden [34, 41].

A 2010 review and international survey by Steinert et al. found similar inconsistencies: in psychiatric hospitals across 12 developed countries, seclusion rates ranged from 3.6% to 15.6%, while restraint use ranged from 1.2% to 8.0% [42]. These findings were further highlighted by a study by Savage et al. that included nine countries: Australia, England, Germany, Japan, Ireland, The Netherlands, USA, Wales, and New Zealand [43]. Several of the measured coercive practices varied by a factor of more than 100 between the countries, for instance, the numbers of mechanical restraints, seclusions, and physical restraints per 100,000 population, as well as the mean admission duration and number of restrictive practice incidents (RPIs) per one million population per day. Japan recorded the highest rates for all these practices, except for physical restraints, as they do not track this category. With regard to involuntary admissions per 100,000 citizens per year, Japan was at the top with 220, whereas Ireland and Wales were at the bottom with 42 and 91, respectively. It is worth noting that while the rates for specific types of coercion differed by a factor of more than 100 between some countries, the RPI, i.e., the overall measure of restrictive practice incidents, differed by a factor of less than 10. This implies that certain types of coercive measures are more frequent than others in different countries. Physical restraint, for instance, is relatively common in Ireland, but quite rare in Germany. For seclusion, the relation is reversed; it is twice as common in Germany as it is in Ireland.

Moving from the national level to the regional level, the variation in rates and prevalences is possibly even higher. A review by Belayneh et al., including 77 studies published between 2010 and 2022, found very different rates both within and between countries [44]. Taking physical restraint as an example, the prevalence ranged from 0.3% in a US study to 53.8% in an Italian one. However, the highest prevalence reported by an American study was 21.6%, and the lowest reported by an Italian study was 7%. Seclusion rates were also fluctuating, with Japan at the top with 55.8% prevalence, and the USA at the bottom with 2.1%. Once again, the rates within a country were highly inconsistent. For instance, Dutch rates ranged from 14% to 41.3%, German rates from 2.9% to 38%, and Canadian rates from 5.7% to 23.2%. Similar findings were made regarding chemical restraint, this time with Norway at the lower end with 2% prevalence, and India at the higher end with 58%. Of course, to some extent, the variability in prevalence rates could reflect actual differences. Nevertheless, the large and inconsistent fluctuations across and within countries suggest that variations in reporting practices and study designs likely contributed to the wide range of estimates. Indeed, there was a highly significant heterogeneity across the 77 studies included ($I^2 > 99\%$), forcing the question whether the studies were suitable for comparison. This does not, however, detract from the fact that this study shows that coercive practices are a relatively common phenomenon in mental health care worldwide, with a pooled proportion of persons being exposed to physical restraints, seclusion and chemical restraints being 14.4%, 15.8%, and 26%, respectively. Moreover, studies from Asian countries generally reported higher proportions of restrictive care practices.

Informal Coercion

Informal coercion refers to a range of strategies used by mental health professionals to encourage patients to accept treatment. These strategies are not based on legal authority and do not involve physical force, yet they still influence a patient's decisions. Examples include persuasion, where a clinician attempts to convince the patient through reasoning and discussion; interpersonal leverage, which uses the therapeutic relationship as a source of influence; inducements, where rewards are offered for compliance; and threats, where potential negative consequences of non-compliance are emphasized. Although these actions may not always be seen as coercive by professionals, they can significantly affect a patient's ability to make independent, informed choices [45]. Informal coercion may also manifest through subtle or even nonverbal cues—such as tone, posture, or institutional rituals—that patients experience as pressure. This reflects the concept of "communicative pressure," where the staff's presence or tone can shape patient behavior without explicit force [46].

Relevance for Substance Use Services

Although much of the research on informal coercion is based in mental health care, this phenomenon is also highly relevant in substance use treatment. People receiving care for addiction may experience various forms of pressure to enter or remain in treatment, including from family members, the justice system, or healthcare professionals. A study from Vancouver found that people who use drugs often felt informally pressured by clinicians and service providers, frequently without experiencing meaningful alternatives. Importantly, this pressure did not lead to improved treatment outcomes. The study suggests that informal coercion may influence patient behavior and expectations but does not necessarily improve health outcomes [47].

Recent research supports these concerns. A systematic review from 2023 examined the effectiveness of involuntary treatment for SUD and found insufficient evidence that coercion leads to better long-term outcomes. Most included studies in the systematic review showed no benefit or only mixed effects, and some pointed to potential harms, such as undermining patient dignity or damaging therapeutic relationships [48]. Similarly, Fischer et al. [49] argue that compulsory drug treatment, even when implemented with therapeutic intent, may not reduce substance use and could contribute to stigma and disengagement from care.

The use of coercion becomes even more complex in the context of co-occurring substance use and mental health disorders. In such cases, informal coercion may intersect with structural vulnerabilities such as poverty, limited-service availability, or legal ambiguity. Individuals with developmental disabilities and co-occurring substance use problems can be considered a particularly vulnerable subgroup in this regard. Norwegian professional sources emphasize that people with developmental disabilities face significant barriers in accessing substance use treatment, and that the current coercion legislation appears overdue for revision [50]. Such structural conditions may contribute to marginalization and increase the risk of involuntary interventions within support systems.

The interplay between coercion and overlapping vulnerabilities, including developmental disability, substance use, and mental health problems, raises important questions about how these dynamics shape experiences of coercion and influence the degree of voluntariness in care. Although coercion is sometimes justified as a means to protect or motivate individuals, research suggests that its effects are limited and may, in some contexts, undermine trust and patient dignity. Taken together, these perspectives highlight the need for critical reflection on how systems and professionals balance protection and autonomy within substance use and mental health care. It can be argued that current practice calls for a stronger rights-based orientation and an increased emphasis on voluntary and individualized approaches, as also advocated in recent Norwegian professional discourse [50].

Relevance in Modern Mental Health Care

Studies suggest that informal coercion is highly prevalent in psychiatric care. According to research, between 29% and 59% of patients report experiencing some form of it [51]. The most common forms include emotional pressure, linking treatment to financial or housing benefits, and suggestions framed as warnings. Importantly, these forms of coercion exist even in systems with strong legal protections, suggesting that formal safeguards alone are not enough to prevent subtle coercion from occurring. In psychiatric settings, informal coercion is often used when patients are hesitant or refuse to engage in treatment. These methods are sometimes seen as preferable alternatives to formal coercion, such as involuntary hospitalization. However, they raise important ethical concerns. For instance, if a patient agrees to take medication solely to avoid eviction from supported housing, can that decision truly be considered voluntary? Research shows that patients often comply without realizing the extent of the pressure they are under [51]. This makes informal coercion particularly challenging, as it is subtle, widespread, and frequently goes unnoticed by both staff and patients. These practices often emerge in the ambiguous space between clinical intention and patient perception, where professionals navigate ethically complex decisions without the legal frameworks that govern formal coercion. This "grey zone" can normalize informal strategies that are difficult to identify, regulate, or challenge [51].

A Spectrum of Influence

To better understand the range of informal coercion, Szmukler and Appelbaum developed a model outlining a "hierarchy of treatment pressures" [52]. At the lower end of this spectrum is persuasion, which respects patient autonomy and involves open discussion. Moving upward, influence becomes more forceful, through emotional appeals, conditional offers, and ultimately threats. At the highest level is formal coercion, such as involuntary hospitalization, which is legally sanctioned and involves clear violations of patient autonomy. Informal coercion, sometimes called "soft coercion," may evolve from benign persuasion into ethically fraught territory, especially when such actions are undocumented and lack scrutiny. Unlike formal coercion, which typically requires legal authorization, soft coercion is often seen as routine and therefore rarely questioned [53].

Three Dimensions of Coercion

The Norwegian psychologist Olav Nyttingnes introduced a useful framework that distinguishes between three types of coercion. First, compulsion refers to legally authorized actions, such as forced hospitalization or medication. Second, informal coercion includes strategies that are not legally mandated but still place pressure on patients—such as implying that refusing treatment could have negative consequences. Finally, experienced coercion is based on how the patient feels about the situation, regardless of the healthcare professional's intent [54].

Two additional concepts are helpful for understanding patients' reactions. The "coercion shadow" [55] refers to how previous experiences with formal coercion can lead patients to perceive even benign interactions as threatening. Likewise, "coercion context" [55] refers to how a person's social environment—such as limited choices, financial dependency, or family pressure—shapes their perception of autonomy. Together, these concepts highlight the psychiatric importance of context, history, and power dynamics in how patients experience psychiatric care.

Informal Coercion Around the World

Informal coercion takes different shapes around the world. In Latin and Southern European contexts—for example, Mexico, Chile, Spain, and Italy—family ties and cultural traditions are central influences. In Mexico, professionals have reported using emotional strategies, including guilt and religious references, and in some cases, hiding medication in food to gain patient compliance [56]. Across these countries, families frequently influence treatment decisions—sometimes pressuring both patients and clinicians. Some studies suggest that professionals in these regions may express less discomfort or ethical tension about the use of informal coercion than those in other cultural settings, indicating that cultural norms could influence how such practices are used and perceived [57].

In Nigeria, patients have reported being deceived about the reasons for visiting a clinic or hospital. Some believed they were attending a job interview or visiting relatives, only to find themselves involuntarily admitted to psychiatric care. Families often take control of these decisions, particularly in the absence of strong mental health infrastructure and legal protection. Health professionals in Nigeria acknowledge these practices, arguing they are necessary due to stigma, resource constraints, and lack of treatment alternatives [58]. These examples reveal how informal coercion is deeply influenced by context. What is considered compassionate or practical in one setting may be viewed as ethically questionable in another. Therefore, cultural awareness and ethical reflection are essential when assessing the use of informal coercion across different healthcare environments.

How Health Professions Use Informal Coercion

Informal coercion is often woven into the therapeutic relationship between healthcare professionals and patients. A psychiatrist might emphasize the benefits of medication. As one participant in an international study described:

> If a young man…doesn't want to take medicine […], then the course of therapy would be to discuss it with him, and try to explain the reason for him taking this medicine […]. In most cases, one way or another at the end they accept. [57]

Similarly, a social worker might express concern about the risks of refusing therapy.

> You know, the more unwell they are, the more likely you're going to use the bigger, more questionable forms of persuasion. "Do this, or you know…" In the hope that they get some insight and their mental health stabilizes. [57]

Although these actions often stem from a sense of responsibility and care, they can create subtle pressure, particularly when patients feel they cannot genuinely decline.

Institutional routines also play a role in informal coercion. When patients are expected to follow strict schedules or abide by rules that are neither explained nor open to discussion, they may experience this as controlling rather than supportive. This is especially concerning in cases of voluntary admission, where individuals may nonetheless feel as though they lack the right to refuse care.

A Norwegian study highlights how such "household rules," though not legally mandated, can significantly impact patients' sense of autonomy and dignity, especially for those admitted voluntarily [59].

The Patient's Perspective

Patients often experience informal coercion as disempowering. In studies conducted in Norway, patients described feeling like they were not being treated as full individuals. Instead, they were often reduced to their diagnosis, with decisions being made for them, not with them [59]. Many reported that they were not included in conversations about their treatment, leading to frustration and a lack of trust.

For patients who have previously experienced formal coercion—such as forced hospitalization or restraint, even well-meaning encouragement can feel threatening.

A suggestion to take medication may be interpreted as a warning or an implicit threat, especially if past experiences were traumatic. This shows how trust, openness, and transparency are essential for maintaining a respectful relationship in mental health care.

Informal coercion is often perceived differently by staff and patients. While professionals may see their actions as supportive or necessary, patients, especially those with past traumatic experiences, may interpret them as controlling or manipulative. This divergence highlights the importance of recognizing how past coercion casts a long shadow over present care [46].

Institutional routines may also contribute to informal coercion. When patients are required to adhere to strict schedules or rules that are neither explained nor subject to negotiation, they may feel controlled rather than supported. This is particularly concerning when individuals are voluntarily admitted but are treated as if they lack the right to refuse.

Autonomy and Power in Psychiatric Care

In discussions of informal coercion, autonomy is often presented as the opposite of paternalism. The assumption often seems to be that when a patient's autonomy is respected, coercion and power are absent. However, this contrast is overly simplistic. In reality, both autonomy and paternalism involve the exercise of power, they just differ in how and why that power is used.

Autonomy, in the context of healthcare, is typically understood as the patient's right to make informed and voluntary decisions about their own treatment. This includes choosing whether or not to accept medical interventions. At first glance, this appears to empower the patient. But this understanding of autonomy, framed as freedom of choice, can be misleading in psychiatric settings.

Patients usually turn to mental health services not as consumers in a marketplace, but as individuals in vulnerable situations. They are seeking support in moments of distress, confusion, or crisis. Their ability to understand, evaluate, or act on options may be compromised by illness, fear, or lack of information. When professionals focus solely on obtaining informed consent, they risk treating autonomy as a checkbox rather than as a meaningful safeguard of the patient's interests.

What's more, the therapeutic relationship in psychiatry is shaped by a fundamental power imbalance. The clinician possesses not only medical knowledge but institutional authority. Even when professionals aim to support patient autonomy, their influence may still be felt as pressure. A patient may consent to treatment not because they truly agree, but because they feel they have no other viable option. In this way, autonomy can become a surface-level reassurance that conceals deeper inequalities in power.

This raises a critical ethical concern: autonomy alone is not enough to protect patients from subtle forms of coercion or manipulation. The fact that a patient agrees to a treatment plan does not automatically mean the decision was made freely or with genuine understanding. The asymmetry of power, between a person in crisis and a professional in control of care, can quietly shape decisions in ways that undermine the spirit of autonomy.

Rather than abandoning the concept, however, we need to rethink how autonomy is applied. It should not be reduced to a legal formality but understood as an ongoing, relational process. Supporting autonomy means creating an environment in which patients feel safe, respected, and informed. It also means acknowledging the power dynamics at play and actively working to balance them through trust, transparency, and collaboration.

In the context of informal coercion, this perspective is especially important. The risk is not only that autonomy is violated, but that it is used as a justification for ethically questionable practices. By viewing autonomy not as the absence of influence, but as the presence of genuine, informed participation, mental health care can better navigate the complex terrain between care and control.

Legal and Ethical Implications

Unlike formal coercion, which is governed by legal standards and subject to oversight, informal coercion often goes unregulated. As a result, staff members must rely on their personal judgment and institutional norms when deciding how to act. Some countries have started using reflection groups and ethical supervision to help professionals navigate this complex area. These approaches encourage self-awareness and provide space for open discussion about the line between supportive care and coercion [45].

Ethical guidelines that clarify how and when different forms of influence are appropriate could help reduce misuse and ensure more respectful treatment. In particular, culturally sensitive approaches are needed to account for how informal coercion is understood and experienced in different societies.

Perceived Coercion

Having addressed both formal and informal coercion, we now turn to perceived coercion. This refers to the subjective experience of being pressured or having one's autonomy restricted, regardless of the legal status of the treatment.

Perceived coercion refers to the individual experience of having one's right to self-determination restricted, regardless of whether any formal legal coercion is applied. Research indicates that there is only a weak to moderate correlation between the formal use of coercive measures and the patient's experience of coercion [60, 61]. This points to a more complex, relational understanding of coercion that extends beyond legal frameworks.

The experience of coercion is just as relevant in SUD treatment as in mental health care. A Norwegian study [62] supports this, showing that patients with SUD, whether admitted voluntarily or involuntarily, frequently reported feeling pressured to enter treatment. Notably, internal pressures like shame or feeling they had no real alternative were common even among those formally admitted of their own will. This highlights that perceived coercion is not primarily about legal status, but about how treatment is experienced.

In this chapter, we examine perceived coercion as a subjective but clinically significant dimension—shaped by how patients are met, involved, and respected throughout the care process.

The Lasting Impact of Past Coercion

Importantly, perceived coercion is not shaped in a vacuum; it is deeply influenced by patients' past experiences. Evidence shows that prior exposure to coercion may leave a psychological imprint that shapes future interactions with mental health care. As supported by Martinez et al. [63], patients with such histories report higher levels of fear and perceived negative pressure even during later voluntary hospitalizations. They also express lower satisfaction, especially when it comes to voicing concerns and being involved in decisions. These findings align with the notion of a "coercion shadow," where earlier experiences color current perceptions and may undermine trust, even in ostensibly voluntary contexts. Recognizing and addressing perceived coercion, therefore, is not only an ethical imperative but also a clinical necessity if we are to build genuine therapeutic alliances and support patient autonomy.

The Relational Nature of Coercion

This insight underscores that reducing formal and informal coercion alone is not sufficient. The experience of coercion is shaped in the therapeutic encounter, through communication, and by the extent to which the patient is given real influence.

Emotional distance from staff and a low degree of participation in decision-making are consistently identified as key contributors to perceived coercion and are also among the lowest-rated aspects of care quality.

Respect and Shared Decisions

There is growing evidence that relational factors can significantly mitigate the experience of coercion [61]. When patients are included in decisions, receive adequate information, and are met with respect and fairness, their perception of coercion decreases, even when formal measures are used.

A study by Silva [60] shows that perceived coercion during admission to mental health services is strongly linked to low treatment satisfaction. Similarly, a Norwegian study found that perceived coercion is associated with lower scores across all dimensions of care quality [61]. This may suggest that perceived coercion significantly influences the treatment process, affecting patient satisfaction and willingness to cooperate.

A Clinical and Ethical Priority

Perceived coercion is not only a matter of legal status but also of how patients are met, involved, and respected in their treatment. Past experiences of coercion may cast a long shadow, shaping fear, mistrust, and satisfaction in later encounters. These insights suggest that reducing harm requires attention not only to formal measures but also to the relational and cultural contexts in which care is provided.

Summary

- International human rights frameworks provide the foundation for understanding coercion, but national laws and practices vary widely.
- Formal coercion includes involuntary admission, restraints and forced treatment, and is regulated by law, yet applied differently across countries.
- Informal coercion consists of subtle pressures such as persuasion, inducements, and threats, shaped by cultural and institutional contexts.
- Patients' experiences of coercion show that treatment may feel pressuring even when formally voluntary, especially when influenced by past experiences.
- Reducing coercion requires more than legal safeguards, calling for respectful communication, transparency, and shared decision-making.
- Coercion in mental health and substance use treatment remains a complex ethical and clinical challenge that requires reflection, cultural awareness, and open dialogue.

Reflection Questions

- Reducing the use of coercion requires knowledge of legal and ethical standards. How can you, in your workplace, contribute to strengthening your own and your colleagues' understanding of rights, laws, and best practices related to coercion?
- Voluntary treatment must be a real and accessible alternative to coercion. What actions can be taken in your service to make voluntary options more available and meaningful for people seeking care?
- A person's experience of coercion is shaped not only by what is done, but by how it is done. How can your workplace reduce the negative impact of coercive practices by focusing on respectful communication and relational safety?
- Involving people with lived experience is essential to improving services. How can you ensure that user perspectives are heard and valued—both in individual care decisions and in broader service development?

- Values, attitudes, and organizational culture play a major role in how coercion is used. How can your team or institution create space for open discussions about power, influence, and ethical dilemmas in treatment?

References

1. International Covenant on Economic, Social and Cultural Rights 1966.
2. Ekeløve-Slydal GM. Hva er menneskerettigheter? [What are human rights?]. Menneskerettigheter En innføring. Oslo: Humanist forlag; 2010.
3. United Nations. Universal Declaration of Human Rights 1948.
4. Collection UNT. Definition of key terms used in the UN Treaty Collection: United Nations; n.d. Available from: https://treaties.un.org/Pages/overview.aspx?path=overview/definition/page1_en.xml#conventions.
5. Vienna Convention on the Law of Treaties. Sect. article 2 (a) (1969).
6. Smith R. International Human Rights Law. 10th ed. Oxford: Oxford University Press; 2021.
7. Ishay M. The history of human rights: from ancient times to the globalization era. University of Calefornia Press; 2008.
8. Hoffmann S-L. Human rights in the twentieth century. Berkeley: Cambridge University Press; 2010.
9. United Nations. About us: United Nations; n.d. Available from: https://www.un.org/en/about-us.
10. Office of the United Nations High Commissioner for Human Rights. Thematic study by the Office of the United Nations High Commissioner for Human Rights on the structure and role of national mechanisms for the implementation and monitoring of the Convention on the Rights of Persons with Disabilities. 2009. Report No.: A/HRC/13/29.
11. United Nations Association of Norway. Konvensjon om rettighetene til personer med nedsatt funksjonsevne [Convention on the Rights of Persons with Disabilities]. United Nations Association of Norway; n.d. [Available from: https://fn.no/avtaler/menneskerettigheter/konvensjon-om-rettighetene-til-personer-med-nedsatt-funksjonsevne.
12. Danbolt IL. Fem fakta om FNs konvensjon om rettighetene til personer med nedsatt funksjonsevne (CRPD) [Five facts about the UN Convention on the Rights of Persons with Disabilities (CRPD)]: United Nations Association of Norway; 2024. Available from: https://fn.no/nyheter/fem-fakta-om-fns-konvensjon-om-rettighetene-til-personer-med-nedsatt-funksjonsevne-crpd.
13. Convention of Rights on Persons with Disabilities. 2006.
14. Office of the United Nations High Commissioner of Human Rights with the United Nations Department for Economic and Social Affairs and the Inter-Parliamentary Union From Exclusion to Equality: Realizing the Rights of Persons with Disabilities. 2007.
15. Steinert C, Steinert T, Flammer E, Jaeger S. Impact of the UN convention on the rights of persons with disabilities (UN-CRPD) on mental health care research - a systematic review. BMC Psychiatry. 2016;16(1):166.
16. World Health Organization. Disability. World Health Organization; n.d. Available from https://www.who.int/health-topics/disability.
17. Convention for the Protection of Human Rights and Fundamental Freedoms. European Convention on Human Rights; 1950.
18. New York State - Office of Mental Health. Mental Hygiene Law. n.d. Available from https://omh.ny.gov/omhweb/forensic/manual/html/mhl_admissions.htm.
19. HR-2023-2018-A [Norwegian Supreme Court judgment in case HR-2023-2018-A], (2023–2018).
20. Swedish Ministry of Health and Social Affairs. Lag (1991:1128) om psykiatrisk tvångsvård 2020 [Act (1991:1128) on Compulsory Psychiatric Care]. 1991.

21. Steinert T., editor An international perspective on the use of coercive measures. 2016.
22. Molodynski A, O'Brien A, Burns J. Key international themes in coercion. BJPsych Int. 2017;14(3):61–3.
23. Human Rights Watch. People with mental health conditions living in chains. 2020.
24. Amnesty International. Philippines: Coercion and abuse disguised as "rehabilitation" at drug detention centres; 2024. Available from: https://www.amnesty.org/en/latest/news/2024/11/philippines-coercion-and-abuse-disguised-as-rehabilitation-at-drug-detention-centres/.
25. Yang J, Giummarra MJ. Compulsory and voluntary drug treatment models in China: a need for improved evidence-based policy and practice to reduce the loaded burden of substance use disorders. Int J Drug Policy. 2021;92:103063.
26. Harm Reduction International. The Death Penalty for Drug Offences: Global Overview 2023. Available from https://hri.global/flagship-research/death-penalty/the-death-penalty-for-drug-offences-global-overview-2023/.
27. Zobel F, Maier L. Chapter 14 Switzerland: moving towards public health and harm reduction. 2018. p. 277–88.
28. RÊGo X, Oliveira MJ, Lameira C, Cruz OS. 20 years of Portuguese drug policy - developments, challenges and the quest for human rights. Subst Abuse Treat Prev Policy. 2021;16(1):59.
29. World Health Organization. Countries move away from using coercive measures in mental health care; 2025. Available from: https://www.who.int/europe/news-room/feature-stories/item/countries-move-away-from-using-coercive-measures-in-mental-health-care.
30. Pasareanu AR, Vederhus JK, Opsal A, Kristensen Ø, Clausen T. Improved drug-use patterns at 6 months post-discharge from inpatient substance use disorder treatment: results from compulsorily and voluntarily admitted patients. BMC Health Serv Res. 2016;16:291.
31. Parhar KK, Wormith JS, Derkzen DM, Beauregard AM. Offender coercion in treatment: a meta-analysis of effectiveness. Crim Justice Behav. 2008;35(9):1109–35.
32. Habermeyer B, Wyder L, Roser P, Vogel M. Coercion in substance use disorders: clinical course of compulsory admissions in a Swiss psychiatric hospital. Swiss Med Wkly. 2018;148:w14644.
33. Israelsson M, Gerdner A. Compulsory commitment to care of substance misusers: international trends during 25 Years. Eur Addict Res. 2012;18(6):302–21.
34. Stefano A, Ducci G. Involuntary admission and compulsory treatment in Europe: an overview. Int J Ment Health. 2008;37:10–21.
35. Sheridan Rains L, Zenina T, Dias MC, Jones R, Jeffreys S, Branthonne-Foster S, et al. Variations in patterns of involuntary hospitalisation and in legal frameworks: an international comparative study. Lancet Psychiatry. 2019;6(5):403–17.
36. Newton-Howes G, Savage MK, Arnold R, Hasegawa T, Staggs V, Kisely S. The use of mechanical restraint in Pacific Rim countries: an international epidemiological study. Epidemiol Psychiatr Sci. 2020;29:e190.
37. World Health Organization. Mental Health, Brain Health and Substance Use 2021. 2021.
38. Hofstad T, Husum TL, Rugkåsa J, Hofmann BM. Geographical variation in compulsory hospitalisation—ethical challenges. BMC Health Serv Res. 2022;22(1):1507.
39. Keski-Valkama A, Sailas E, Eronen M, Koivisto AM, Lönnqvist J, Kaltiala-Heino R. A 15-year national follow-up: legislation is not enough to reduce the use of seclusion and restraint. Soc Psychiatry Psychiatr Epidemiol. 2007;42(9):747–52.
40. Raveesh BN, Lepping P, Palmstierna T. Eastern and Western approaches to coercion in mental health. In: Hallett N, Whittington R, Richter D, Eneje E, editors. Coercion and violence in mental health settings: causes, consequences, management. Cham: Springer Nature Switzerland; 2024. p. 27–39.
41. Salize HJ, Dressing H. Epidemiology of involuntary placement of mentally ill people across the European Union. Br J Psychiatry. 2004;184:163–8.
42. Steinert T, Lepping P, Bernhardsgrütter R, Conca A, Hatling T, Janssen W, et al. Incidence of seclusion and restraint in psychiatric hospitals: a literature review and survey of international trends. Soc Psychiatry Psychiatr Epidemiol. 2010;45(9):889–97.

43. Savage MK, Lepping P, Newton-Howes G, Arnold R, Staggs VS, Kisely S, et al. Comparison of coercive practices in worldwide mental healthcare: overcoming difficulties resulting from variations in monitoring strategies. BJPsych Open. 2024;10(1):e26.
44. Belayneh Z, Chavulak J, Lee DA, Petrakis M, Haines TP. Prevalence and variability of restrictive care practice use (physical restraint, seclusion and chemical restraint) in adult mental health inpatient settings: a systematic review and meta-analysis. J Clin Nurs. 2024;33(4):1256–81.
45. Engerdahl IS, Moljewijk A, Pedersen R. Etiske utfordringer ved bruk av tvang i psykisk helsevern [Ethical challenges in the use of coercion in mental health care]. Tidsskrift for Norsk psykologforening. 2016:102–10.
46. Aluh DO, de Almeida JMC, Richter D, Whittington R. Coercion in contemporary mental health services: key concepts, historical development and contextual factors. In: Hallett N, Whittington R, Richter D, Eneje E, editors. Coercion and violence in mental health settings: causes, consequences, management. Cham: Springer Nature Switzerland; 2024. p. 67–92.
47. Pilarinos A, Barker B, Nosova E, Milloy MJ, Hayashi K, Wood E, et al. Coercion into addiction treatment and subsequent substance use patterns among people who use illicit drugs in Vancouver, Canada. Addiction. 2019:115.
48. Bahji A, Leger P, Nidumolu A, Watts B, Dama S, Hamilton A, et al. Effectiveness of involuntary treatment for individuals with substance use disorders: a systematic review. Can J Addict. 2023;14(4):6–18.
49. Fischer B, Hall W, Jutras-Aswad D, Le Foll B. Involuntary treatment for severe substance use disorders—issues, evidence and considerations for its use. Can J Psychiatry. 2025;70(8):597–9.
50. Vagle BR, Storvik M. Utviklingshemming og rus: Tvangslovverket er overmodent for revidering [Intellectual disability and substance abuse: The coercion legislation is long overdue for revision]. 2025. Available from: https://fontene.no/fagartikler/utviklingshemming-og-rus-tvangslovverket-er-overmodent-for-revidering-6.47.1161767.fdcccccf2f.
51. Hotzy F, Jaeger M. Clinical relevance of informal coercion in psychiatric treatment-a systematic review. Front Psychiatry. 2016;7:197.
52. Szmukler G, Appelbaum PS. Treatment pressures, leverage, coercion, and compulsion in mental health care. J Ment Health. 2008;17(3):233–44.
53. Allison R, Flemming K. Mental health patients' experiences of softer coercion and its effects on their interactions with practitioners: a qualitative evidence synthesis. J Adv Nurs. 2019;75(11):2274–84.
54. Nyttingnes O. Patients' experience of coercion in mental health care. Oslo: University of Oslo; 2018.
55. Szmukler G. Compulsion and "coercion" in mental health care. World Psychiatry. 2015;14(3):259–61.
56. García Cabeza I, Calcedo A, Márquez Mendoza O, Mundt A, Valenti E. Cultural differences in the use of covert coercion among mental health professionals of Latin culture: a focus group study. Ethical Hum Psychol Psychiatry. 2021;23:EHPP-D.
57. Valenti E, Banks C, Calcedo-Barba A, Bensimon CM, Hoffmann KM, Pelto-Piri V, et al. Informal coercion in psychiatry: a focus group study of attitudes and experiences of mental health professionals in ten countries. Soc Psychiatry Psychiatr Epidemiol. 2015;50(8):1297–308.
58. Aluh DO, Ayilara O, Onu JU, Grigaitė U, Pedrosa B, Santos-Dias M, et al. Experiences and perceptions of coercive practices in mental health care among service users in Nigeria: a qualitative study. Int J Ment Heal Syst. 2022;16(1):54.
59. Mantila JCH, Johnson T, Nyttingnes O, Hammer J. Utforsket pasienters opplevelse av tvang [Explored patients' experiences of coercion]. Sykepleien forskning (Oslo); 2019.
60. Silva B, Morandi S, Bachelard M, Bonsack C, Golay P. Pathways to experienced coercion during psychiatric admission: a network analysis. BMC Psychiatry. 2024;24(1):546.
61. Fossum SØ, Larsen MØ, Thorsen GM, Agneta S, Skundberg-Kletthagen H. Investigating the associations between patient-reported quality of care and perceived coercion: a Norwegian cross-sectional study. Issues Ment Health Nurs. 2024;45(8):784–93.

62. Opsal A, Kristensen Ø, Vederhus JK, Clausen T. Perceived coercion to enter treatment among involuntarily and voluntarily admitted patients with substance use disorders. BMC Health Serv Res. 2016;16(1):656.
63. Martinez D, Brodard A, Silva B, Diringer O, Bonsack C, Morandi S, et al. Satisfaction and perceived coercion in voluntary hospitalisations: impact of past coercive experiences. Psychiatr Q. 2022;93(4):971–84.

Encounters with Violence and Suicidality 10

Jan Aasen

Abstract

In clinical work with patients with elevated risk of committing violence or self-harm in outpatient and domestic patient settings, our capability to assess and manage harms risk is vital for keeping both ourselves and our patients safe. Understanding the causal mechanisms of aggressive behaviors is key to preventing unwanted and hazardous events. When caregivers seek to understand aggressive behaviors and meet violence with knowledge, we move from working against the patient's behavior to working with the patient's coping strategies as an integrated part of supporting the patient's recovery. In this chapter, we will look at the risk factors associated with violence and self-harm specific to individuals with co-occurring substance use and mental disorders (SUD/MH). We will also look at how we may manage violence risk in outreach and domestic healthcare SUD/MH services. Much is overlapping between suicide and violence when it comes to triggering factors and risk. We will see that many of the neurobiological and cognitive mechanisms behind suicide, reactive violence, and self-harm are overlapping and that many of the preventive strategies are similar.

Keywords

Violence risk · Suicide risk · Safety planning · Safety management

J. Aasen (✉)
DPS Elverum/Hamar, Innlandet Hospital Trust, Hamar, Norway

Research Centre for Substance Use Disorders and Mental Illness, Innlandet Hospital Trust, Hamar, Norway

VID Specialized University, Oslo, Norway
e-mail: jan.aasen@sykehuset-innlandet.no

T. W. Lie, L. Lien (eds.), *Integrated Treatment of Co-occurring Substance Use and Mental Health Disorders*, https://doi.org/10.1007/978-3-032-20049-5_10

People with substance use and mental disorders (SUD/MH) are a highly vulnerable group of patients. Many live their lives with insecure living conditions, long-term psychosocial distress, mental disorders, and addiction. Altogether, these risk factors reinforce each other and constitute an unpredictable and potent risk complex for violence, self-harm, and suicide [1–3]. A life in chaos with violence and crime as part of everyday life is common for many individuals with SUD/MH, both as perpetrators and victims [4, 5].

The incidence of violence-related work absence among health and social workers within mental health and social services has been high and increasing over the past decade. In line with the shift from inpatient to outreach and mobile services, there has been a particular increase in violence incidents in mental healthcare and SUD treatment [6–8]. At the same time, health services are developing toward less inpatient treatment and more outreach and homecare treatment [9, 10]. Health and social workers in mobile and homecare health services are at particularly high risk of being subjected to work-related violence [6, 11, 12]. Additionally, there is significantly increased mortality among individuals with SUD/MH. Suicide is found to be significantly elevated in people with SUD/MH compared to the suicide rate in the general population. Next to overdose deaths, suicide is the most common cause of early death in this patient group [2].

Various strategies for predicting, preventing, and managing violence have been extensively researched in hospital environments since the 1980s, and a variety of different models for managing violence risk have been developed [13–15]. Most models focus mainly on various communication skills, regulation of own behavior, and various physical and mechanical control measures. However, these are based on professional and legal guidelines adapted to the controlled environment in psychiatric wards or prisons [16, 17].

Recent research on violence risk management has shown that different clinical settings, different patient groups, different healthcare tasks, and different types of violence require different approaches to risk management [14]. Measures to predict, prevent, and manage violence need to be specifically adapted to the clinical setting they are to be used in [15]. In outreach substance use and mental health services, violence is a complex phenomenon with a wide spectrum of risk factors, causes, and forms. Managing violence risk in outreach health services thus requires risk assessment strategies to manage many different types of risk situations [8]. Despite the deinstitutionalization of mental health care over the past decade, there is scarce research on violence between users and staff in clinical settings outside the controlled environments of inpatient wards [15, 18].

What Is Violence?

To get a better understanding of violence risk management, we need to clarify what violence really is, and how we may comprehend the causal mechanism behind violence and aggression. First and foremost, it is vital to understand violence as a variety of different phenomena. Some use violence and threats to achieve their own advantages, some use violence to control and punish others. Some use violence to compensate for their own vulnerability, some use violence and threats as a coping strategy when they become scared, and others use violence because they enjoy it. Violence can be physical, with punches, kicks, scratching, pinching, etc. Violence can be psychological through threats, both directly and via social media or through control, manipulation, and sexual abuse [19]. Violence can primarily be understood as either proactive or reactive, and one distinguishes whether the violence is about overcoming or defending against negative emotions, or whether it is driven by the desire to harass, harm, or kill others [20].

Proactive violence is violence, threats, or aggression that is carried out intentionally, with a goal to kill, harm, manipulate, or harass others. This is called functional violence, which can be sorted as predatory violence; "*predatory aggression,*" and pleasure-driven violence; "*appetitive aggression.*" Predatory violence is about power, manipulation, revenge, or gain and is about appropriating material benefits, robbing, stealing, harming, or killing to achieve social status. This type of violence is motivated by external reward. This is also called instrumental violence, as it is planned, has a conscious intention, and a calculated outcome.

Pleasure-driven violence is motivated by an inner desire, appetite for violence, sadism, and cruelty [19–22]. The underlying cognitive mechanisms behind proactive violence are linked to the lack of empathy, guilt, and low affect [22]. The neurobiological mechanisms behind proactive violence are not fully mapped but are linked to GABA and glutamine influence in the hypothalamus. These are the same mechanisms that regulate hunger and are also thought to be linked to hunting instinct and the brain's reward systems for food intake [22, 23].

Reactive violence is impulsive, spontaneous, and directed at those who are perceived as threatening or frightening. Reactive violence is based on a reactive defense mechanism where aggression is triggered by a spontaneous defense reaction to an event, situation, threat, or danger that triggers negative emotions such as fear, anxiety, anger, or dread. Reactive violence is therefore also called defensive aggression. This is violence that is driven by the inherent defense mechanisms to avert, flee from, or fight out of a dangerous situation [20, 21, 24]. Reactive violence is triggered when fear reactions in the limbic system exceed the inhibitory capacity in the frontal lobe, so that violent impulses are not stopped. These mechanisms are regulated by serotonergic signals in the limbic structures of the brain [24].

Why Is Violence and Suicide So Prevalent Among People with SUD/MH?

Psychosis, depression, anxiety, trauma disorders, and personality disorders are the most common mental illnesses found among SUD/MH patients. Violence and suicide have a higher prevalence in this group than in patient populations with similar diagnoses who do not use substances. This means in practice that mental disorders in themselves do not explain why we find such high occurrences of violence and suicide among dual diagnosis patients. In a study by the National Epidemiologic

Survey on Alcohol and Related Conditions (NESARC) in the US, with 34,000 respondents, it was found that the most important risk factors for violence were previous violence, physical abuse, juvenile delinquency, SUD, parental crime, relationship breakdown, unemployment, and victimization [25]. All these factors have been found to be overrepresented among people with mental disorders [25, 26]. Surveys from the United States, the United Kingdom, and the Netherlands show significantly increased occurrences of physical and sexual abuse among SUD/MH patients compared to the general population [27–33]. In these surveys, it was found that between 45% and 99% of SUD/MH patients struggle with post-traumatic disorders. This is also reflected in surveys among youth with SUD/MH, where it has been found that between 50% and 90% of the youth have trauma experience [34–36].

Additionally, those who are not traumatized before they develop addiction often end up with traumas through violence, threats, and exploitation in the substance user communities [37]. Regardless of diagnoses, the combination of trauma experiences and drug use is found to be the biggest risk factor for both violence and suicide. Moreover, previous experiences of violence as a perpetrator further increase the risk. We will take a closer look at what makes trauma disorders and SUD lead to increased risk of violence.

Upbringing, Attachment, and Trauma

Those who have been exposed to traumatic stress in early childhood have more severe adverse experiences, earlier debut of substance use, more polydrug use, higher degree of substance dependence, and more treatment attempts than those who have trauma experiences from adulthood. It has also been found that childhood traumatization causes more severe disorders, with poorer mental and physical health, poorer functional level, poorer work ability, and poorer treatment results than adult traumatization [31].

There is much to suggest that mental abuse, maltreatment, and serious neglect also cause serious traumatization [29, 38–41]. Growing up with sexual, violent, or mental abuse leads to self-development and attachment that is not functional in relationship formation with real caregivers and friendly people [38]. In addition, adults who initially have established secure attachment can have this destroyed by traumatizing experiences. Especially in interpersonal traumatization in close relationships, with long-term trauma loads and repeated traumatization, ambivalent, and disorganized attachment is developed. This makes it difficult to establish safe relationships for the rest of life [42].

Drugs and Risk of Violence

Drugs provide psychoactive effects because they chemically resemble natural neurotransmitters in the brain and cross the blood–brain barrier. Different substances provide different intoxication effects depending on which neurotransmitters they structurally resemble, to what extent they cross the blood–brain barrier and to what extent they bind to the transmitter receptors in the brain. The neurotransmitters particularly involved in processes that make us experience intoxication effects are serotonin, which regulate mood and happiness and gastrointestinal activity; dopamine, which regulates mood, attention, reward, learning, and sexual satisfaction; and norepinephrine, which is involved in regulating cardiovascular activity (pulse and blood pressure), attention, and fear response. Drug use increases the prevalence of violence both in the general population and among the mentally ill, with a particularly increased risk in the patient group with SUD/MH [1]. The connection between violence and drugs is particularly linked to dopamine and serotonin. We will look a little closer at violence risk mechanisms related to specific substances.

Alcohol

Alcohol increases aggressiveness by suppressing inhibitory activity in the frontal lobe and by disrupting the cognitive capacity to regulate impulse actions and emotional reactions.

Central Stimulants

These substances are often seen in connection with impulse control failure and violent episodes. Especially in combination with alcohol, these substances seem to increase the risk of violence. The acute intoxication effect of central stimulants increases self-confidence, impairs judgment, paranoid delusions, hyperactivity, cognitive disturbances, and emotional dysregulation. Chronic use can trigger changes in both noradrenaline and serotonin levels in the limbic structures. High doses and long-term use are often seen in connection with intense psychosis symptoms, with severe delusions and hallucinations. Dose reduction in long-term use leads to prolonged deprivation of serotonergic nerve signals and gives withdrawal reactions that also lead to increased aggressiveness and impaired impulse control [1].

Cannabinoids

Cannabinoids are usually little associated with violence and aggression. However, it has been found that long-term use leads to a chronic intoxication state that leads to both anxiety, paranoia, and increased aggressiveness [43–45]. Both long-term use and withdrawal reactions from cannabis are associated with violent episodes. In recent years, new cannabis concentrates, such as "shatter," "crumble," and "wax" with 80–90% THC, have emerged. These cannabis products can be so potent that even acute cannabis intoxication can increase the risk of violence.

Synthetic Cannabinoids

Today, there are many different synthetic cannabinoids, with a large number of different chemical substances that are structurally different but have in common that they bind to the cannabinoid (anandamide) receptors in the brain. Synthetic cannabinoids are usually somewhere between 4 and 45 times as potent as natural THC, but there are also substances, such as HU-210, which are between 100 and 800 times as potent as natural THC. There have been a number of serious acute mental reactions, such as intense hallucinations, severe psychosis, violent agitation, paranoia, and suicide in connection with the intake of these substances [46].

Opioids

Opioids are best known as a sedative drug but can also lead to increased risk of violence. Particularly, withdrawal reactions have been associated with violent episodes where the user experiences pain sensitization, anxiety reactions, agitation, aggression, nausea, and sleep deprivation. There is also a clearer connection between heroin use disorder, incrimination crime, and psychosocial problems. Prescription opioids, such as tramadol and oxycontin, may also lead to severe withdrawal symptoms that can lead to aggressive behaviors [1].

Benzodiazepines

Can cause paradoxical reactions with agitation, irritability, and aggression even within therapeutic doses. Such reactions are most common with mixed substance use, in the elderly, and in patients with brain injuries. Benzodiazepines can also suppress inhibitory activity in the frontal lobe, but can also lead to aggressive reactions, such as alcohol. Aggressive withdrawal reactions have also been seen in patients with benzodiazepine addiction [1].

New Psychoactive Substances (NPS)

NPS encompasses synthetic cannabinoids, synthetic cathinones, phenethylamines, tryptamines, aminoindanes, piperazines, phencyclidine-type substances, plant-based substances, and other substances [47]. NPS can cause intense intoxication effects with violent hallucinations and extremely aggressive behavior. These are very toxic substances, with very small differences (nanograms) between intoxicating and lethal doses. There is particular concern about violence, outbursts, and overdoses related to the development of synthetic stimulants such as geranamine, mephedrone, MDPV, desoxypipaprol, synthetic cations, various imitations of sidenafil, and synthetic sedatives such as methylmetaqualone and premazepam [48].

There have been many cases of brutal violence, murder, suicide, and overdoses in connection with the use of these substances [1, 49].

Read more about drug use and addiction in Chap. 6.

Can We Predict Violence and Suicide?

As helpers, we must understand violence as phenomena with complex causes, and with a wide range of consequences [8]. Hence, we need knowledge about what both increases individuals' intrinsic risk of violence and what increases the risk of violence in particular situations. We must deal with both suicide risk assessments, violence risk investigations, and violence risk assessments.

Violence risk assessment is a structured clinical investigation to assess the danger of future violence, and how to design measures that reduce violence and promote personal growth. Violence risk assessments are also used to justify decisions about security measures, compulsory admissions, and control measures [50]. These are assessments based on structured instruments, such as HCR20V3 and V-Risk-10 (the instruments can be found at hcr-20.com and sifer.no/verktoy/v-risk-10). These instruments provide a prognosis of future risk of violence, based on client-related variables, such as previous violence, serious mental illness, substance use, personality pathology, and psychosocial factors. Violence risk assessments are done interdisciplinary and should be validated by a doctor or psychologist with specific training. A screening of individual risk factors for violence should be done by everyone with SUD/MH. This is important in the work to include measures against violence in integrated treatment of SUD/MH. It is better to work with the prevention of violent incidents, than dealing with the aftermath of such incidents. However, these violence risk assessments are based on linear risk modeling with static risk factors and therefore do not give us any basis for assessing situational or relational risk factors. Violence risk assessments thus tell little about the present danger of violence in a given here-and-now situation, where a given set of different risk factors influence each other and may lead to several possible outcomes [50, 51]. In everyday clinical life outside the hospital wards, one must always relate to violence as a present risk instead of something that may occur at some future point in time. In concrete risk situations, one must assess both individual and situation-dependent risk factors in the context of the cause factors' interactions with each other in the specific situation one is in. Then we must work with risk assessments in addition to the violence risk assessments.

Violence Risk Assessments

In outreach and domestic SUD/MH services, the staff work in patients' homes or local communities where the actual risk of violent incidents in a given here-and-now situation will consist of a multivariable mix of individual, situational, relational, and context-related risk factors, many of which are present for limited periods of time, in specific situations, or under certain circumstances. Hence, the given set of risk factors varies from different times and different situations with the same individual patient [51]. Altogether, this leads to a multivariable, reciprocal risk complex that is much less predictable than static, linear risk factors.

When one encounters violence risk in outreach services, one must weigh risk against vulnerability. In the present context, we may understand risk as an assessment of whether violent incidents may occur, what kind of consequences that may follow the incidents, and how harmful these consequences may be.

Vulnerability in this context may be understood as our ability to anticipate and reduce the risk of violent incidents before they occur, and our capacity to handle and endure violent incidents if they occur. We will look a little closer at how one can relate to this in practice. When the patient becomes insecure, scared, or triggered in a way that triggers aggression, signs of emotional affect will be present before the patient becomes aggressive. The Brøset Violence Checklist (BVC, see frenzs.org/bvc-broset-violence-checklist) provides a summary of the most typical signs of emotional reactions that can lead to aggression and is a good starting point for individual-related violence risk assessment. However, the BVC is developed for and used in hospital departments and is a linear risk assessment model. BVC lacks assessments of substance-related, situation-related, and environmental risk factors. However, we need to consider this in all patient-related work outside the ward as it is not given that we have control over the surroundings around us or the patient's substance use. Ideally, the BVC should be scored on a form, but this is both impractical and difficult in ongoing situations. The time aspect is also completely different when we work ambulatory. Inside the psychiatric wards, the patient is observed around the clock, and with active use of the BVC, one has a good insight of the patient's inner emotional pressure before meeting them. In outreach and homecare practice, no one has observed the, and we must make risk assessments quickly and before it is too late.

The degree of violence risk can never be determined exactly. Reactive violence risk will always be a result of stress exposure and impulse control and can change quickly [24]. In outreach and ambulatory practice, it will therefore be more appropriate to arrange early signs on a fluid scale as shown in Fig. 10.1.

This way of assessing violence is quick and effective in here-and-now situations and gives us immediate indications of which measures one can resort to in the situation.

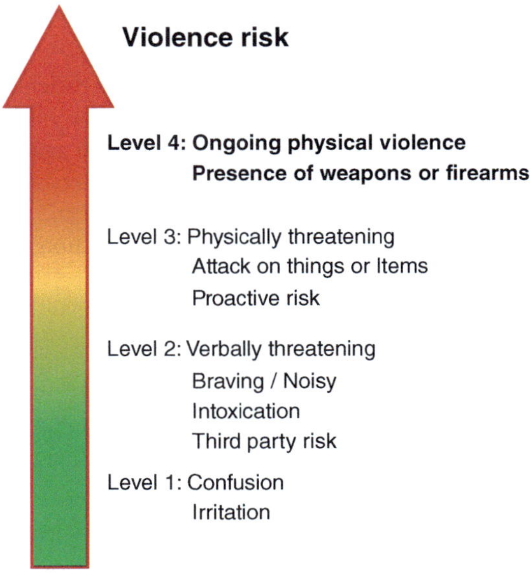

Fig. 10.1 Increasing degree of violence risk. (Figure by author)

How Can We Handle Violence Risk?

Outside hospital wards, our options for exercising physical force are restricted. Our focus must therefore be preventive and focused on breaking the escalations of situations that can end with violence, before the violence occurs. Our communication and interaction in meeting with aggressive patients can both trigger aggression and trigger violence and help patients with downregulating affect and breaking situation escalation [52]. There are many different models, variants, and descriptions of conflict-reducing communication. Here is a list of the most important principles:

- Break the situation as early as possible.
- Seek contact and promote dialogue.
- Take your time, give the patient time to calm down, give the patient space.
- Act calmly, speak slowly, and in a low voice.
- Accept and tolerate the patient's feelings, give the patient the opportunity to vent verbally.
- Do not give messages before the patient makes contact.
- Take your time with communication.
- Try to understand the patient's problem experience, and help the patient to verbalize and explain the reasons for the aggression.
- Be very careful about proximity and distance. Some patients find comfort in being close, but patients with attachment difficulties can become very insecure if you get too close. Withdraw to a safe distance in the event of escalating aggression.

- Work with a solution-oriented approach, find out how we can help, look for compromises, and highlight opportunities.
- Be clear about what you can meet the patient on, and what you cannot contribute.
- Be honest rather than making promises you cannot keep.
- Do not give messages before you have made contact with the patient.
- Do not give more instructions than necessary.
- Do not give more than one instruction at a time.
- Give the patient time to follow instructions/requirements.
- Help with carrying out instructions.
- Always give positive feedback when instructions are carried out.
- Always monitor exits and be ready to withdraw from the situation if necessary.

It is important to be honest with your own feelings. Our own feelings appear very clearly in our nonverbal expression, and we always regulate ourselves up against each other. Active regulation of our own feelings is therefore important. It is okay to be insecure yourself, and express it, but it is important to withdraw if you feel your own aggression and can't regulate it appropriately. In the early stages of an escalating outburst situation, it is important not to act authoritative and forceful as this may trigger more aggression. If the situation escalates, however, we must dare to be assertive enough. It is also important that we do not reject the patient and withdraw from a situation where the patient needs help.

Many are also very scared and vulnerable when they are aggressive and are as scared of helpers as the helpers are of the patient. Many of the SUD/MH patients have traumatic experiences with violence and abuse from the past, and also negative experiences with compulsory treatment. In addition, many are afraid of our reactions in the situation and sanctions after situations. Many have also experienced rejection from the aid apparatus in the aftermath of situations with loss of control and are afraid of losing self-control. It is also not uncommon to be traumatized by one's own violence [19]. Therefore, it is very important to maintain the patient relationship during and after such situations.

Mapping risk factors and planning safety measures in advance is crucial to work safely and securely in risk situations. A key factor in this is to meet specific risk factors with specific measures to reduce risk and create safety in the situation we are in. A safety plan that also includes factors and measures in the surroundings and situation is necessary to make quick safety assessments and avoid injuries when working with aggression-reducing measures outside controlled environments in the department. We will take a closer look at such measures.

Safety Planning

A safety plan follows the risk levels in the risk assessment and can be set up as in Table 10.1. Here, individual adjustments must be made, together with the patient.

Table 10.1 Safety plan

Level 1	«STAY&PLAY»
Meet the user with understanding, empathy, and comfort Tolerate the user's emotions. Work therapeutically with aggression-reducing communication Be careful to regulate proximity and distance to the patient Control exits Regulate your own behavior, and remember that we are also triggers Always check out the cause of confusion; this can be a symptom of serious head injuries and intoxication It is okay to continue the conversation if we can downregulate irritation and the situation is otherwise okay	
Level 2	«EXIT & WAIT»
Keep a safe distance from the patient Give clear feedback on the perceived risk Calmly advise the patient to calm down and promote dialogue Withdraw from the user, create distance, and give space Call for help from colleagues and do not be alone with the patient Give the patient the opportunity to calm down and give time Give positive feedback if the patient is able to calm down on their own Withdraw from the situation and agree to return in a while if the user does not calm down Wait until the patient has calmed down or is out of the acute effects of intoxication before re-entering the situation In the event of situational risk, ask the patient to remove risk factors themselves, give some time, and come back again later Make a new appointment with the patient Talk to the user about the situations afterward, what was the problem, what went well, and how will we solve it next time ALWAYS report the incident Implement preventive safety measures according to the department's safety plan	
Level 3	«ESCAPE & RETURN»
The patient has too high an aggression level or the situational risk is unacceptable WITHDRAW FROM THE SITUATION Call colleagues Consider whether you can change the situational conditions or secure the surroundings Request assistance from the police and provide security in the situation. If you can establish sufficient preparedness, you may consider entering the situation to try to assist the patient to calm down and resolve the situation in collaboration with the user If threats are directed at specific people, they should be removed from the situation It is important to re-establish contact with the patient, show that we do not accept violence and threats, but that we do not reject the patient after an outburst of anger Always report threats	
Level 4	«EVACUATE & EVALUATE»

(continued)

Table 10.1 (continued)

EVACUATE EVERYONE IN THE IMMEDIATE PROXIMITY
Move away from the situation (completely out of the apartment, house, area...)
Call the police and possibly an ambulance if there is a risk of personal injury
Bring injured people to safety and provide first aid if necessary
Ensure the care of all involved
Notify the unit manager
Inform the employee's relatives if necessary
Always personnel defusing, incident evaluation
Follow-up with systematic debrief in the group and individual personnel follow-up afterward
OVERDOSE/INTOX
Assess the risk of lethal intoxication, type of substance, method of administration/amount/mixed intake
Take to a doctor, if necessary, give naloxone if opiate overdose is suspected
If breathing/circulation/consciousness is affected, call an ambulance
Consider the need for detoxification

Coping Plan

The coping plan is the patient's own plan for affect management and behavior control. When working with aggressive patients, this may be a good tool for patient cooperation before one is at risk of violent incidents. An important point in this is that coping plans are to be developed in collaboration with the patient. In this collaborative process, you agree on how to deal with the patients' aggressive behaviors in advance and how to help the patient break the escalation of aggression. The coping is written with the patient's own language is used the action point descriptions. Clarification of words and expressions, and dialogue in advance, promotes predictability, cooperation, and safety in situations of aggression and prevents misunderstandings in the situation. The development of the coping plan gives the patient ownership and responsibility for resolving situations with aggression, and the patient is reassured about our role. When this is done together with the user, conflict-reducing communication has already started long before the aggression has started. This makes it much easier to get in a position to help the patient out of aggression later. See Table 10.2 for an example of an aggression management plan.

The implementation of written plans contributes to us being well prepared if we end up in a demanding situation. Through the planning process itself, we will gain insight into the need for competencies, resources, and assistance. This gives us the opportunity to acquire the resources we need, prepare for appropriate solutions, and increase our capability to handle situations before they arise. Being well prepared is crucial for handling risk situations properly. We should take with us a few important points in this:

Table 10.2 Coping plan

What is happening?	What am I experiencing?	What can I do?
I don't do what I'm asked to do I am not able to what I'm asked to do I don't ask for help I don't want to listen to an explanation I don't get what I want I don't get it the way I want it I'm not understood I don't get help I'm not allowed to do what I want I have to stop what I'm doing	I get angry I get scared I get ashamed I get frustrated I get pissed off	Explain what I'm experiencing Go outside for a short walk and calm down Ask for an explanation of a demand/message
What is happening?	What am I experiencing?	What can i do?
I can't calm down I'm still angry I'm still insecure I want to scare someone I want to break something I'm thinking about hitting someone I want to punish someone	I'm about to black out I'm angry I'm pissed off I'm scared I'm scared of myself I'm scared of you	Explain how I feel. Ask for distance and space Ask to be alone Explain how I want help to calm down
What is happening?	What am i experiencing?	What can I do?
I lose control I threaten and intimidate others I break things I attack people	I black out I'm furious I'm terrified	STOP aggressive behaviours STEP OUT of the situation Ask others to move away

- It is important that everyone who works with the patient implements the program equally.
- It is important that those who implement the program with the patient also have responsibility for, and influence on how the measures are designed.
- Patient and family involvement is crucial for the effectiveness of the measures.
- All plans must be implemented consistently and purposefully.
- Plans and measures that are not working should be terminated.

Suicide Risk Assessment

The link between suicide and SUD/MH is complex. The suicide risk for mental disorders such as bipolar disorder, schizophrenia, depression, and anxiety is elevated, the suicide risk for substance use disorders is elevated, and the suicide risk for complex disorders is even higher. In addition, comorbidity and substance use in itself increase suicide risk [2, 3, 25]. Causes of suicide are often very complex and originate from both predisposing and situational factors. Structured clinical algorithms can to some extent predict suicide risk, but there are studies suggesting that 83% of suicide deaths are unexpected or avoidable [25]. Thorough and comprehensive clinical mapping and assessment of situational risk factors are necessary to prevent suicide. Efficient treatment of the underlying disease is still the best way to prevent suicide.

Traditionally, one distinguishes between acute, dynamic risk factors and static risk factors that are weighed against protective factors in suicide risk assessments. There are no specific risk assessment algorithms designed for SUD/MH patients who are not admitted to specialist clinics. Thorough mapping of risk factors is important to arrive at good preventive measures that are effective for the person concerned. However, a large registry study has been conducted in Norway, where all suicides during and after contact with interdisciplinary specialized SUD treatment from 2009 to 2017 have been reviewed. Some of the main findings from this survey give us an indication of what may be important situational risk factors:

- The majority (43%) of the people in contact with specialized SUD/MH treatment the year before suicide died because of hanging, or strangulation, while 23% died of intoxication. In addition, there may be underreporting, especially regarding intoxications.
- A significant proportion (64%) had contact with mental health services during their last year of life.
- Over 90% of those who died within one year after contact with SUD/MH care services had had outpatient contact during the last year, but the number of contacts per patient was relatively low with a median of 6 outpatient contacts.
- A large proportion (68%) had one or more overnight stays last year: 40% in SUD services and 49% in mental healthcare services.

The admissions were mainly short-term: In SUD services, 30% of admissions were under 7 days, while 50% of admissions in mental healthcare wards were under 7 days. The majority (91%) were diagnosed with a substance use disorder last year. Of these, alcohol use disorder was the most common diagnosis (45.6%), followed by polysubstance use (27.7%) and opioid addiction (22.1%). One-third (32.9%) of the men and almost half (46.9%) of the women in the sample had been diagnosed with a depression or anxiety disorder in addition to a substance use disorder last year [2].

When we combine these findings with findings from other studies that have examined clinical risk factors in substance use populations, and what we know about impaired cognitive and inhibitory mechanisms in substance use, then the most serious risk factors for suicide in complex substance use and mental disorders can be summarized as shown in Table 10.3.

Table 10.3 The most serious risk factors for suicide in substance use and mental disorders

Dynamic risk factors	Static risk factors	Situational risk factors
• Current suicidal ideation • Current suicide plan • Preparation for suicide • Acute symptoms of mental illness • Severe psychological anxiety • Anxious rumination • Persistent insomnia • Psychosis with delusions of poverty or doom • Alcohol addiction, opiate addiction and polysubstance use • Mixed alcohol and opiate addiction • Co-occurring SUD and bipolar disorders • Unipolar affective disorders, Depression, Schizophrenia, Anxiety • Withdrawal reactions	• Family history • Unmarried status • Living alone • Lack of social support • Somatic illness • Unemployment • Fall in social or economic status • Rejection by spouse or partner	• Previous suicide attempts • Difficulty controlling anger and impulsivity • Anniversary of significant loss Diagnosed with alcohol use disorder, poly substance use disorder, or opiate addiction in the past year • Diagnosed depression or anxiety disorder in addition to substance use disorder in the past year • Little follow-up after admission in SUD/MH treatment in the past year Several short hospital admissions
Preventive factors • Reasons for living • Sobriety • Participates in support groups • Religious affiliation and/or internalized spiritual teachings against suicide • Presence of a child in the home and/or child-rearing responsibility • Intact marriage • Trusting relationship with a therapist, doctor, psychologist, or other service provider • Work • Long-term and close follow-up after admission to specialist services • Trusting therapist relationship • Had contact with mental healthcare services within the past year		

Managing Acute Suicide Risk

The most important thing initially in the acute phase of admission in psychiatric wards is to detect and handle conditions that immediately pose a threat to life and health. Acute stabilization will often be about detoxification and reducing self-destructive behavior and aggression in a ward with a level of security and competence that enables the implementation of stabilizing measures in a safe way. The overall goal in an emergency situation is to treat specific symptoms with specific measures, so that aggression and suicidal issues are quickly brought under control, in order to establish a collaborative relationship between the patient and staff as soon as possible. The further focus in acute treatment of suicide risk is directed toward treating and changing the dynamic risk factors that can be changed. In the discharge phase, it is important to develop a strategy for long-term treatment of the patient. This involves decisions about further treatment, whether the patient can be discharged, the need for follow-up, further treatment in an open or closed ward, and the need for further diagnostic investigations.

Most suicides occur within a year after treatment, often after short stays of less than a week and often when there has been little follow-up after admission. Thorough planning of discharge from the department, establishing a safety plan, and close follow-up after admission are therefore paramount in preventing suicide. After the acute follow-up phase, one must address the risk factors that take time to change. Long-term measures aimed at suicide risk should be set up as part of the patient's integrated treatment in further follow-up. It is important to involve relatives and close family in follow-up and in the safety plan. Many are familiar with crisis plans in connection with suicide prevention. A safety plan is a more specific type of crisis plan that follows its own method and is scientifically validated. Safety plans have proven to be an effective measure in preventing suicide [53].

Suicide Safety Plan

The suicide safety plan is the patient's own self-help tool just like the coping plans for violence. Safety plans must be developed early in the treatment course before discharge and should be developed in collaboration with the patients. The suicide safety plans are also built-up step by step, like the coping plan. However, in the development of the suicide safety plan, one must map a little differently. It is important that this is done together with the patient, and that the safety plans are established as the patient's own plan.

The following points should be included in the safety plan:

A—Recognize Danger Signals

Early signs, such as feelings of hopelessness, discouragement, and despair. Also, compensatory behavior, such as isolating oneself, staying in bed, increasing substance use, etc. It is important to describe specific and concrete feelings and behaviors with the patient's own words.

B—Use Internal Coping Strategies

The patient's own strategies for self-regulation and distraction. Use simple, practical measures aimed at the senses for distraction. For example, watching TV, listening to music, taking a shower, going for a walk, exercising, cooking, etc. Coping strategies are identified together with the patient. Those that are easiest to implement and work best are put at the top of the list.

C—Use External Coping Strategies

External coping strategies are aimed at contact with other people to dissolve feelings of loneliness and isolation when suicidal thoughts become intrusive. This can be to call friends/family, visit friends/family, and invite someone to visit. Here, one can also use strategies for visiting public places with other people, such as going to a café, shopping mall, cinema, gym, etc., to counteract the feeling of exclusion. It may be wise to involve relatives/friends/family in the planning.

D—Professional Helpers Who Can Be Contacted

It is important that the patient has a direct number to a therapist they trust, and who can be called if everything else fails. Here, you also include other services that the patients themselves want help with in an acute situation.

E—Limit Available Methods

Here, you discuss with the patient what can be done to remove access to aid in the local environment. These can be weapons, medications, ropes, tools, etc. It is important to remove the means that the patient has thought of, to delay impulsive actions and gain time to regain self-control. Method limitation is discussed after the coping strategies are established [53].

Quality and Leadership in Risk Practice

The best strategies for preventing both violence and suicide are to work purposefully with integrated treatment of both SUD, mental illness, violence, and suicide in a holistic process. Treatment of violence and suicide risk should therefore always be an integrated part of the treatment plans, along with measures aimed at affect management and self-regulation. Integrated treatment and recovery-oriented follow-up are described in the other chapters of this book, and need not be repeated, but we should take with us that the risk of both violence and suicide will always follow us when we work with this patient group. Follow-up of people with SUD/MH especially outside the hospital also involves working to create safe frameworks for both the users and ourselves. We will therefore look at how we can work to create safety margins at the system level in our work.

The causes of violence against health personnel in outreach and ambulatory practice have also been shown to be linked to the health personnel themselves [8], to the work environment, and to leadership [54]. Violence is always the perpetrator's responsibility, but as helpers, we should be part of the solution and not part of the problem. Understanding our role in this is therefore a key factor. A key point is that violence against health personnel can be understood as events that have occurred because we have misjudged the situation and not withdrawn in time or have failed to de-escalate the situation. It is very difficult to assess ongoing situations on the spot, and people make mistakes all the time, particularly under pressure. Understanding what influences human decision-making processes, action choices, behaviors, skills, and communication in risk situations is therefore a key factor in understanding how violent incidents occur and are prevented.

"The Swiss Cheese Model" is a well-known model for understanding risk and safety that describes four layers of safety levels, where there must be breaches through all four layers to lead to unwanted events [55]. This model can be operationalized into an understanding of risk factors and preventive measures at the system level, as shown in Table 10.4.

Management and quality improvement in the health and care sector require safety management and internal control as well. This requires a separate safety management plan aimed at managing violence risk on an organizational level. A safety management plan related to complex SUD and violence risk can be implemented if one follows up individuals where several risk factors are present, or if one has had episodes of aggression. In such situations, it can be very useful to start early by establishing plans, initiating training, and clarifying as much as possible before serious incidents occur. A safety plan on a system level may look like this (Table 10.5):

Table 10.4 Vulnerability risk

Individual risk factors in staff for risk management		
Psychological risk factors	Physical risk factors	Mental and physical limitations
Overfocusing on tasks excessive self-confidence or complacency Poor/lack of concentration Mental exhaustion Haste and lack of alertness distraction Lack of motivation Stress/time pressure	Illness Injuries Reduced or inhibited physical capacity Physical exhaustion Lack of sleep	Physically unfit for planned activity lack of self-competence for implementing measures Mentally unfit for the task Lack of insight into/recognition of own limitations Denial of own limitations medical/mental/emotional stresses SUD
Risk factors in staff communication and interaction		
Risk factors in team cooperation	Systemic risk factors in staff relations	
Lack of agreements and clarifications for activities and measures Failure to utilize available resources Lack of team leadership Misunderstandings in communication Lack of safety planning and preparation	Lack of belonging in the work environment ongoing conflicts in the work environment Weak and negative contact between colleagues Weak trust between colleagues Unclear standards for desired practice Unclear consequences for rule violations and deviations Unfamiliar with each other's expertise	

(continued)

Table 10.4 (continued)

Risk factors in team management		
Inefficient team management	Inefficient team leadership	
Lack of staff supervision and guidance Lack of information and compliance with safety recommendations and procedures Lack of control and overview Lack of ability to provide training Lack of feedback / communication Inappropriate pair / team composition	Failed error correction in safety plans Undetected risk accumulation in the patient failed or missing error correction in safety measures Lack of reporting and/or feedback on risk culture Lack of reporting of adverse events and mishaps	
Inappropriate team management	Failing team leadership	
Providing insufficient information Providing insufficient time for preparation and planning Plan not in accordance with safety procedures Lack of safety equipment control Lack of safety preparedness Lack of/errors in risk assessment Lack of plan adjustment to changes in conditions	Promote peer pressure for unsafe practices sanctions instead of guiding in case of unnecessary risk or danger Failed/ineffective enforcement of safety regulations and procedures Sanctions instead of guiding/following up/taking care of unqualified/inexperienced personnel	
Administrative and organizational influence on risk management		
Human resources (HR)	Structure	Administration
Staffing recruitment education/competence-raising/ training	Management line delegation of authority and responsibility communication Formalized clarifications of responsibilities	Activity load Time pressure Qualification requirements Objectives/evaluations Schedules
Financial management	Policies	Quality development
Excessive cost cuts Lack of income or funding	Personnel policy Hiring and firing promotions Follow-up of staff substance use Absence follow-up	Procedures Standards Map defined goals Documentation Instructions Research Knowledge and evidence anchoring

Table 10.5 Example: safety plan on system level

Goals	
1	Staff experience security in meeting with users
2	Staff experience trust, belonging, and security in the staff group
3	Staff experience clarity and predictability in the purpose of the service
4	Staff have sufficient competence to fulfill the purpose of the service
5	Staff experience clear and trustworthy management
Measures	
1	Develop safety plans A long-term treatment plan aimed at reducing the risk of violence is developed in collaboration with therapists and patients The measures in the plans are quality assured and evaluated weekly
2	Implement preventive measures Do not be alone with the patient, meet the user outside, in the office, or other arenas in controlled environments Increase follow-up and intensify treatment
3	Develop safety plan and the patient's coping plan Crisis plan is prepared and presented/discussed, and trained with the staff
4	Staff supervision The staff group is offered regular supervision Department management is offered regular supervision
5	Skill-building measures Introduce/review procedures for aggression-reducing communication and safety preparedness Implement training in physical self-defense for the staff Safety procedures are briefed/reviewed and trained with the staff group
6	Measures to promote workplace belonging Conduct weekly staff meetings Individual follow-up of employees Increase the frequency of performance appraisals Arrange social activities in the staff group

Summary

- The combination of SUD and childhood trauma provides the greatest risk for violence.
- We must be better at talking to users about violence and integrate measures to prevent violence in patient treatment.
- We must be better at planning discharges and follow up closely over time to prevent suicide.
- We must work actively to reduce violence risk all the time.
- We must work systematically and structured with safety plans and coping plans with measures that are aimed at both patients, caregivers, employees, and at the system level.

Reflection Questions

- How can you take care of the user's need for safety, security, and care when they are aggressive?
- How can you help patients tolerate and make use of the aid apparatus's measures when they are aggressive?
- How can you ensure user participation in violence prevention work?
- How can you rebuild trust in the patient relationship after violent episodes?
- How can you ensure and take care of the relatives of patients who commit violence?
- How can you rebuild the patient relationship after suicide attempts?

Recommended Literature

- Coercion and Violence in Mental Health Settings. Causes, Consequences, Management (Springer Nature, 2024).

References

1. Schifano F, Zangani C, Chiappini S, Guirguis A, Bonaccorso S, Corkery JM. Substance-use disorders and violence. In: Carpinelli B, Vita A. and Menacci C, editors. Violence and mental disorders. Cham: Springer2020. p. 95–114.
2. Walby FA, Myhre MØ, Kildahl AT. Selvmord under og etter kontakt med tverrfaglig spesialisert rusbehandling 2009 til 2017—En nasjonal registerstudie [Suicide during and after contact with interdisciplinary specialized substance abuse treatment 2009–2017—a national register study]. Oslo; 2020.
3. Hesse M, Thylstrup B, Seid AK, Skogen JC. Suicide among people treated for drug use disorders: a Danish national record-linkage study. BMC Public Health. 2020;20(1):146.
4. Randby M. Å leve med alvorlige rus-og psykiatriproblemer: På vei mot en bedre hverdag [Living with severe substance use and psychiatric problems: towards a better everyday life]. Oslo: Kommuneforlaget; 2010.
5. Chermack ST, Bonar EE, Ilgen MA, Walton MA, Cunningham RM, Booth BM, et al. Developing an integrated violence prevention for men and women in treatment for substance use disorders. J Interpers Violence. 2017;32(4):581–603.
6. Hagen I. Vold og trusler–et stort arbeidsmiljøproblem i helse-og sosialsektoren. [Violence, threats and harassment in the health and welfare sector]. Oslo: Fafo og FO; 2019.
7. The Norwegian Health Directorate. Kartlegging av vold mot helsepersonell og medpasienter IS-2618 [Mapping violence victimation in healthcare professionals and fellow patients IS-2618]. Oslo; 2017.
8. Konttila J, Pesonen HM, Kyngäs H. Violence committed against nursing staff by patients in psychiatric outpatient settings. Int J Ment Health Nurs. 2018;27(6):1592–605.
9. Hove IH. Flere pasienter og færre senger [More patients and fewer beds] Statistics Norway; 2020. Available from: https://www.ssb.no/helse/artikler-og-publikasjoner/flere-pasienter-og-faerre-senger.
10. The Norwegian Health Directorate. Nasjonalhelse-og sykehusplan [National Norwegian health and hospital plan]. Oslo: Helse-og omsorgsdepartmentet; 2019.

11. National Institute of Occupational Health. Nasjonal statistikk om arbeidsmiljø og helse [National Norwegian Statistics on work environment and health]. Oslo; 2017.
12. Hawkins D, Ghaziri ME. Violence in health care: trends and disparities, bureau of labor statistics survey data of occupational injuries and illnesses, 2011–2017. Workplace Health Safety. 2022;70(3):136–47.
13. Hallett N, Dickens GL. De-escalation of aggressive behaviour in healthcare settings: concept analysis. Int J Nurs Stud. 2017;75:10–20.
14. Pompeii L, Benavides E, Pop O, Rojas Y, Emery R, Delclos G, et al. Workplace violence in outpatient physician clinics: a systematic review. Int J Environ Res Public Health. 2020;17(18):6587.
15. Provost S, MacPhee M, Daniels MA, Naimi M, McLeod C. A realist review of violence prevention education in healthcare. Healthcare. 2021;9(3):339.
16. Engel RS, McManus HD, Herold TD. Does de-escalation training work? A systematic review and call for evidence in police use-of-force reform. Criminol Public Policy. 2020;19(3):721–59.
17. Nag T, Engen M, Eldhammer G, Svenning B. Et samlet fagmiljø står bak MAP-programmet for forebygging av vold [A united professional community support the MAP program for the prevention of violence]. Sykepleien. 2021;109(86110):86110.
18. Konttila J, Holopainen A, Pesonen HM, Kyngäs H. Occurrence of workplace violence and the psychological consequences of it among nurses working in psychiatric outpatient settings. J Psychiatr Ment Health Nurs. 2021;28(4):706–20.
19. Isdal P. Meningen med volden [Meaning of violence]. Oslo: Kommuneforlaget; 2000.
20. Elbert T, Schauer M, Moran JK. Two pedals drive the bi-cycle of violence: reactive and appetitive aggression. Curr Opin Psychol. 2018;19:135–8.
21. Halevy N. Preemptive strikes: fear, hope, and defensive aggression. J Pers Soc Psychol. 2017;112(2):224.
22. Peterson JB, Shane MS. The functional neuroanatomy and psychopharmacology of predatory and defensive aggression. In: Beyond Empiricism. Routledge; 2017. p. 107–46.
23. de Boer SF. Animal models of excessive aggression: implications for human aggression and violence. Curr Opin Psychol. 2018;19:81–7.
24. Lickley RA, Sebastian CL. The neural basis of reactive aggression and its development in adolescence. Psychol Crime Law. 2018;24(3):313–33.
25. Esang M, Ahmed S. A closer look at substance use and suicide. Am J Psychiatr Resident. 2018;13:6.
26. Elbogen EB, Johnson SC. The intricate link between violence and mental disorder: results from the National Epidemiologic Survey on Alcohol and Related Conditions. Arch Gen Psychiatry. 2009;66(2):152–61.
27. Liebschutz J, Savetsky JB, Saitz R, Horton NJ, Lloyd-Travaglini C, Samet JH. The relationship between sexual and physical abuse and substance abuse consequenses. J Subst Abus Treat. 2002;22:121–8.
28. Najavits LM, Norman SB, Kivlahan D, Kosten TR. Improving PTSD/substance abuse treatment in the VA: a survey of providers. Am J Addict. 2010;19(3):257–63.
29. Wu NS, Schairer LC, Dellor E, Grella C. Childhood trauma and health outcomes in adults with comorbid subtanceabuse and mental heath disorders. Addict Behav. 2009;35:68–71.
30. Nordfjærn T. Patients with substance use disorders: an investigation of relapse, substance use and recovery. Trondheim: Norges teknisk-naturvitenskapelige universitet; 2011.
31. Farrugia PL, Mills KL, Barrett E, Back SE, Teesson M, Baker A, et al. Childhood trauma among individuals with co-morbid substance use and post-traumatic stress disorder. Ment Health Subst Use. 2011;4(4):314–26.
32. Rosenberg L. Addressing trauma in mental health and substance use treatment. J Behav Heal Serv Res. 2011;38(4):428–31.
33. Dass-Brailsford P, Myrick AC. Psychological trauma and substance abuse: the need for an integrated approach. Trauma Violence Abuse. 2010;11(4):202–13.

34. Greenbaum PE, Prange ME, Friedman RM, Silver SE. Substance abuse prevalence and comorbidity with other psychiatric disorders among adolescents with severe emotional disturbances. J Am Acad Child Adolesc Psychiatry. 1991;30(4):575–83.
35. Greenbaum PE, Foster-Johnson L, Petrila A. Co-occurring addictive and mental disorders among adolescents: prevalence research and future directions. Am J Orthopsychiatry. 1996;66:52.
36. Rounds-Bryant JL, Kristiansen PL, Hubbard RL. Drug abuse treatment outcome study of adolescents: a comparison of client characteristics and pretreatment behaviors in three treatment modalities. Am J Drug Alcohol Abuse. 1999;25(4):573–91.
37. Øverlien C, Hauge M-I, Schultz J-H. Barn, vold og traumer: møter med unge i utsatte livssituasjoner [Children, violence and trauma: encounters with young people in vulnerable life situations]. Oslo: Universitetsforlaget; 2016.
38. Herman JL. Trauma and recovery. USA: Basic Books; 1997.
39. Nordanger D, Braarud H, Albæk M, Johansen V. Developmental trauma disorder: En løsning på barnetraumatologifeltets problem? Tidsskriftet For Norsk Psykologforening. 2011;48:1086–90.
40. Karterud S, Wilberg T, Urnes Ø. Personlighetspsykiatri [Personality psychiatry]. Oslo: Gyldendal akademisk; 2010.
41. Braarud HC. Kunnskap om små barns utvikling med tanke på kompenserende titak iverksatt av barnevernet [Knowledge of young children's development with a view to compensatory measures implemented by child welfare services]. Norges Barnevern. 2012;89(3):152–67.
42. Golier Julia ea. The relationship of borderline personality disorder to posttraumatic stress disorder and traumatic events. Am J Psychiatr onlineorg [Internet] 2003. Available from: https://ajp.psychiatryonline.org/cgi/reprint/160/11/2018.
43. Lundqvist T, Ericsson D, Jensen HJ, May J. Ud af hashmisbrug: en ambulant behandlingsmodel. 2.udgave. ed. København: Schønberg; 1999.
44. Hall W. What has research over the past two decades revealed about the adverse health effects of recreational cannabis use? Addiction. 2014;110:19.
45. Lin C-H, Chan C-H. Cannabis-induced psychosis presenting to a psychiatric emergency department: a case series. J Subst Abus. 2021:1–4.
46. AAPCC. Syntethic Marjiuana 2012. Available from: https://www.aapcc.org/alerts/synthetic-marijuana/
47. Drugs UNOo. World drug report 2024. Stylus Publishing, LLC; 2024.
48. Boyce N. Bath salts and other newer drugs: Ontario HIV and substance abuse program; 2012. Available from: https://www.slideshare.net/NickBoyce/bath-salts-and-other-newer-drugs-june-2012?qid=72ed3840-741a-4bc0-b620-e083cbf8b039&v=qf1&b=&from_search=5
49. Tamama K. Synthetic drugs of abuse. Adv Clin Chem. 2020;103:191–214.
50. Callaghan P, Grundy A. Violence risk assessment and management in mental health: a conceptual, empirical and practice critique. J Ment Health Train Educ Pract. 2018;13:3.
51. Hollnagel E, Wears RL, Braithwaite J. From Safety-I to Safety-II: a white paper. The resilient health care net: published simultaneously by the University of Southern Denmark, University of Florida, USA, and Macquarie University, Australia. 2015.
52. Lillevik OG, Øien L. Miljøterapeutisk arbeid i møte med vold og aggresjon [Therapeutic work in the face of violence and aggression]. Oslo: Gyldendal akademisk; 2014.
53. University of Oslo. Sikkerhetsplan- en metode med forebyggende effekt [Safety plan- a method for preventing suicide]. Oslo; University of Oslo; 2021. Available from: https://www.med.uio.no/klinmed/forskning/sentre/nssf/aktuelt/aktuelle-saker/2021/sikkerhetsplan%2D%2D-en-metode-med-selvmordsforebyggen.html
54. Stevenson KN, Jack SM, O'Mara L, LeGris J. Registered nurses' experiences of patient violence on acute care psychiatric inpatient units: an interpretive descriptive study. BMC Nurs. 2015;14(1):1–13.
55. Reason J. Human error. Cambridge university press; 1990.

Mental Healthcare in Prison

11

Tore Willy Lie and Lars Lien

Abstract

Inmates with co-occurring substance use disorders and mental disorders (SUD/MH) often struggle with a number of health challenges, but they often lack equal rights or access to mental health services compared to the general population. If they formally have equal rights, it might not practically be the case. Political willingness to invest in prison health care, resource prioritization, juridical regulation of substances, lack of compliance to human rights, and moral judgments are among factors that can negatively affect how this is handled in each country. This chapter explores the inmates' rights to care, barriers to adequate care, and describes an approach for integrated treatment in prison, including a proposal for a new treatment model: Integrated Prison Team.

Keywords

Forensic mental health services · Integrated Prison Team · Criminal justice system · Integrated treatment

T. W. Lie (✉)
Department of Health and Nursing Sciences and Section for Mental Health and Rehabilitation, University of Inland Norway, Elverum, Norway
e-mail: tore.lie@inn.no

L. Lien
Department of Health and Nursing Sciences and Section for Mental Health and Rehabilitation, University of Inland Norway, Elverum, Norway

Research Centre for Substance Use Disorders and Mental Illness, Innlandet Hospital Trust, Hamar, Norway
e-mail: lars.lien@inn.no

T. W. Lie, L. Lien (eds.), *Integrated Treatment of Co-occurring Substance Use and Mental Health Disorders*, https://doi.org/10.1007/978-3-032-20049-5_11

The prevalence of substance use and mental disorders (SUD/MH) among incarcerated populations is substantially higher than in the general community [1, 2]. For example, around half of the prison population with nonaffective psychosis or major depression have a comorbid SUD [2], and among people released from prison, SUD/MH is associated with an increased risk of injury [3]. Another important and specific point is women prisoners' needs that demand gender-aware care in view of their high rates of mental health problems, including their vulnerability and histories of trauma [4], and interventions aimed at preventing reoffending must take into account demonstrated gender differences [5]. Despite this and more, correctional systems are typically under-resourced, with limited staff training, support and guidance, scarce therapeutic programs, and fragmented care pathways—leaving individuals at heightened risk of self-harm, suicide, overdoses and relapse upon release [6], and more. This gap reflects not only systemic neglect but also issues in addressing SUD/MH before incarceration. Another challenge, related to the time after release, is services or personnel who feel insecure and afraid, and thereby reluctant or ambivalent to follow up someone who is considered or expected to have a high risk of violence (read about follow-up related to violence in Chap. 10), who also might be diagnosed with ICD-11 moderate or severe personality disorder, with dissocial traits. This can affect the willingness to closely cooperate or contribute to an ecosystem of parties that seem to be needed in order to help someone to a better life. Particularly challenging are inmates who are considered to be too ill to be in prison and at the same time are rejected by or transferred quickly back to prison by the specialist services (e.g., acute ward). This group of inmates has a high risk of being caught in a "nonresponsibility back-and-forth loop" between the prison and alternate ways of serving time, or being in prison without satisfactory health care. Some countries are better than others, but often there is a lack of structured transition between prisons and the community, coordination seems random and left to individual initiatives and information transfer is patchy at best.

Prison sentences should be intended to rehabilitate people with SUD/MH to a better functional level. It's a naive idea to think that the punishment itself (being incarcerated) for inmates with severe mental illness—with lack of stable social network on the outside, lack of employment or meaningful activities, lack of proper housing, and not being offered proper assessment and treatment, will make sure that many of these citizens won't have contact with the criminal justice system again or use less health services than before the incarceration.

Further, staying in prison should not be a break from comprehensive, integrated rehabilitation, neither for the convict himself nor for the health services on the outside. Instead, the correctional service comes in addition to those responsible for contributing to rehabilitation from the municipality, specialist service, and other services. The work toward a life where drugs and illness do not dominate their daily life must continue while people are in prison. If you do start working toward a drug-free life at the end of or after serving, relapse into (more severe) substance use when the serving ends is very high. In summary, in an international perspective, the need for comprehensive and integrated SUD/MH treatment in prisons is urgent.

Human Rights in Prisons

There are several international guidelines that emphasize the obligation to provide healthcare equivalent to that available in the community. These guidelines underline the importance of continuity of care upon release—that are shown to reduce recidivism, improve well-being, and support reintegration. Yet, the implementation of these principles into practice remains inconsistent and scarce, from an international perspective. Two of these guidelines are the United Nations Standard Minimum Rules for the Treatment of Prisoners (the Nelson Mandela Rules) and the European Prison Rules.

To set a global minimum standard of treatment of prisoners globally, The Nelson Mandela Rules were published in 1955, revised in 2015 [7], and adopted by the UN General Assembly. They are defined as universally agreed minimum standards for health care and many other themes in prison. The rules are only "soft law," meaning they are not legally binding. National law takes precedence. Many UN Member States have incorporated the provisions of the rules into their domestic laws or are in the process of doing so. Furthermore, the judiciary in each country may use the rules as a secondary source when adjudicating the constitutionality of national prison practices [8].

The other guideline, The European Prison Rules, was developed by the Council of Europe, set out standards on the management of prisons and the treatment of people in prison. They apply in all 47 Council of Europe countries and provide critical guidance to prison staff on how to protect and safeguard the human rights of people in prison [9]. They cover everything from basic living conditions to prison management and the rights of prisoners, where the purpose is to ensure that imprisonment respects human rights and human dignity, in line with the European Convention on Human Rights (ECHR) [10].

Clear Roles in a Regulated, Strict Context

The prison context poses some extra challenges when organizing mental healthcare services. The different roles, prison guards, and healthcare workers implicate the need for a cooperating and supporting atmosphere to optimize each role's mandate. Security and associated daily routines might need to be prioritized over health-related follow-up in certain prisons. In other cases, where there are few healthcare personnel available, prison guards with a caring attitude, but with varying or no formal mental health competency, practically end up having an added mental health worker-like role. It can be both task and role conflicting, and might wear them out, especially if there are too few people working at each shift.

Symptom Expressions

Caricatured, it is tempting to say that prisons are organized for the benefit of the largest population of inmates; healthy, tough, relatively young men born in the respective country. This involves opportunities for education, job training, physical activity, living training, sobriety, rehabilitation like programs and other activities tailored to this group. Prisons can be mentally challenging environments that require the incarcerated to draw on personal capacities, like resilience and adaptive (interpersonal) skills to cope with the context. The social dynamics between the incarcerated, where acting tough might be seen as beneficial among inmates, can hinder expression of the individuals' actual suffering. See Box 11.1 with examples about why prison can be seen as a pathogenic environment. These factors vary a lot internationally, and some countries are obviously better than others.

Box 11.1 Examples of Why Prison Can Be Seen as a Pathogenic Environment

- Overcrowding and poor conditions (stress, noise, lack of privacy)
- Poor hygiene
- Exposure to aggression from peers and staff
- Institutional coercion and discipline
- Absence of stimulation, monotonous environment
- Limited access to care

Further, types of offense can also be a normating factor between inmates, related to social exclusion or other consequences. You can be forced to socialize with strangers (whom you may not necessarily like) in common areas and activities, are deprived of freedom, experience lack of comfort, adhere to strict rules that regulate what you can or need to do when, eat "institutional food," may have a prohibition against contact with others, etc. For some, the frames in prison help them in an otherwise chaotic, unstable, and unpredictable life. For others, however, it is very stressful, where isolation in the prison cell and more is contributing to worsening the overall condition.

Sometimes, prison inmates become so sick—or desperate—that they resort to self-harm or suicide attempts. This will typically be related to the various mental difficulties that can arise. The prison services are often not equipped to care for severely ill people, and if someone is severely ill, a specialist ward is often the most suitable place. Whether a person who self-harms or threatens suicide should be in a hospital or prison is often a dilemma. If inmates are obviously seriously ill (e.g., severely depressed), they might be cared for in a hospital. On the other hand, psychiatric wards will not necessarily admit the severely ill, while the prison is not equipped to help them.

Ableness to Serve

In a country, there might be provisions that certain people cannot be punished for otherwise punishable acts. For example, this can apply to those who were underage at the time of the act, people who are severely mentally retarded (e.g., IQ < 60), and people who at the time of the act had a strongly deviant mental state. It can be questioned the usefulness of sentencing people with an IQ of around 60 and a huge lack of adaptive behavior, who are considered to be accountable for their actions and pose a danger to society, and at the same time have no or little follow up from mental health services during incarceration. Add the fact that some of them might not have a clue of why they are locked in in this context. Other relevant aspects related to ableness are severe somatic conditions, for example, cancer. Read more about somatic illness and lifestyle habits in Chap. 7. In summary, there is an obvious need to have other options than regular sentencing for several groups of incarcerated individuals with severe mental health conditions.

Assessments in Prison

Early in the incarceration, ideally on entry, there should be a mapping health status, including systematic screening of SUD/MH. When the inmate is ready for it, an assessment of SUD/MH should be conducted if it hasn't been done recently before incarceration. How comprehensive the assessment can be in each case will vary because of available resources, competency, but it should strive for an approach and content as described in Chap. 3. It might be feasibility issues related to the context or the inmate sometimes. On the other hand, imprisonment offers a unique possibility to do an assessment of what might be otherwise, from an outpatient clinic perspective, not feasible. You get more flexibility with the possible length and amount of sessions, and more time to get an alliance—depending on working conditions (capacity) for available health personnel.

The Role and Needs of Caregivers

As in other treatment and rehabilitation contexts, caregivers are an important resource for a better life during and after serving the sentence. It should be generally natural to involve caregivers in treatment plans in the same way as for people who are not in prison. Caregivers can be very important for several reasons, among them:

- Continuity of care: Caregivers can have a role in bridging the gap between prison-based treatment and community health services after release, and in different ways help to ensure that medication, therapy, and relapse-prevention plans continue outside prison. In such cases, it is important to underline that it is the services' responsibility to make sure the services work together in a proper manner.

- Emotional support: Having strong social and emotional ties reduces the risk of recidivism, relapse, and deterioration of mental health, including providing a sense of belonging and stability.
- Motivation for treatment: Family engagement can back up and stimulate the encouragement of the (formerly) incarcerated to be an active participant in their own recovery.
- Advocacy: Caregivers can advocate for appropriate treatment inside prison and help navigate complex justice and healthcare systems.
- Reintegration: Upon release, caregivers often provide housing, financial support, and structure, which are vital in reducing reoffending and relapse risk.

On the other side, the services also need to help the caregivers, related to possible negative aspects. For example, stress in terms of shame and guilt (e.g., among parents of inmates), fear (perhaps especially for children of inmates), despair and worry for the future, often for the partner of inmates. In some cases, it can be highly stressful for a caregiver who has been repeatedly exposed to physical or psychological violence by her/his partner before, when the inmate has been or is about to be released. Read more about the role of caregivers in Chap. 13.

A New Treatment Model: Integrated Prison Team

In Norway in recent years, Lars Linderoth and Tore Willy Lie (2022–2024, then representing the Norwegian National Advisory Unit on Concurrent Substance Abuse and Mental Health Disorders), along with representatives from the Directorate of the Norwegian Correctional Service and the Norwegian Health Directorate, developed an initial framework of a treatment model: Integrated Prison Team (IPT) [11]. This model can be further assessed in each country, to be eventually piloted and evaluated, depending on the official authorities' political willingness and resources to do so in each country.

The purpose of IPT is to reduce the major challenges in the community that people with severe mental disorder or SUD/MH represent, who are also in touch with the correctional services. Such teams can be a good supplement to, for example, existing FACT teams, who also include those with the greatest challenges and who represent the highest socioeconomic costs. IPT is not yet another inclusion-limited team (only for people with SUD, the elderly, high violence risk, sentenced to treatment, etc., which primarily works outreach in an open context in the community). It is a multidisciplinary team, with broad inclusion, adapted to clinical work in the prison context—with FACT (read more about FACT teams in Chap. 12) and IDDT (read more about IDDT in Chap. 2) elements. See Box 11.2 for an overview of the team composition. The full range and form of specific, relevant expertise may not be available in every team at all times or from the start, for various reasons. However, it is something expected and targeted to build on, including having a management-based plan for competence development (training, guidance) and recruitment, with ongoing optimization of the service according to, for example, an IPT fidelity scale (that needs to be developed).

Box 11.2 Team Composition in IPT

- Psychiatrist
- Psychologist
- Social worker
- Nurse/social educator
- Peer consultant (who has earlier been convicted)
- SUD specialist
- Employment specialist
- Prison officer

An ordinary FACT team (or other "hard to reach" assertive teams) cannot be regularly available to people in a physically closed and regulated context like prison. In addition, the assertive team belonging to the inmate's hometown may be far away. However, collaboration with such teams and others in individuals is an important element (before-during-after serving time). IPT can also, if feasible, contribute actively and in a committed manner for a period after release, together with other local services. This ensures better continuity, as well as closer, safer, and more mutually committed follow-up from all parties in the transition phase. Such teams can be called a kind of organizational hybrid, an integration between health/social and correctional services' responsibilities/regulations, and would thus be a formal and financial sectoral collaboration between all parties.

The target group for IPT is people with severe mental illness who have a great need for services over time, medium or high risk of recidivism (including people with low probability would be too expensive to include). They may have co-occurring SUD, somatic illness, and other difficulties. Severe mental illness is defined as in FACT, that is, not a psychosis criterion for admission. In summary, the IPT model harmonizes with several of the 2024 statements by the UNODC-WHO Informal Scientific Network, the UN Commission on Narcotic Drugs. Among them, treatment for individuals should follow a continuum of care that includes broader health and social services to strengthen success upon return into the community and drug use prevention, including children and family members of incarcerated persons [12].

Probable Gains

A team composed of several professional groups with a satisfactory vacancy rate will be able to follow up flexibly, professionally, and competently in relation to a number of challenges and needs that concern the inmates' quality of life, both during sentence, in preparation for and after release. Further, better working environment and safer prison guards (less negative stress and strain, less work-related absence and turnover), and increased cooperation and more guidance between services inside and outside the prisons. See Box 11.3 with snippets of probable gains with IPT:

Box 11.3 Probable Gains with IPT During Sentence and After Release

During sentence:

- Significant increase in fulfilled rights to health care among inmates, and better health and quality of life
- An officer employed in the team will limit personnel resource challenges related to trips out of prison (e.g, health care related trips), and will have an important "mental health worker-associated" officer role, who at the same time can be a support for other officers.
- "Outreach" in the prison, and over time attempts are made to establish an alliance with inmates who are not necessarily interested in- or very ambivalent about contact/follow-up initially (even if they have a very poor level of functioning/suffer a lot).
- The amount of potential (and time needed for) effectful follow-up will be increased per person who needs health care.
- Less use of coercion (holding, locking up/security cell, medical restraint).
- Less isolation, less suicide (attempts), self-harm and acting out.
- Less use of acute admissions in the specialist service.

After release

- Available work capacity among those who have served time.
- Less recidivism.
- Less relapses and improvement of SUD/MH.
- Better psychosocial conditions (meaningful activity, socializing).
- Limit/avoid breaks in established health service related follow-up (continuity and group dynamics, maintain common goals and responsibility).

To make this work, established support systems should be close at hand in a very vulnerable phase after release. Someone from the IPT can accompany the released individual to their hometown if necessary and feasible, and collaborate with local parties to achieve a best possible transition. In some cases, local services might be ambivalent or reluctant to follow up on an individual, based on their history (physical violence, serious threats, knowing what the person has done to others in the local community). This needs to be openly addressed between all associated service parties, in order to find common ground for proper co-operation dynamics and treatment planning.

You can read more about the IPT model here (in Norwegian, use the translation option in your web browser or other methods): https://www.integrertbehandling.no/forside/integrert-fengselsteam

Summary

- Inmates should have the same rights and access to health care as the rest of the population.

- Systematic screening of SUD/MH should be done at entry, and comprehensive assessment should be offered during the sentence (when feasible).
- The criminal justice system and healthcare services should strive for clear roles and train on how they handle and prevent difficult situations when they are present together, to make sure that the inmates get proper health care, other recovery-related follow-up and security is handled accordingly.
- Staff support and training should be provided for both healthcare personnel and prison officers, to ensure proper quality of care and prison conditions.
- When the inmates' health condition is so severe that they are not suitable to be in prison, the criminal justice system should consider alternate solutions, for example, admission to psychiatric hospital or SUD/MH institution, transfer to other ways of serving the sentence or sentence interruption.
- Rehabilitation to a dignified, law-abiding life should be the main purpose of incarceration for people with SUD/MH, no matter the type of sentencing and prisons.
- Further development and country-wise adaptation of the model Integrated Prison Team is recommended, and further piloted and evaluated.

Reflection Questions

- How can healthcare workers maintain a helper role in a prison, in co-operation with prison guards, to help the inmate make the most out of the potential for recovery during incarceration?
- What characterizes a good process between the criminal justice system and healthcare, before and after release, in order to avoid/limit relapse and recidivism, and offer proper follow-up of practical needs related to daily life and SUD/MH treatment?

Recommended Literature

- Handbook of mental health assessment and treatment in jails. Oxford: Oxford University Press; 2023.

References

1. Baranyi G, Fazel S, Langerfeldt SD, Mundt AP. The prevalence of comorbid serious mental illnesses and substance use disorders in prison populations: a systematic review and meta-analysis. Lancet Public Health. 2022;7(6):e557–68. https://doi.org/10.1016/S2468-2667(22)00093-7. PMID: 35660217; PMCID: PMC9178214.
2. Fazel S, Seewald K. Severe mental illness in 33,588 prisoners worldwide: systematic review and meta-regression analysis. Br J Psychiatry. 2012;200(5):364–73. https://doi.org/10.1192/bjp.bp.111.096370.
3. Young JT, Heffernan E, Borschmann R, Ogloff JRP, Spittal MJ, Kouyoumdjian FG, Preen DB, Butler A, Brophy L, Crilly J, Kinner SA. Dual diagnosis of mental illness and substance use disorder and injury in adults recently released from prison: a prospective cohort study.

Lancet Public Health. 2018;3(5):e237–48. https://doi.org/10.1016/S2468-2667(18)30052-5. Epub 2018 Apr 18.
4. Bartlett A, Hollins S. Challenges and mental health needs of women in prison. Br J Psychiatry. 2018;212(3):134–6. https://doi.org/10.1192/bjp.2017.42.
5. Kjelsberg E, Friestad C. Social adversities in first-time and repeat prisoners. Int J Soc Psychiatry. 2008;54(6):514–26. https://doi.org/10.1177/0020764008091406.
6. National Institute on Drug Abuse. Criminal Justice DrugFacts; 2020. Available at https://nida.nih.gov/publications/drugfacts/criminal-justice
7. United Nations Office on Drugs and Crime. The United Nations standard minimum rules for the treatment of prisoners (the Nelson Mandela Rules); 2015. https://www.unodc.org/documents/justice-and-prison-reform/Nelson_Mandela_Rules-E-ebook.pdf. Accessed 15 Aug. 2025.
8. United Nations Office on Drugs and Crime. The Nelson Mandela Rules. The History of the rules. https://www.unodc.org/unodc/en/justice-and-prison-reform/nelsonmandelaruleshistory.html. Accessed 27 Sept 2025.
9. Council of Europe. European Prison Rules Short guide; 2021. https://cdn.penalreform.org/wp-content/uploads/2021/09/PRI_Short-guide-to-the-European-Prison-Rules_WEB.pdf. Accessed 27 Sept 2025.
10. Council of Europe. European Convention on Human Rights; 2020. https://www.echr.coe.int/documents/d/echr/convention_eng. Accessed 27 Sept 2025.
11. Lie TW. Integrert fengselsteam [Integrated prison team]. https://www.integrertbehandling.no/forside/integrert-fengselsteam. Accessed 27 Sept 2025.
12. Volkow ND, Scoppetta O, Busse A, Poznyak V, Krupchanka D, Campello G, the UNODC/WHO Informal Scientific Network. Treatment of substance use disorders in prison settings: statement by the UNODC-WHO Informal Scientific Network, UN Commission on Narcotic Drugs. World Psychiatry. 2024;23(2):294–5. https://doi.org/10.1002/wps.21210.

Assertive Community Treatment (ACT and Flexible ACT)

12

Anne Landheim and Hanne Clausen

Abstract

In this chapter, we will describe the challenges faced by people with co-occurring substance use disorder and mental illness (SUD/SMI) and key guidelines from the health authorities to meet the service needs of this population. The ACT and FACT models are two service delivery models that aim to provide integrated and individually tailored services. The models will be described, including how they are adapted to the typical needs of this group. This will be followed by a presentation and discussion of research on ACT and FACT and experiences and challenges of these models for clients, in general, and for those with SUD/SMI, in particular. Finally, there will be a summary and some conclusions on the benefits of ACT and FACT.

Keywords

Flexible assertive community treatment · Assertive outreach · Integrated care · Co-occurring substance use disorder and mental illness

A. Landheim (✉)
The Research Centre for Substance Use Disorders and Mental Illness, Innlandet Hospital Trust, Hamar, Norway

Faculty of Health and Nursing Sciences and Section for Mental Health and Rehabilitation, University of Inland Norway, Elverum, Norway
e-mail: anne.signe.landheim@sykehuset-innlandet.no

H. Clausen
The Research Centre for Substance Use Disorders and Mental Illness, Innlandet Hospital Trust, Hamar, Norway

The R&D Dept. in Mental Health and Addiction Services, Akershus University Hospital, Lørenskog, Norway
e-mail: hanne.kristin.clausen@sykehuset-innlandet.no

T. W. Lie, L. Lien (eds.), *Integrated Treatment of Co-occurring Substance Use and Mental Health Disorders*, https://doi.org/10.1007/978-3-032-20049-5_12

People with substance use disorder and mental illness (SUD/SMI) often have complex problems and need services from many different providers. They are faced with an extensive system of services in both primary and specialist health care. The main challenge is often that the services do not interact and are not sufficiently coordinated. To address this problem, health authorities in many countries have invested strongly over the past decade in models designed to improve collaboration between primary and specialist health care. Assertive Community Treatment (ACT) and Flexible Assertive community Treatment (FACT), two models developed in the United States and the Netherlands, have been particularly emphasized and recommended. The main aim of these models is that the ACT/FACT team will provide most of the services, which will enable clients to experience that care and support are holistic and coordinated. To ensure this, ACT and FACT in Norway must consist of a binding collaboration between primary and specialist health care. ACT and FACT are both programs for people with severe mental disorders, often co-occurring substance use disorders, and who have extensive, complex, and long-term service needs. ACT and FACT aim to help people in the target group to live their lives in the community as well as possible. A further aim is to empower them to cope with life on the basis of their needs and wishes, and suitable care and support services are created in collaboration with clients.

People with Co-Occurring Disorders Often Have Extensive, Complex Service Needs

People with severe SUD/SMI often have substantial, complex needs. These can include problems with physical health, employment, meaningful everyday activities, accommodation and living conditions, finances, social functioning, social networks, and a sense of belonging to society and the local community. Figures from the Norwegian (5.5 million inhabitants) "Service User Plan" (BrukerPlan) show that there are around 5000–6000 people with severe co-occurring SUD/SMI who have very poor functioning in many of these areas at the same time [1, 2]. In addition, there are people with less severe disabilities, but who may also need care and support from several primary care providers and to some extent from specialist care services. The figures indicate about 13,000 people in this group. They often find it difficult to access the help and support they need and may perceive services as fragmented and inadequate. Many clients have difficulty in attending treatment and utilizing traditional care services. Poor continuity of care can be a challenge. In the literature, these individuals are often described as "hard to reach and hard to treat" [3]. This refers to clients who are difficult to engage and stay in contact with, and for whom traditional services are unable to adequately and appropriately meet their needs. The service system in Norway is insufficiently adapted to the complexity of its individual needs. Figure 12.1 is an illustration of the variety of needs and the number of services that a person with severe SUD/SMI may be involved with. The example is of a patient receiving services from an integrated care team for people with SUD/SMI.

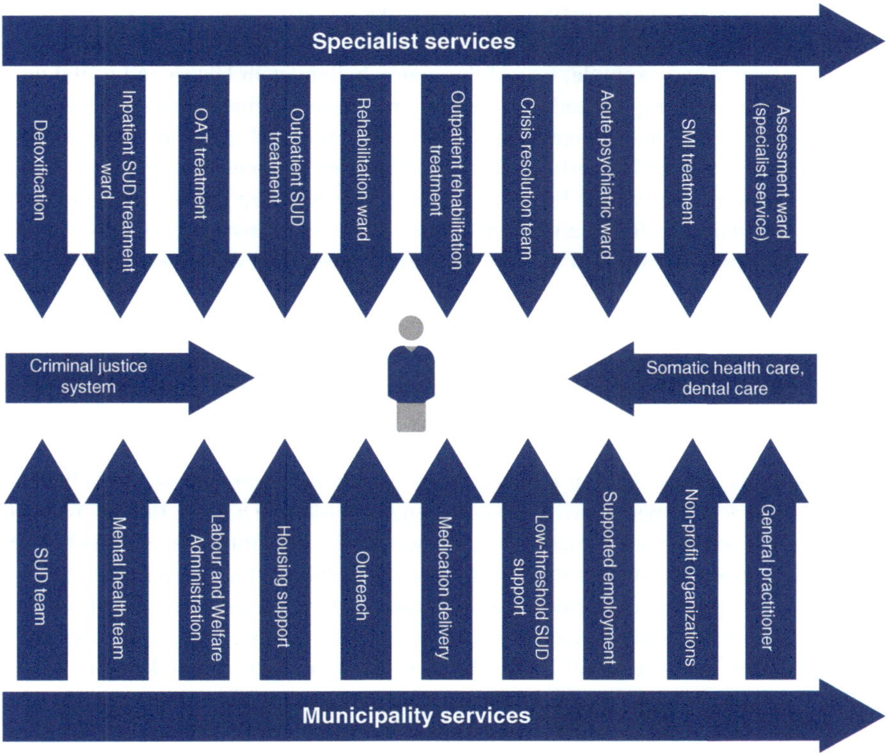

Fig. 12.1 All the services that people with SUD/SMI may be in contact with. (Based on an illustration by Bård Grønstøl)

It is not unusual to find that people with a severe substance use disorder, often in combination with severe mental illness, have physical problems and conditions, no or inadequate housing, no regular income, no paid work, and no meaningful everyday activities. Further, they may have lost contact with their parents or other relatives. With so many challenges, they will need services from a wide variety of providers. They often must coordinate the services themselves, and it can be difficult to know which service provider has the main responsibility. Is it the SUD counselor in primary care, the therapist at the department of addiction treatment, or the general practitioner? They may forget or may be unable to meet for appointments at the clinic, and they might have difficulties paying the patient contribution. There is thus a great need for holistic and coordinated services provided on the basis of a common treatment plan for clients in this target group.

A Complex and Fragmented Service System

Using Norway as an example, one of the main challenges in health and social care is the complex and fragmented service system. There are many services, and they often appear to be uncoordinated and poorly integrated [4–8]. The "coordination reform" was introduced as early as 2009, emphasizing the need for services to interact, both between and within levels of care [4]. Primary care services were to have greater responsibility for treatment and care, while specialist care was to provide services to a greater extent in clients' local environment, in collaboration with primary care. The need for collaboration and improved coordination of services within and between levels of care for people with co-occurring SUD/SMI has been emphasized in several national policy documents [5, 7, 8]. It was also pointed out in a report by the National Audit Office of Norway (2021), which argued that people with SUD/SMI did not have equal access to services and that the quality of services varied according to geographical location [9]. The National Audit Office of Norway also stated that almost 30% of municipalities do not have outreach services that can enable contact with people with co-occurring disorders. There is thus a risk that many people who do not contact services themselves will not receive the help they need [9]. A more recent report from the National Audit Office General states that 42% of municipalities responded that they did not have access to FACT/ACT, and that the programs should be expanded for people with co-occurring disorders [10]. They consider that FACT/ACT, as one of the few models adapted to this client group, appears to have insufficient capacity. This means that many clients who could benefit from such programs are unable to access them. As these government documents point out, it has been argued for several decades that there is a clear need to coordinate services for people with SUD/SMI who have complex needs. The challenges at the systemic level indicate a need for coordinated services for this client group that cover all their various needs, including outreach programs.

Measures to Provide Holistic and Coordinated Services

In order to address these challenges, the Norwegian health authorities have in recent decades encouraged various models to improve coordination between and within levels of care [4, 6–8]. The aim is to ensure that people with SUD/SMI and complex needs receive long-term, comprehensive, and coordinated health and social care. Services that are comprehensive and coordinated will clearly be better integrated. The national guideline for the assessment, treatment, and care of people with co-occurring disorders [5] contains the following recommendations:

- Treatment of co-occurring disorders should be integrated and based on an overall plan, preferably anchored in an individual plan (recommendation 38).
- Collaboration between and within levels of care should take place through formal collaboration agreements. For individual clients, the individual plan speci-

fies the collaboration. Collaboration agreements should be drawn up between the units involved in individual patients (recommendation 89).
- Outreach teams such as ACT teams with members from both primary and specialist health care should be considered for people with complex needs and poor functioning (recommendation 92).

These recommendations thus emphasize that services should be provided simultaneously and in an integrated manner, that coordination should be determined by individual plans, interdisciplinary coordination teams, and collaboration agreements and that care and treatment in the form of outreach should be considered. The aim is to avoid providing parallel services that are not coordinated. A guideline for rehabilitation, individual plans, and coordinators points out that an individual plan is a legal requirement and should be offered to all clients with complex needs [11]. This also applies to the establishment of an interdisciplinary coordination team, which must be composed of staff from different service providers and include the client. Interdisciplinary coordination teams often develope and follow up individual plans. Collaboration agreements between municipalities and regional health authorities are another means of realizing the coordination reform. The purpose of these collaboration agreements is to encourage coordination between the parties by specifying the division of tasks and responsibilities between primary and specialist healthcare services. Such an agreement must also describe effective procedures in various areas of collaboration. The agreements should help ensure that patients and clients experience coordinated services and have a clear understanding of who is responsible for delivering each type of service. Another scheme is case management, which aims to assist clients with complex needs by coordinating the various services they require [12]. According to statistics in the "Service User Plan" [1], only 14% of clients with severe co-occurring problems (substance use problems and mental health problems) and 12% of those with less severe co-occurring disorders have an individual plan. Forty percent of all clients with substance use problems have an interdisciplinary coordination team. There is thus a large proportion of the target group with neither an individual plan nor an interdisciplinary coordination team. The figures also show that the case management scheme is little used in Norway. Clients still have to deal with several different service providers, even though a case manager should be familiar with the services and coordinate them. The various service providers do not necessarily know what the others are providing, and to enable holistic and coordinated services, the providers should follow a common plan. Thus, even with the different schemes mentioned here, there is still a need for better coordination of service provision.

ACT and FACT in Norway, a national initiative

Since 2009, there has been a national focus on Assertive Community Treatment (ACT), and since 2013 on Flexible Aassertive Community Treatment (FACT). This was because the evaluation of the "Escalation Plan for Mental Health" [13] included a recognition that there was a group of people in society who fell outside the regular care and treatment system and who needed an alternative to traditional services [14]. The ACT model was familiar from the United States, and research showed that clients benefited greatly from care and treatment provided by an ACT team [3, 15–17]. In Norway, the two service models are organized as a binding collaboration between primary and specialist care, where the main aim is to provide most services on an outreach basis, using a single interdisciplinary team. An ACT or FACT team ensures that services for clients are coordinated and holistic [3, 18, 19]. These two models are primarily targeted at people with severe mental health disorders, often substance use disorders and with complex needs. There are recommendations to use ACT and FACT in several guidelines, escalation plans, and grant schemes from the Norwegian Directorate of Health [5, 8, 20]. The health authorities have encouraged the testing and establishment of ACT and FACT through a grant scheme called "People with Extensive and Complex Service Needs" [21]. In addition, the Norwegian Resource Centre for Community Mental Health (NAPHA) and the National Advisory Unit on Concurrent Substance Abuse and Mental Health Disorders (NKROP) have provided a national training program, translated and revised manuals and fidelity scales, conducted fidelity assessments, and established and managed team leader networks and regional networks for members of ACT and FACT teams.

Unlike other measures to enhance collaboration, such as interdisciplinary coordination teams, individual plans, and case management, ACT and FACT provide most services from a single team. In cases where others contribute, the team will coordinate the services and have overall responsibility for care and treatment. ACT and FACT provide services in the client's local community. These service models are thus an example of the coordination reform in practice. ACT is an evidence-based model that is highly beneficial for people with severe mental disorders, often substance use disorders, and complex needs [15]. The piloting of ACT also adhered to the recommendations for integrated care and treatment in the guideline for co-occurring disorders.

ACT and FACT in Norway is a binding collaboration between primary and specialist health care:

- There must be a collaboration agreement between primary care and the regional health authority.
- Primary and specialist healthcare services must both contribute staff and/or financial resources to the ACT/FACT team.
- With staff from both levels of care, teams will work in accordance with both the Specialist Health Services Act and the Municipal Health and Care Services Act.
- Team members will have access to medical records from both levels of care.
- Team members will be involved with both primary and specialist healthcare services.

ACT and FACT two Service Models for Integrated Care

Assertive Community Treatment (ACT) was developed in the United States in the early 1970s and was aimed at people with severe mental disorders, primarily psychosis. Flexible Assertive Community Treatment (FACT) is a version of ACT developed in the Netherlands, mainly based on practical experience with the ACT model [18, 19]. The FACT model aims to provide services to an expanded target group, that is, people with a wider variety of severe mental illnesses, such as severe anxiety and depression or severe personality disorder, and is thus not restricted to those with psychotic disorders or severe bipolar disorder. Both programs are designed to provide outreach-based, simultaneous, and holistic services to people with severe mental illness, often substance use disorders/problems, and complex needs, who do not benefit from traditional services. ACT and FACT will provide outreach-based, simultaneous, and holistic services to people with severe mental illness, often combined with substance use problems/disorders.

Assertive Community Treatment (ACT)

An important goal when establishing ACT was to enable people who had spent many years in psychiatric institutions to live their lives in the community instead of in an institution. The model was originally called "Training in Community Living," and its primary aim was to enhance people's ability to thrive in their local communities by supporting independent living [3]. Here, it was important to focus on more than medication to treat symptoms, as many of these people had poor social and practical functioning, they lacked work, meaningful activities and a social network, and they generally lived on the margins of society. ACT teams were designed to support clients in various ways based on their needs and problems, such as in housing, finances, paid work, meaningful activities, the creation or maintenance of a social network, contact with their family, and a sense of belonging to the local community. An important principle was that support should be provided in the form of *outreach* to where clients lived their lives, in their home and their local community. Furthermore, therapists in the ACT team should have an *active, assertive approach*, using a variety of methods to try to establish contact with people who did not necessarily want help and support. By offering care and treatment locally and using methods to establish contact and build relationships, the desired therapeutic relationship could be achieved. An important point was that contact with a client would be continuous, even during admissions and inpatient treatment [22]. A key aspect of the ACT model is the intensive support and care provided to clients. People in the target group are expected to need an average of three or more direct contacts each week [23]. Stein and Test [3] described the importance of a team approach and shared caseload. ACT team members should have in-depth knowledge of each client and address the client's various needs through an interdisciplinary team approach. The whiteboard method should be used to ensure that all team members were familiar with each client and that the team worked in an interdisciplinary manner. Further, ACT teams should use the recommended evidence-based methods for the target group, including psychotherapy, support work, or integrated dual disorder treatment. Since the 1970s, the ACT model has evolved, particularly through updating the evidence-based methods used. Among the programs included in ACT are "individual placement and support," "housing first," and "integrated dual disorder treatment." There has also been an increased focus on the recovery perspective, and it is emphasized that the care and treatment provided by the ACT team should be based on the client's resources, wishes, and goals [24].

An ACT team primarily targets hard-to-reach people with psychotic disorders, often with substance use problems, who have had many long-term treatment programs in traditional mental health care, often involving coercion, but do not benefit from the usual care and treatment options [25]. ACT clients will need intensive support for a long period of time. It has been suggested that about 1% of the Norwegian population needs the services of an ACT team. With a maximum of 100 clients per team, a catchment area of at least 100,000 inhabitants is required [24]. The recommended caseload (ratio of staff to clients) in an ACT team is 1:10.

Flexible Assertive Community Treatment (FACT)

As mentioned, the FACT model is largely based on the ACT model [18, 19]. These models were established due to the realization in the Netherlands that services outside psychiatric hospitals were inadequate for people with severe mental disorders. Case management had been tried but was found to be inadequate and unsustainable [26]. People with SUD/SMI benefited little from traditional services, and many were homeless or in prison. There was a great need for community-based mental health care, and in the early 2000s ACT teams were established to reach the most unstable and vulnerable people. Following the experience with ACT, some adaptations were made for the Dutch context. The ACT model was not well suited to areas with low population density, but by expanding the target group, teams could also be established in more thinly populated areas. There was also a need to provide community-based mental health care from a single team to more people than those with psychosis. The target group was therefore expanded to include people with severe mental health disorders apart from psychosis. Further, variation was found in client needs for long-term intensive services; not all clients needed the typical intensity of ACT. During stable periods, clients needed less intensive care and treatment, which would then be provided by the case manager in the team. Conversely, during periods when clients needed intensive services, for example, relapses or crises, the full team provided the care and treatment. The term "flexible" in FACT indicates the difference between the two models and is a core quality of FACT. In brief, flexibility in FACT can be described as serving a broader target group than in ACT and involving variation in the intensity of care and treatment depending on the needs of the individual client. Apart from this, FACT is based on the same principles as the ACT model. A local FACT team will support 100 people in a region with 40,000–50,000 inhabitants, where one therapist will have the main responsibility for a maximum of 10 clients. For further information, see the Norwegian description of the FACT model [27].

Common Features of ACT and FACT

Table 12.1 presents an overview of the aims and principles of ACT and FACT. Each model has its own fidelity scale. The scales are used to assess the organization and operation of the teams and the content of the care and treatment [23, 28]. Both models have a common set of values based on a recovery approach. This implies that clients should participate actively in their recovery process, and the role of the team is to provide support to enable them to live a better life in accordance with their wishes. Empowerment is a key concept that involves providing care and treatment in line with each client's resources, wishes, and needs. In this approach, the services provided must cover a variety of needs. The aim is for clients to live as well as possible with the problems they have. A further key feature of both models is that clients are involved in designing their own treatment plan [26].

In Table 12.2, we describe the most important elements of the ACT and FACT models in terms of the organization and content of care and treatment.

Care and treatment provided by an ACT or FACT team should be evidence-based and adapted to the target group for each model. National guidelines are also used as a basis for care and treatment. ACT and FACT clients have complex needs, and the evidence-based methods used must be related to these needs. Clients may need help to find work or integrated treatment of their SUD/MH; they may need psychotherapy, help with family members and social networks, and support in many other areas. Regarding the content of the ACT and FACT models, the main evidence-based methods recommended are summarized in the points below:

- *Integrated treatment of SUD/SMI ("integrated dual disorder treatment" or IDDT)*

This implies simultaneous and integrated assessment and treatment of the SUD/SMI. See the next page for further details.

- *Work rehabilitation based on the individual placement and support model (IPS)* IPS is the most evidence-based and successful model to enable people with severe mental illness, with or without substance use disorders, to find regular

Table 12.1 Aims and principles of ACT and FACT

The aims of ACT and FACT: To strengthen the client's ability to live as well as possible in society To enhance the client's quality of life To improve the client's functioning To decrease the number of days the client needs to spend in inpatient mental health care and the number of long-term hospitalizations To decrease the number of involuntary admissions and inpatient days in mental health care	ACT and FACT will provide integrated care and treatment by: Ensuring that clients receive holistic services (to meet their various needs) Ensuring that services are provided in a consistent and coordinated manner based on a common treatment plan

Table 12.2 Core areas of the organization of ACT and FACT teams

The team provides services in the form of outreach in the local community, in clients' homes or in areas of society where clients want to succeed.
The team provides services round the clock, seven days a week. The aim is to deal with any crises that may arise, and to support clients in various ways in the afternoons, evenings, and weekends. Leisure activities often take place in the afternoons and evenings, and many clients also need support in such situations.
The team is interdisciplinary and consists of a mental health nurse, a social worker, a social educator, a psychologist, and a psychiatrist. The team should also include a vocational specialist, a substance abuse specialist, and a peer specialist. The interdisciplinary nature of the team ensures that clients receive the services they need. The FACT team must also include a case manager who provides care and support to clients during periods when they do not need intensive service provision.
The team provides integrated and practical support. It provides comprehensive care and treatment and individual support based on clients' needs and wishes. This may include leisure activities, contact with other service providers, physical health care, help with finances and social security payments, support in the home, at work and in meaningful activities, and contact with the client's family, social network, and neighborhood to provide a sense of belonging in the local community, in addition to medication and psychotherapy.
In principle, all services are provided by one team. Instead of having to deal with several agencies, clients receive almost all the services and help they need from the team.
The team functions as a team, not as individual therapists. All the team members know and provide care to all clients needing intensive support. The whiteboard method helps to ensure the implementation of the team approach. All clients who need intensive services from the team are listed on the whiteboard. The team starts the day with a whiteboard meeting where the members review the status of each client and the support the client will receive from the team during the week. In FACT, clients who are not on the whiteboard (FACT board) are followed up by the case manager, who keeps the other team members informed and involves them as necessary. The case manager also involves and coordinates services outside the team. Treatment plans for clients are also presented and decided upon by the team.

paid employment [29, 30]. The aim of IPS is to help clients to find regular paid work as soon as possible after being accepted for ACT or FACT. This should be work that the client wants to do, and the IPS consultant or the team provides long-term support, including guidance and assistance at the workplace. Several ACT and FACT teams include an IPS consultant. Read more about IPS in Chap. 5.

- *Evidence-based psychotherapy*

The team provides individual or group psychotherapy based on clients' needs, goals, and treatment plans. Recommended methods are cognitive behavioral therapy, metacognitive behavioral therapy, and dialectical behavioral therapy.

- *Psychoeducation for the client*

Team members teach clients about various forms of SUD/SMI. They initiate a dialogue about problem-solving strategies, relapse prevention, and involvement of family members. In some cases, group psychoeducation is provided (exchange of knowledge and experience).

- *Psychoeducation for family members of clients*

The team members inform family members about SUD/SMI where applicable. They provide advice and guidance on the role of family members and on how they can handle difficult situations. They also provide information about support groups that family members can contact. In some cases, the team will offer group psychoeducation (exchange of knowledge and experience) and follow the family psychoeducation model (single-family or multifamily groups).

- *Physical health care*

The team should be aware of clients' physical health, facilitate annual check-ups, and offer physical health screening. The team also ensures that clients attend appointments and treatment for physical illnesses.

- *Medication treatment (psychotropic medication)*

The team ensures that clients are given psychotropic medication in accordance with recommendations in guidelines. It also provides information about the recommended use of different medications and their effects and side effects. Clients should participate in decisions on medication. The team also systematically records and monitors clients' symptoms, side effects, and interactions between medications [23, 31].

Integrated Treatment of SUD/SMI (IDDT)

Integrated treatment of SUD/SMIs must be based on the principles of the integrated dual disorder treatment (IDDT) model. This implies that the two conditions must be considered together, and that treatment and interventions must be stage-based and based on the client's motivation to change. In some cases, the goal of the treatment will be harm reduction, while in other cases it will be to achieve abstinence from substances. Treatment of SUD/SMI must be integrated and phase specific. The main elements are as follows:

1. A systematic and comprehensive assessment of the interaction between a client's substance use and mental health symptoms.
2. To identify, monitor, and document the phase of the change process a client is in, and use this knowledge to determine the appropriate treatment.
3. To be proactive and use motivational interviewing.
4. To use cognitive behavioral therapy to prevent relapse.
5. Interventions and treatment should be adapted to the phases of the change process.

There should be one or two substance abuse specialists in an ACT or FACT team. Their role in the team is to be aware of substance use issues, be familiar with evidence-based methods of treatment and care, and supervise the other team members on IDDT. They should also coordinate services from external providers according to the individual client's needs. Read more about IDDT in Chap. 2.

A Typical Working Day for a FACT Team

We have flexible working hours and our first team meeting is a whiteboard (FACT board) meeting at 8.30. Telephone calls are answered between 8 and 3, Monday to Friday. Some team members like to start the day early by writing in client records or doing other paperwork, while others come to the meeting at 8.30.

It is now 8.30, and we are all here together with our coffee and tea for today's whiteboard meeting. The moderator welcomes us all and asks if anyone has any matters to raise after the meeting. The peer support worker and the vocational specialist have one item for discussion and one information item. The moderator then asks if there are any more clients to put on the whiteboard. Today, there are none and the meeting begins. We are given a brief status report on the clients already on the whiteboard. We decide on new actions and check that they fit the targets for the "whiteboard period." Risk assessments are made as to whether it is safe to visit clients alone. We then decide who will go on home visits. Cars are allocated to those who need them.

After the review of the clients on the whiteboard, it is time to discuss problems or any other matters relevant to the team. The lived experience consultant says that she is not yet in a position to help Steffen in his home. His flat is dirty and untidy. There are also holes in the cupboard door in the kitchen and piles of bags of rubbish. Steffen said he would tidy up ready for the next visit from FACT, but nothing has changed. We reflect on this and share our experiences. The consultant wants to take a nurse with her to assess whether Steffen's symptoms have increased and whether he may need more intensive support. We also conclude that we need to contact the caretaker as there is damage to the flat. Perhaps there will be a new client on the whiteboard tomorrow. The vocational specialist informs us that she will be on a course on Wednesday. If there are any cases that cannot wait until Friday, we can contact one of her colleagues at the Labour and Welfare Administration for assistance. She will send us an email with the contact details.

At 9.30, only the team leader and a case manager (Tone, a nurse) are left in the office. The others are on their way out for appointments and home visits. Tone has a meeting in the interdisciplinary coordination team at 10. The client will arrive before then to have an injection and the observation time will be included in the meeting.

We have lunch at 11.30. During lunch, we try to give ourselves 20 min without any talk about work. It is good for us to talk to each other about everyday things that are unrelated to our FACT work. After 20 min, we are allowed to bring up problems or work-related matters. The leader emphasizes to the team members that they should, as far as possible, prioritize coming in for lunch.

At 12.15, the team members are on their way out again to meet clients. The leader gets a phone call from the housing service asking us to join an emergency call to the flat of a FACT client. A disturbance has been reported and bags of rubbish have been thrown out of a window on the third floor. There are probably several people in the flat and loud music can be heard from the street. The leader contacts the client's case manager and asks him to make an appointment to visit the flat with the housing service. This is a high-priority task, and planned visits have to be postponed or canceled.

Several FACT clients live in 24-hour staffed housing. FACT is responsible for coordination with the housing facility, and clients' individual plans explain which areas

FACT is in charge of, and which responsibilities and support belong to the housing facility. Today, a case manager and lived experience consultant will provide guidance to the staff of a housing facility.

The father of a client comes in and is dissatisfied with the help his daughter is receiving. The team leader sits down and listens.

We have received a message from the hospital about a patient ready for discharge, and the leader replies.

A case manager works on a treatment plan and updates a coping plan with a patient. These plans will be reviewed at a treatment meeting next week.

A client comes in to borrow a phone to call his lawyer.

A psychologist has individual counseling with the lived experience consultant.

A psychologist has a meeting in town with a client receiving exposure therapy.

It is now almost 3 o'clock, and the office is filling up again with team members. Some go and sit in the meeting room to talk to a colleague about an unpleasant home visit where a despairing client shouted insults. Others are writing in their client records and answering emails.

The team leader receives a call from a case manager who is on his way to the emergency ward with a suicidal client who needs to be assessed by a doctor. The case manager decides that there is no need for two team members and says that he will be able to continue working after office hours.

Text: Dagrunn Sømme, FACT Sandnes

International Research on ACT and FACT

International Research on the ACT Model

The assertive community treatment (ACT) model has been documented as a beneficial and cost-effective way of organizing outreach services to enable the most severely mentally ill to live outside psychiatric institutions [3, 25]. A systematic Cochrane review shows that intensive case management including ACT compared to standard treatment reduces the number of inpatient days and results in a higher score on the social functioning scale of the Global Assessment of Functioning (GAF), greater patient satisfaction, a higher proportion who make and maintain contact with services/the team, and a better living situation. The higher the model fidelity, the better the outcome in terms of reducing the number of inpatient days [15]. In the review mentioned above, people with co-occurring substance use disorders are also included (around 40%). Patients with and without substance use disorders were not compared in the review. The authors recommend that ACT should be targeted at patients with frequent and prolonged hospitalizations for mental health disorders and those who have a high need for services but are difficult to engage through traditional mental health care. The ACT model has been expanded to include people with SUD/SMI [32, 33].

Studies of ACT and related models of intensive case management in Europe (particularly the United Kingdom and the Netherlands) have not all shown similar results to those from the United States and Australia [34–37]. There are various explanations as to how this can be understood. It may be due to different patient samples, varying degrees of fidelity to the ACT model, or the fact that mental health care in European countries has become largely based on outpatient care and partly on outreach psychosis teams (community mental health teams), which involved less change when ACT teams were introduced [38–40]. Based on current knowledge of ACT, we can conclude that the model shows good evidence of successful treatment for people with severe mental disorders, although there is some variation, particularly from European studies. Questions have been raised about which elements of the ACT model are most effective [41]. Tom Burns conducted a meta-analysis of 64 randomized controlled trials of ACT teams where the outcome measure was a reduction in admissions and in days spent in inpatient mental health care [41]. The results of this meta-analysis show that model fidelity (total score) is important in reducing admissions and days spent in inpatient care. Burns also showed that organizational elements of the model, such as an interdisciplinary approach, outreach activities, and regular contact with clients, had an impact on outcomes. However, the intensity of service provision and the use of highly specialized teams had no effect on the outcome. Burns argues that the organizational elements of ACT are the most important aspects [41].

Few studies have been conducted researching the *benefits and effects of ACT for people with a substance use problems or disorder in addition to severe mental illness*. A systematic review from 2023 examined substance use among people receiving ACT [42]. The review included 23 studies published up to April 2021, both randomized controlled trials and cohort studies. It revealed little or no change in substance use or in the proportion of people with substance use problems during ACT, but there appeared to be an improvement related to the stage of change in the treatment.

There have also been three systematic reviews focusing on other outcome measures. These reviews partly overlap [43–45]. The most recent review from 2019 included 11 studies using a randomized controlled trial design and showed the following results for people with SUD/MH receiving treatment and care from an ACT team [43]:

- Higher treatment engagement in ACT in four data sets.
- Higher number of contacts with ACT services in one data set.
- A greater reduction in substance use in four studies, and one study found that this was associated with higher fidelity to the ACT model.
- Two studies found a reduction in admissions, while one study found fewer admissions in the control group. A reduction in admissions and inpatient days appeared to be associated with higher ACT fidelity.
- This systematic review [43] included studies up to 2017. Individual studies conducted since then show similar results, particularly regarding treatment engagement and frequency of contact with clients [46, 47].
- Overall, the studies reviewed above show that treatment and care provided by ACT teams is a promising approach for people with severe SUD/SMHI.

International Research on the FACT Model

Some research has been conducted on the FACT model with regard to the effectiveness for clients [48–58], mostly observational or pre-post studies. All of these studies except one show a reduction in admissions and inpatient days in mental health care, while one study only shows a reduction in inpatient days following both voluntary and involuntary admission [48, 50–52, 59]. A recent study from Denmark comparing results from FACT with clients receiving care from municipal mental health teams also shows a decrease in mental health admissions, but no decrease was found in the number of inpatient days following voluntary or involuntary admission [55]. Several of the studies also showed that FACT clients had better quality of life, psychosocial functioning, and empowerment [48, 50, 56, 58]. A study from Denmark that compared different outcome measures between FACT and ACT clients one year from baseline showed that the FACT clients had lower personal and social functioning [57]. It is important to point out that these 11 studies had different designs and target groups, and observation periods of different lengths. In the studies with a control group, this often consisted of patients receiving different types of care and treatment. There is thus a limited evidence base for the effectiveness of FACT, although most studies show a reduction in the number of admissions and inpatient days and an improvement in clients' quality of life and social functioning. The research described above does not compare clients with and without co-occurring substance use disorders. It is important to note that this group is also represented in the FACT programs included in the studies mentioned here.

What Does Research Show About of ACT and FACT in Norway?

In connection with the piloting of ACT and later FACT in Norway, a research based evaluation was conducted of the first 12 ACT teams and the first 7 FACT teams [60, 61]. The results presented here are taken from the two final reports, which were mainly written by the authors of this chapter [60, 61]. We will also refer to findings from articles based on data from the evaluation of the Norwegian ACT teams [62–77], and of the first FACT teams in Norway [59, 78–80].

Research on ACT in Norway

The evaluation of the first 12 ACT teams showed that they had succeeded in implementing many of the core elements of the model, and that the use of ACT in Norway could be justified. The Norwegian teams were largely organized in accordance with the main principles of the ACT model. The teams had a community-based outreach approach, were interdisciplinary, and functioned as a team. They provided a wide variety of services, such as psychotherapy medication administration, planning of treatment or interventions, various types of practical help with housework and accommodation, psychotherapy, family counseling, activities to improve social contact, and training in social or practical skills. The teams also interacted with other services in meetings and accompanied clients to relevant services. All teams were organized as a binding collaboration between primary care and a specialized mental health center. However, none of the Norwegian ACT teams were available 24 hours a day, 7 days a week. They mainly kept regular office hours on weekdays. Responsibility for dealing with crises thus fell on the usual crisis and emergency services, which meant that the teams had low model fidelity in this area. With regard to the use of evidence-based methods, the teams used elements of IDDT and most of them included a substance abuse specialist. The individual placement and support (IPS) model was rarely used, and many of the teams found it difficult to collaborate with the Labour and Welfare Administration. Strengthening clients' recovery and self-determination was implemented to a moderate extent. The teams demonstrated potential in creating treatment plans for each client and encouraging clients to participate in the process [61].

Key Results of the Evaluation

- Based on the ACT teams' catchment areas and estimated figures for the target group, the teams recruited people with severe mental disorders who generally did not benefit traditional services. Around 60% of clients also had substance use disorders.
- The ACT teams were able to reach clients that traditional service providers had previously found hard to reach. They were also able to maintain contact and provide long-term, continuous care and treatment.
- After 2 years of treatment and care from ACT teams, clients showed improvements in several important areas of their lives. Their housing conditions had improved, several had a stable income in the form of disability benefits and more were in employment programs and education. However, there were few clients in regular jobs.
- Clients' symptoms and functioning showed improvement, and there was a trend towards better overall quality of life. Clients were also more satisfied with their

housing and living conditions after receiving ACT for 2 years and showed greater treatment engagement.

- Clients who had received ACT for 2 years had a 50% reduction in mental health inpatient days following voluntary and involuntary admission, compared to the 2-year period before ACT. They were admitted just as often as before, but for shorter periods. The reduction in inpatient days was considerably greater than the national change.
- People with SUD/SMI had fewer inpatient days following involuntary admission, despite ongoing problematic substance use. However, clients without substance use problems showed no change in this area.
- Clients with SUD/SMI showed the same changes as those without substance use problems. The substance use group was less satisfied with life both before and after becoming an ACT client.
- ACT clients who had substance use problems at baseline showed no significant change in substance use after receiving ACT for 2 years. However, despite continued problematic substance use, they improved in the areas mentioned above. Most of the clients with substance use problems received integrated treatment (IDDT).

Clients described ACT as better than previous treatment. They felt that their health had improved after coming into contact with the ACT team. They were generally more satisfied with the help they received from the ACT team than clients receiving traditional services in Norway and ACT clients in several other countries [66]. They emphasized their good relationship with their main therapist and were highly satisfied with the specific working methods in ACT. They placed particular emphasis on meeting staff at home or outdoors rather than in the health service, relating to several team members rather than a single therapist, and receiving all or most services from one team instead of having to seek help from various service providers	*Family members* of ACT clients were generally satisfied with the ACT teams' efforts to help the client and themselves. They were satisfied with the extent of support, with the way the team visited clients at home or where they were, and with the fact that several team members provided care and support. They felt that ACT teams showed much more openness in areas of importance to them than they had experienced in other mental health services. Family members' experience of co-operation and shared responsibility was also better with ACT teams than with other health care services [81]

The research group concluded that the piloting of ACT teams in Norway was successful and that the model should be extended to other regions of the country [61]. However, several questions were raised in connection with the piloting and evaluation of ACT teams in Norway. Firstly, primary care providers felt that the target group of the ACT teams was too narrow, and that there were people in the community who needed a collaborative care team but did not receive one. Secondly, it emerged that the ACT teams, which were meant to provide holistic integrated services, did so to varying degrees. Clients were still receiving primary care services, and it was sometimes unclear who should provide which services to a particular client. Thirdly, ACT requires large catchment areas of at least 100,000 inhabitants.

Many municipalities have a much smaller population, and it was questioned how widespread the ACT model could become in Norway. FACT teams were then established in response to some of these questions. The rationale for establishing FACT teams was that they would reach more people with severe mental illness, including those who needed less intensive care and treatment than ACT clients. Further, the model could be used in a smaller catchment area and was therefore better adapted to the Norwegian context. FACT teams are not intended to replace ACT teams, and in large catchment areas there may be a need for both models.

Research on FACT in Norway

The evaluation of the first seven FACT teams in Norway showed that the teams were successful in implementing many of the core elements of the model. The FACT teams were largely outreach-based, providing integrated and practical care and treatment. The teams were interdisciplinary, cooperated on support for individual clients and shared responsibility for their clients. The teams were organized in different ways, but all teams had members with experience from primary and specialist healthcare services. This enabled clients to receive both health care and social care. Areas for improvement for the FACT teams were similar to those for the ACT teams; they included a lack of 24-hour availability, a lack of full responsibility for crisis and emergency services, and insufficient client involvement in treatment plans in many cases. The team approach and more intensive care and treatment had room for improvement in relation to the requirements of the FACT model [60].

Key Results of the Evaluation

- The target group for FACT teams in urban areas was mainly people with psychotic disorders. FACT teams in less densely populated areas had a broader target group.
- People with SUD/SMI were well represented in FACT at between 25 and 100% of clients.
- The FACT teams were able to maintain contact with their clients and ensured continuity of care and treatment.
- Partners of the FACT teams, particularly from primary care, called on the teams to expand their target group. This was particularly relevant for people with substance use problems, poor functioning, and complex needs.
- Clients showed improvement in various areas of their lives 2 years after treatment and care provided by the teams. Those with SUD/SMI achieved the same positive changes (unpublished data).
- No decrease was seen in the number of *admissions* to inpatient mental health care after 2 years of receiving FACT compared to the 2 years before FACT. However, there was a decrease in the number of involuntary admissions.
- The total number of *inpatient days* in mental health care decreased by 34% 2 years from baseline compared to the previous 2 years.

- The number of inpatient days following involuntary admission fell by 43% after 2 years of receiving FACT. The sharp decline in inpatient days, in general, and in involuntary treatment, in particular, differs from national figures for the same period [59, 82].
- There was a 33% reduction in costs of the total number of inpatient days in the 2-year period after baseline, compared with the 2-year period before baseline, while the costs of inpatient days in involuntary treatment decreased by 42% [59].

Client Experiences of FACT

Clients were satisfied with the quality and extent of the services they received from the FACT team. They were satisfied with the interdisciplinary and outreach approach, and they did not feel that the team had been too pushy or intrusive. Many clients emphasized positive, long-lasting relationships with team members. Areas for improvement pointed out by clients were information provision, participation in decisions on medication, and access to medical records. The majority would return to FACT if they needed support again and would recommend FACT to a friend who needed similar care and support [83].

> It's really great that they come to my home. Then I don't have to go anywhere. It's easier to find solutions to problems when I'm in my own surroundings.
>
> *(FACT client)* [60]

> I feel that they take me seriously. They believe in me: they make me responsible for looking after myself.
>
> *(FACT client)* [60]

Family Members' Experiences of FACT

Family members of clients were satisfied with the care and support provided by the FACT teams and emphasized that this way of organizing services *had to* continue. They found it particularly important that they could call the FACT team and discuss problems and share responsibility with them. They felt that the FACT team was more accessible and provided more comprehensive care with greater continuity. FACT had a positive impact on their safety and health. Family members pointed out that they would like more information about the team's role and responsibilities. They also wanted more training and support for their role as family members, particularly how to deal with challenging situations. Several family members wanted the team to have longer opening hours to enable them to help in crisis situations. Further, they expressed a desire and need for better coordination and easier transitions between different providers, especially in a crisis [84].

> Now at least we have somewhere to contact, and we think that makes things much easier. First of all, we trust each other, and we don't have to repeat ourselves. (…) We get to the point faster, they know what it's all about.
>
> *(Father of client)* [60].

Summary

The results of the evaluation showed that FACT provided useful services to people in the target group, in comparison with the services they had received previously. The goal of providing more comprehensive and coordinated services (IDDT) had been largely achieved. The FACT teams appeared to provide multidisciplinary services based on client needs and many of the services were provided by the team itself. However, there are some services that FACT teams cannot provide, such as Labour and Welfare Administration services (employment, benefits), and some primary care services such as providing housing and extensive support in the client's home. Physical health care must also be offered by other providers, and here the general practitioner is an important partner. In order to provide integrated care, FACT teams need to know which services are provided by other agencies, they need to coordinate their work with these and accompany clients to other service providers as necessary. This implies that the teams also function as a case manager. To enable teams to have in-depth knowledge of the other services their clients are receiving, they need access to medical record systems and communication systems in primary and specialist healthcare services. However, they do not always have access, which makes it more difficult to see the whole picture. They can therefore only partly fulfill their intended role as coordinators. However, the team members did report that they were generally familiar with most of the services of other providers and that they had a coordinating role. Further, a key aim of integrated services is to prevent clients from receiving competing services or the same type of services from the FACT team as they receive elsewhere, such as primary mental health or SUD services. If this does occur, clients will receive parallel instead of integrated services. Most FACT teams make efforts to avoid providing parallel services and provide as many services as they can themselves

We can conclude that Norwegian ACT and FACT are broadly successful in providing holistic and integrated services, and that both of them are the most suitably adapted models for people in Norway with mental illness, substance use disorders, and complex needs [10].

> Clients get better care and support because moving services to where they live is more effective.
>
> We are impressed by how they cope with challenging patients.
>
> The teams offer something different from ordinary services, they are outreach-based and they provide practical help. That is the fundamental attitude of the team. They provide key services. They do outreach and handle everyday events to establish trust with patients. They accept clients as they are. They relate to people at home, not on a ward.
>
> *(Collaborating partners of FACT teams)* [60]

- ACT and FACT provide services to people with severe mental disorders and complex needs who do not benefit from traditional services. People with SUD/SMI are recruited to both ACT and FACT programs.
- ACT and FACT help clients to live a better life in the community. The teams provide a variety of services based on client needs, such as practical assistance in their everyday life, housing, finances, work, meaningful activities, IDDT, and psychotherapy.

- ACT and FACT provide many benefits to clients. They function better in everyday life, and many have a stable income, better housing, and a more meaningful life following care and treatment in ACT and FACT. They spend far fewer days in inpatient mental health care, especially during involuntary admission. These results apply to clients with and without substance use problems.
- Although many clients with co-occurring disorders still have substance use problems after follow-up by an ACT team or a FACT team, they live their lives in a better way.
- ACT and FACT differ from other mental healthcare models in that care and treatment are mainly provided by a single team instead of by different service providers. ACT and FACT appear to provide and support a holistic and coordinated range of services for people with mental illnesses, often substance use problems, and complex service needs.
- Norwegian ACT and FACT teams represent binding collaboration between primary and specialist health care. This means that the team members relate to two sets of legislation and have access to two medical record systems. This commitment can potentially enhance interaction between the two levels of care.
- The ACT and FACT models emphasize that the teams should be interdisciplinary and that the members should draw on each other's expertise, professional background, and personal qualities. The whiteboard method with daily team meetings and joint treatment meetings enables team members to know every client and use each other's expertise. In this way, the team ensures that their efforts to help clients are coordinated and aimed at a common goal.
- Team members work together and within the same framework and are located in the same place. This makes it easier to achieve a common understanding of the individual client than if they belonged to different agencies.
- ACT and FACT teams should have access to digital communication systems in both primary and specialist care in order to gain insight into other services provided to clients and to coordinate these services.
- In Norway today, ACT and FACT appear to be the best service models to provide integrated care and treatment to clients with mental illness, substance use disorders, and complex needs.

Reflection Questions

- Reflect on the aim of ACT and FACT: how does it differ from the aim of care and treatment in the traditional service system?
- How do ACT and FACT enable clients to receive integrated services?
- How useful do you consider the team approach in ACT and FACT in comparison with teamwork in interdisciplinary coordination teams?
- What is integrated treatment (IDDT) for FACT clients with co-occurring disorders, and how useful do you consider IDDT?
- What would you highlight as important aspects of the ACT and FACT models for people with co-occurring disorders?

Recommended Literature and Online Resources

- Certification Centre for ACT and Flexible ACT (CCAF): ccaf.nl/fact-facts/english.
- European Assertive Outreach Foundation (EAOF): eaof.org
- FACT-FACTS. A website with information about Flexible Assertive Community Treatment or Flexible ACT (FACT)): fact-facts.nl.
- Assertive Community Treatment (ACT) Evidence-Based Practices (EBP) KIT (SAMHSA): library.samhsa.gov/product/assertive-community-treatment-act-evidence-based-practices-ebp-kit/sma08-4344

References

1. Hustvedt I, Bosnic H, Håland M. Brukerplan årsrapport 2019. Tjenestemottakere med rusproblemer og psykiske helseproblemer i kommunen. [Service User Plan Annual Report 2019. Service users with substance use problems and mental health problems in the municipality]. Stavanger: KORFOR—Helse Stavanger, Norway; 2020.
2. Håland M, Lie T, Nesvåg S, Stevenson B. Brukere med rus-og psykiske helseproblem i norske kommuner. BrukerPlan—statistikk 2015 [Clients with substance abuse and mental health issues—userplan statistics 2015]. Stavanger, Norway: KORFOR—Helse Stavanger; 2016.
3. Stein LI, Test MA. Alternative to mental hospital treatment: I. Conceptual model, treatment program, and clinical evaluation. Arch Gen Psychiatry. 1980;37(4):392–7.
4. Helsedepartementet (Department of Health). Samhandlingsreformen—rett behandling på rett sted til rett tid [The coordination reform proper treatment—at the right place and right time]. Oslo; 2008–2009.
5. Helsedirektoratet (Directorate of Health). Nasjonal faglig retningslinje for utredning, behandling og oppfølging av personer med samtidig ruslidelse og psykisk lidelse—ROP-lidelser: sammensatte tjenester—samtidig behandling [National guideline for assessment, treatment, and follow-up for persons with co-occurring substance disorder and mental illness]. Oslo, Norway; 2012.
6. Helsedirektoratet (Directorate of Health). Sammen om mestring. Veileder i psykisk helsearbeid for voksne [National guide for community mental health work]. Oslo, Norway 2014.
7. Helsedirektoratet (Directorate of Health). Veileder om oppfølging av personer med store og sammensatte behov [nettdokument]. In: National guide: care for persons with complex needs. Oslo, Norway; 2017.
8. Helse- og omsorgsdepartementet (Department og health and welfare services). Fremtidens primærhelsetjeneste—nærhet og helhet [The primary health and care services of tomorrow—localised and integrated]. Oslo, Norway; 2015.
9. Riksrevisjonen (Office of the Auditor General). Riksrevisjonens undersøkelse av psykiske helsetjenester—Dokument 3:13 (2020–2021) [The office of the auditor general's investigation of mental health services—document 3:13 (2020–2021]. Oslo, Norway; 2021.
10. Riksrevisjonen (Office of the Auditor General). Helse- og velferdstjenester til personer med samtidige rusmiddellidelser og psykiske lidelser (Health and welfare services to persons with concurrent substance use disorders and mental illness). Oslo, Norway; 2025.
11. Helsedirektoratet (Directorate of Health). Veileder om rehabilitering, habilitering, individuell plan og koordinator [National guide to rehabilitation, habilitation, individual plan and coordinator] Oslo, Norway; 2015.
12. Lukersmith S, Millington M, Salvador-Carulla L. What is case management? A scoping and mapping review. Int J Integr Care. 2016;16(4):2.

13. Sosial og helsedepartementet (Ministry of Social Affairs and Health). Om opptrappingsplan for psykisk helse 1999——2006 Endringer i statsbudsjettet for 1998 [Escalation plan for mental health 1999–2006. Amendments to the fiscal budget FOR 1998]. Oslo, Norway; 1998.
14. Huus G, Storm-Olsen B, Herheim Å. Mennesker med alvorlige psykiske lidelser og behov for særlig tilrettelagte tilbud [People with severe mental illness and the need for specially adapted services]. Oslo, Norway; 2008. Contract No.: IS-1554.
15. Dieterich M, Irving CB, Bergman H, Khokhar MA, Park B, Marshall M. Intensive case management for severe mental illness. Schizophr Bull. 2017;43(4):698–700.
16. Dieterich M, Irving CB, Park B, Marshall M. Intensive case management for severe mental illness. Cochrane Database Syst Rev 2010(10):CD007906.
17. Marshall M, Lockwood A. Assertive community treatment for people with severe mental disorders. Cochrane Database Syst Rev 2000(2):CD001089.
18. van Veldhuizen J, Bahler M. Manual: Flexibel assertive community treatment: vision, model, practice and organization. Groningen, The Netherlands: CCAF; 2013.
19. van Veldhuizen JR. FACT: a Dutch version of ACT. Community Ment Health J. 2007;43(4):421–33.
20. Helsedirektoratet (Directorate of Health). Utredning, behandling og oppfølging av psykoselidelser [Assessment, treatment and follow-up of patients with psychotic illness]. Oslo, Norway; 2013. Report No.: 9788280812421.
21. Helsedirektoratet (Directorate of Health). Tilbud til voksne med langvarige og sammensatte tjenestebehov—Tilskudd [Grants for services for adults with long-term and complex needs]. Oslo, Norway; 2019.
22. Bachrach LL. Continuity of care and approaches to case management for long-term mentally ill patients. Psychiatr Serv. 1993;44(5):465–8.
23. Monroe-DeVita M, Moser LL, Teague GB. The tool for measurement of assertive community treatment (TMACT). In: McGovern MP, McHugo GJ, Drake RE, Bond GR, Merrens MR, editors. Implementing evidence-based practices in behavioral health. Chapell Hill, NC: University of North Carolina (UNC) at Chapel Hill School of Medicine, Department of Psychiatry, Center for Excellence in Community Mental Health; 2013.
24. Monroe-DeVita M, Teague GB, Moser LL. The TMACT: a new tool for measuring fidelity to assertive community treatment. J Am Psychiatr Nurses Assoc. 2011;17(1):17–29.
25. Allness DJ, Knoedler WH. A manual for ACT start-up: based on the PACT model of community treatment for persons with severe and persistent mental illnesses. National Alliance for the Mentally Ill; 2003.
26. Aakerholt A. ACT-håndbok (Inkludert en beskrivelse av FACT-modellen) [Handbook for assertive community treatment (act), (including a description of the FACT model)]. Hamar, Norway; 2013.
27. Aakerholt A. Fact Modellbeskrivelse (Fact handbook—Norwegian). Trondheim, Norway; 2023. Available from: https://napha.no/multimedia/12114/FACT-modellbeskrivelse
28. Bähler M, Van Veldhuizen R, Van Vugt M, Delespaul P, Kroon H, Lardinois J, et al. Fidelity scale FACT Woerden: Certification Centre for ACT and FACT; 2010 [.
29. Becker D, Drake R, editors. A Working Life for People with Severe Mental Illness. Oxford University Press; 2003.
30. Bond GR, Drake RE, Becker DR. Generalizability of the individual placement and support (IPS) model of supported employment outside the US. World Psychiatry. 2012;11(1):32–9.
31. Smith LF, Drake RE, Mueser KT, Brunette MF, Becker DR, McGovern MR, et al., editors. Integrated dual disorders treatment (IDDT)—expanded and updated edition. Dartmouth: Hazelden; 2010.
32. McHugo GJ, Drake RE, Teague GB, Xie H. Fidelity to assertive community treatment and client outcomes in New Hampshire dual disorders study. Psychiatr Serv. 1999;50(6):818–24.
33. Cleary M, Hunt G, Matheson S, Siegfried N, Walter G. Psychosocial interventions for people with both severe mental illness and substance misuse. Cochrane Database Syst Rev 2008(1):Cd001088.

34. Killaspy H, Bebbington P, Blizard R, Johnson S, Nolan F, Pilling S, et al. The REACT study: randomised evaluation of assertive community treatment in North London. BMJ: Br Med J 2006;332(7545):815–820.
35. Killaspy H, Johnson S, Pierce B, Bebbington P, Pilling S, Nolan F, et al. Successful engagement: a mixed methods study of the approaches of assertive community treatment and community mental health teams in the REACT trial. Soc Psychiatry Psychiatr Epidemiol. 2009;44(7):532–40.
36. Burns T, Catty J, Dash M, Roberts C, Lockwood A, Marshall M. Use of intensive case management to reduce time in hospital in people with severe mental illness: systematic review and meta-regression. BMJ: Br Med J 2007;335(7615):336.
37. Sytema S, Wunderink L, Bloemers W, Roorda L, Wiersma D. Assertive community treatment in The Netherlands: a randomized controlled trial. Acta Psychiatr Scand. 2007;116(2):105–12.
38. Burns T, Fioritti A, Holloway F, Malm U, Rossler W. Case management and assertive community treatment in Europe. Psychiatr Serv. 2001;52(5):631–6.
39. Rosen A, Mueser KT, Teesson M. Assertive community treatment--issues from scientific and clinical literature with implications for practice. J Rehabil Res Dev. 2007;44(6):813–25.
40. Johnson S. So what shall we do about assertive community treatment? Epidemiol Psichiatr Soc. 2008;17(2):110–4.
41. Burns T. The rise and fall of assertive community treatment? Int Rev Psychiatry. 2010;22(2):130–7.
42. Abufarsakh B, Kappi A, Pemberton KM, Williams LB, Okoli CTC. Substance use outcomes among individuals with severe mental illnesses receiving assertive community treatment: a systematic review. Int J Ment Health Nurs. 2023;32(3):704–26.
43. Penzenstadler L, Soares C, Anci E, Molodynski A, Khazaal Y. Effect of assertive community treatment for patients with substance use disorder: a systematic review. Eur Addict Res. 2019;25(2):56–67.
44. De Witte NA, Crunelle CL, Sabbe B, Moggi F, Dom G. Treatment for outpatients with comorbid schizophrenia and substance use disorders: a review. Eur Addict Res. 2014;20(3):105–14.
45. Fries HP, Rosen MI. The efficacy of assertive community treatment to treat substance use. J Am Psychiatr Nurses Assoc. 2011;17(1):45–50.
46. Drummond C, Gilburt H, Burns T, Copello A, Crawford M, Day E, et al. Assertive community treatment for people with alcohol dependence: a pilot randomized controlled trial. Alcohol Alcohol. 2017;52(2):234–41.
47. Ruppelt F, Rohenkohl A, Kraft V, Schöttle D, Schröter R, Gaianigo J, et al. Course, remission and recovery in patients with severe psychotic disorders with or without comorbid substance use disorders: long-term outcome in evidence-based integrated care (ACCESS II study). Schizophr Res. 2020;222:437–43.
48. Drukker M, Maarschalkerweerd M, Bak M, Driessen G, a Campo J, de Bie A, et al. A real-life observational study of the effectiveness of FACT in a Dutch mental health region. BMC Psychiatry. 2008;8:93.
49. Drukker M, Visser E, Sytema S, van Os J. Flexible assertive community treatment, severity of symptoms and psychiatric health service use, a real life observational study. Clinical practice and epidemiology in mental health: CP & EMH. 2013;9:202–9.
50. Nugter MA, Engelsbel F, Bahler M, Keet R, van Veldhuizen R. Outcomes of FLEXIBLE assertive community treatment (FACT) implementation: a prospective real life study. Community Ment Health J. 2016;52(8):898–907.
51. Firn M, Hindhaugh K, Hubbeling D, Davies G, Jones B, White SJ. A dismantling study of assertive outreach services: comparing activity and outcomes following replacement with the FACT model. Soc Psychiatry Psychiatr Epidemiol. 2013;48(6):997–1003.
52. Firn M, White SJ, Hubbeling D, Jones B. The replacement of assertive outreach services by reinforcing local community teams: a four-year observational study. J Ment Health. 2018;27(1):4–9.

53. Sood L, Owen A, Onyon R, Sharma A, Nigriello J, Markham D, et al. Flexible assertive community treatment (FACT) model in specialist psychosis teams: an evaluation. BJPsych Bulletin. 2017;41(4):192–6.
54. Neijmeijer LJ, Korzilius HPLM, Kroon H, Nijman HLI, Didden R. Flexible assertive community treatment for individuals with a mild intellectual disability or borderline intellectual functioning: results of a longitudinal study in The Netherlands. J Intellect Disabil Res. 2019;63(8):1015–22.
55. Nielsen CM, Hjorthøj C, Killaspy H, Nordentoft M. The effect of flexible assertive community treatment in Denmark: a quasi-experimental controlled study. Lancet Psychiatry. 2021;8(1):27–35.
56. Svensson B, Hansson L, Lexén A. Outcomes of clients in need of intensive team care in flexible assertive community treatment in Sweden. Nord J Psychiatry. 2018;72(3):226–31.
57. Munch Nielsen C, Hjorthøj C, Arnfred BT, Nordentoft M. Patient outcomes of flexible assertive community treatment compared with assertive community treatment. Psychiatr Serv. 2023;74(7):695–701.
58. Mueller-Stierlin AS, Becker T, Greve N, Hänsel A, Herder K, Kohlmann A, et al. Results from a randomized controlled trial investigating effectiveness of a community-based intervention on empowerment of people with severe mental illness. Soc Psychiatry Psychiatr Epidemiol. 2025;60:2135.
59. Brekke E, Lamu AN, Angeles RC, Clausen H, Landheim AS. Changes in inpatient mental health treatment and related costs before and after flexible assertive community treatment: a naturalistic observational cohort study. BMC Psychiatry. 2025;25(1):164.
60. Landheim A, Odden S. Evaluering av FACT-team i Norge—Sluttrapporten. In: Evaluation of FACT teams in Norway—final report. Hamar, Norway; 2020.
61. Landheim A, Ruud T, Odden S, Clausen H, Heiervang KS, Stuen HK, et al. Utprøving av ACT-team i Norge—Hva viser resultatene? In: Evaluation of act teams in Norway—key findings. Hamar, Norway; 2014.
62. Pettersen H, Ruud T, Ravndal E, Havnes I, Landheim A. Engagement in assertive community treatment as experienced by recovering clients with severe mental illness and concurrent substance use. Int J Ment Health Syst. 2014;8(1):40.
63. Pettersen H, Ruud T, Ravndal E, Landheim A. Walking the fine line: self-reported reasons for substance use in persons with severe mental illness. Int J Qual Stud Health Well-being. 2013;8:21968.
64. Pettersen H, Ruud T, Ravndal E, Landheim A. Searching for sobriety: how persons with severe mental illness experience abstaining from substance use. 2014.
65. Lofthus A-M, Weimand BM, Ruud T, Rose D, Heiervang KS. "This is not a life anyone would want"—a qualitative study of Norwegian ACT Service users' experience with mental health treatment. Issues Ment Health Nurs. 2018;39(6):519–26.
66. Lofthus A-M, Westerlund H, Bjørgen D, Lindstrøm JC, Lauveng A, Clausen H, et al. Are users satisfied with assertive community treatment in spite of personal restrictions? Community Ment Health J. 2016;52(8):891–7.
67. Lofthus AM, Westerlund H, Bjorgen D, Lindstrom JC, Lauveng A, Rose D, et al. Recovery concept in a Norwegian setting to be examined by the assertive community treatment model and mixed methods. Int J Ment Health Nurs. 2018;27(1):147–57.
68. Stuen HK, Landheim A, Rugkåsa J, Wynn R. How clinicians make decisions about CTOs in ACT: a qualitative study. Int J Ment Health Syst. 2018;12:51.
69. Stuen HK, Landheim A, Rugkåsa J, Wynn R. Responsibilities with conflicting priorities: a qualitative study of ACT providers' experiences with community treatment orders. BMC Health Serv Res. 2018;18(1):290.
70. Stuen HK, Rugkåsa J, Landheim A, Wynn R. Increased influence and collaboration: a qualitative study of patients' experiences of community treatment orders within an assertive community treatment setting. BMC Health Serv Res. 2015;15:409.

71. Odden S, Landheim A, Clausen H, Stuen HK, Heiervang KS, Ruud T. Model fidelity and team members' experiences of assertive community treatment in Norway: a sequential mixed-methods study. Int J Ment Health Syst. 2019;13:65.
72. Clausen H, Landheim A, Odden S, Heiervang KS, Stuen HK, Killaspy H, et al. Associations between quality of life and functioning in an assertive community treatment population. Psychiatr Serv. 2015;66(11):1249–52.
73. Clausen H, Landheim A, Odden S, Saltyte Benth J, Heiervang KS, Stuen HK, et al. Hospitalization of high and low inpatient service users before and after enrollment into assertive community treatment teams: a naturalistic observational study. Int J Ment Health Syst. 2016;10:14.
74. Clausen H, Ruud T, Odden S, Benth JŠ, Heiervang KS, Stuen HK, et al. Improved rehabilitation outcomes for persons with and without problematic substance use after 2 years with assertive community treatment—a prospective study of patients with severe mental illness in 12 Norwegian ACT teams. Frontiers in Psychiatry. 2020;11:1387.
75. Clausen H, Ruud T, Odden S, Saltyte Benth J, Heiervang KS, Stuen HK, et al. Hospitalisation of severely mentally ill patients with and without problematic substance use before and during assertive community treatment: an observational cohort study. BMC Psychiatry. 2016;16:125.
76. Israel P, Ruud T, Weimand B. Carer involvement in the assessment of personal recovery: a naturalistic study of assertive community treatment in Norway. Front Psych. 2023;14:1135135.
77. Ruud T, Selle ML, Clausen HK, Heiervang KS, Odden S, Stuen HK, et al. Clinical outcomes and outcome predictors of two-year assertive community treatment in Norway: an explorative prospective pre-post study. BMC Psychiatry. 2024;24(1):729.
78. Trane K, Aasbrenn K, Rønningen M, Odden S, Lexén A, Landheim A. Flexible assertive community treatment teams can change complex and fragmented service systems: experiences of service providers. Int J Ment Health Syst. 2021;15(1):38.
79. Trane K, Aasbrenn K, Rønningen M, Odden S, Lexén A, Landheim A. Integration of Care in Complex and Fragmented Service Systems: experiences of staff in flexible assertive community treatment teams. Int J Integr Care. 2022;22(2):17.
80. Trane K, Aasbrenn K, Rønningen M, Odden S, Lexén A, Landheim AS. Flexible assertive community treatment in rural and remote areas: a qualitative study of the challenges and adaptations of the model. Front Public Health. 2022;10:913159.
81. Weimand B, Tembjerg P, Ruud T. Pårørende og ACT-team. En undersøkelse om pårørendes erfaringer med ACT-team, og ACT-teamlederes erfaringer med samarbeid med pårørende [Relatives and act-team. a study on relatives' experiences with act team, and act team leaders' experiences with collaboration with relatives]. Lørenskog, Norway; 2014.
82. Helsedirektoratet (Directorate of Health). Tvang i psykisk helsevern IS-2812 [Coercion in mental health care IS-2812]. Oslo, Norway; 2019.
83. Kvam EA, Oddli HW, Landheim AS. Anker i normalitet [Ancored in normality]. Tidsskrift for Norsk Psykologforening. 2019;56(3):166–77.
84. Martinsen R, Landheim AS, Bronken BA. A turning point after FACT: a qualitative study of family members' experiences and follow-up provided by flexible assertive community treatment. BMC Health Serv Res. 2025;25(1):1254. https://doi.org/10.1186/s12913-025-13485-z.

Caregivers: Burdened Yet Essential 13

Anne Kristine Bergem

Abstract

Caregivers of people with co-occurring substance use disorder and mental disorder (SUD/MH) are a group with great burdens. Young carers are particularly vulnerable.

At the same time, caregivers are not involved and supported enough in the health services.

Involving the whole family in the work around people with SUD/MH is important and necessary and has a positive effect both for the person who is sick/dependent, for adult caregivers, children, and health personnel.

Caregivers are a heterogeneous group, and there is not one good way to take care of and cooperate with caregivers. But recognition, information, inclusion, and cooperation are key words. More important than which method or model one uses is that as health personnel identify both adults and children who are caregivers and ensure that relevant caregivers are involved and become a natural part of the work around the person who needs support and treatment. In addition, caregivers need support for their own sake.

There are many services for caregivers, and as health personnel, one should know these.

As a helper, it is important to know oneself and one's own reactions in meeting with caregivers. One can seek support and guidance among colleagues and from experts in the field.

A. K. Bergem (✉)
Center for Next of Kin and Carers, (Pårørendesenteret), Stavanger, Norway

The Norwegian Psychiatric Association, Oslo, Norway
e-mail: akbergem@me.com

T. W. Lie, L. Lien (eds.), *Integrated Treatment of Co-occurring Substance Use and Mental Health Disorders*, https://doi.org/10.1007/978-3-032-20049-5_13

Keywords

Caregivers · Carers · Dependents · Next of kin · Family · Support · Childcare · Addiction · Mental health

In this chapter, I will use the term *caregivers* to refer to adults and *dependents* to refer to children. The term *dependents* inherently reflect the dependency children have on their parents. The term *young carers* will also be used where appropriate.

Basic and Everyday Hope

All people need hope. The hope that life will someday get better can be what makes people endure when life is difficult. The one who is sick needs hope. Those who are close need hope. Hope can revolve around survival, that the situation will change for the better or that life will feel a little less difficult. It can be demanding to hold on to such hope for people affected by SUD/MH. At times, it may therefore be that the caregivers must hope on behalf of the one who is sick in addition to carrying their own hope.

A saying goes "hope is the last thing to die" and emphasizes the strength of hope. However, it is not a given that people are able to maintain hope when life is difficult. The surroundings can have a great significance for whether it is possible to maintain hope for caregivers. Guilt and shame can stand in the way [1]. For caregivers' hope to survive and live, the guilt that many carry must be reduced. Shame and guilt among caregivers to people with SUD/MH are greatly influenced by attitudes in society.

Many of the attitudes in society are linked to prejudices, ignorance, and morality. To support caregivers and caregivers' hope requires attitude changes in society to how one views addiction and mental disorders.

For most caregivers, the encounter with the support system will have a great significance. Caregivers must experience being met, recognized, and taken care of in the healthcare system if they are to manage to hold on to the hope for themselves and their family.

Sælør and Biong [1] describe two types of hope caregivers need, basic hope and everyday hope. The basic hope is a life prerequisite akin to love and faith, and changes little over time. Being there for a close person who needs support rests on this basic hope. Everyday hope is about accepting one's life situation, among other things by processing guilt, forgiving oneself and finding realistic goals in everyday life. Everyday hope is greatly influenced by the surroundings, including the professionals caregivers meet. The expression of hope for the one who is sick by the professionals is of great importance. Furthermore, cooperation between caregivers and professionals means a lot for everyday hope. Both through reflection around difficult feelings like shame and guilt and through being "co-hopers," health personnel and other support personnel can be important for caregivers.

Caregivers: Who Are They?

Between 16% and 30% of the Norwegian population today are caregivers in some capacity [2, 3]. There is no reason to think this differs from other countries. If anything, there will be more family caregivers in countries with poorer healthcare services than in Norway. Young people are caregivers, young adults are, adults and elderly are too. The Norwegian government's caregiver strategy from 2020 was named "We—the caregivers" because most people are or become caregivers during life. Some are caregivers to people they live with, while others have their loved ones in an institution or care home. Some have daily and extensive care tasks for a long time, while others contribute and support now and then.

Caregivers can be closest family, relatives, friends, or others. Not everyone necessarily has the same legal rights or responsibilities, but everyone who *feels* affected is affected. It is the caregivers themselves and the person who is sick who knows who is affected. "Next of kin" is mentioned in the legislation, and those who are designated as next of kin have their own rights and roles. The right to information, the opportunity in special situations to consent on behalf of the person who is sick, opportunities for access to medical records, and the right to complain are among them [4]. The legislation and rights of next of kin may vary from country to country. Healthcare professionals have a duty to familiarize themselves with the legislation applicable in the country where they work.

Caregivers of People with SUD/MH

In a national survey of caregivers in Norway in 2021, it was found that of all caregivers, 24 percent were caregivers to a person where substance addiction was the cause of the need for help and 23% were caregivers to a person where mental illness was the cause. How many are caregivers to people with both health problems at the same time is not apparent from the report, but there is reason to believe that it is a significant proportion [3].

Caregivers of people with SUD/MH have a particularly burdensome responsibility, which is both extensive and complex. They experience to a much greater extent than other caregivers that the person who is sick does not want or cannot accept help. Even though caregivers do not always spend a lot of time physically contributing to everyday life, the role of being a caregiver is perceived as burdensome. Part of the burden is precisely that caregivers do not get the opportunity to provide the support and care that they would like to give [3].

Being a caregiver to a person with SUD/MH can be exhausting and affect one's own life, whether it be health-wise, financially, in social networks, and family relationships. Their own health is assessed as worse, and caregivers of people with SUD/MH have to a greater extent than other caregivers themselves asked for or received health help for ailments related to the role of being a caretaker. Depression, anxiety, and irritation are common emotional reactions. Caregivers often have reduced quality of life, challenges in their social life, and experience a lot of stress.

They also have an increased risk of being subjected to violence in close relationships as well as their own substance use [3, 5].

Caregivers of people with SUD/MH assess the services to the person they are related to as poorly coordinated and spend a lot of time navigating the system. This group of caregivers also experiences less opportunity for participation than other caregivers and to a lesser extent to participate in the design of the services [3]. Caregivers of people with SUD/MH experience that collaboration, interaction, and co-production are nice words, but far from what they themselves experience [6].

Bereaved After Overdose Deaths

Globally, around 185,000 people die annually from overdoses, according to estimates from the World Drug Report 2023, published by the United Nations Office on Drugs and Crime (UNODC). This figure includes deaths related to both illicit drugs and prescription medications such as opioids [7]. In connection with one person's death, many affected and bereaved are left behind. It is more burdensome to be bereaved in such deaths than in other types of deaths. Unexpected and dramatic deaths also increase the risk of more serious and long-term grief reactions [8]. The bereaved can be divided into two groups: those who know about the drug problems beforehand and those who do not. The first group seems to reconcile with death to a greater extent than the last group. Those who do not know about drug use beforehand often feel anger, guilt, and helplessness. But all the bereaved experience their health as weakened after a death.

For caregivers who are aware of drug problems, constant worry and fear of a fatal outcome of the drug use will be present. Many experience not being taken seriously in the health service when it comes to the fear of death, even though some also have positive experiences. Caregivers find that health personnel justify the lack of information and contact with confidentiality. Caregivers understand the duty of confidentiality, but there is something about the way situations are handled that gives caregivers a feeling of being excluded, when what they want is to contribute. The worry also includes concerns about where the family member is and how it will be possible to get help. Caregivers themselves express a desire for a place to turn with their concerns.

Some experience the time around deaths related to the relevant illegal drugs as a period of increasing problems. Caregivers describe the time leading up to the death as a particularly demanding period, both psychosocially and physically for the person who is sick, while other caregivers have experienced their close person as "lighter" due to hospitalization or recently completed treatment. This last group naturally experiences the death as a greater shock.

After an overdose death, several caregivers experience a deterioration of their own health and an increased need for help and support, while negative attitudes from the surroundings to illegal drug use are an additional burden. It can also be demanding to have to talk about the death to friends and acquaintances due to fear of reactions to the cause of death. Overdose deaths are perceived as taboo. Many caregivers also experience little understanding from the surroundings and expectations that the grief should pass quickly.

For some, such a death of a close one triggers existential questions about their own worth. Many are left with unanswered questions and painful memories. These reactions come on top of the fact that many caregivers are already exhausted. Many wait a long time for help, and few are offered help without having to ask for it themselves [9].

Children as Dependents

It is estimated that a significant number of children worldwide live with at least one parent who has a mental health disorder or substance use disorder. According to data from the Substance Abuse and Mental Health Services Administration, in the United States alone, around 12% of children live in households with at least one parent who has a past-year alcohol use disorder, while 3% of children live with a parent with a past-year illicit drug use disorder [10]. The children themselves tell of upbringings characterized by chaos, fear, physical/psychological violence, and abuse. Children in families with substance use problems are in critical life situations with a need for help to cope with everyday life. The children's challenges are many, including difficulties sleeping due to noise and unrest in the house, and not getting enough food or having to prepare food themselves [5].

Children growing up with substance-dependent or mentally ill parents have a higher risk of developing health problems themselves, both mental, social, and behavioral [10]. The children also have a higher risk of experiencing family conflicts, less functional parents, and violence, abuse, and traumatic life events [10–15]. Symptoms such as aggression, concentration difficulties, attention difficulties, problems with self-regulation and their own emotions, rule-breaking, and depressive disorders, anxiety, stress, physical ailments, withdrawal, and poor self-image are common, and many feel lonely.

These children generally have worse living conditions than other children. Substance use problems in the family often contribute to a worse living situation, more crime, fewer friends, worse economy, and worse family cohesion. Such factors are again related to how the children manage their schoolwork and how they are at school. For some, school is a sanctuary, while others struggle there [5].

Children in families with substance use problems must take care of themselves. In addition, many must care for siblings and their parents. Children are worried about their parents and that they might get hurt. Taking care of their parents is the most demanding task, along with the fear that the parents will harm themselves [5].

Based on the burdens children may experience when they are caregivers, it was legislated in Norway in 2010 that health personnel have a duty to assess whether adult patients have care for children under 18 years, and in 2018 the duty was extended to apply to minor siblings and survivors [16]. Several countries have similar laws and frameworks that recognize children as next of kin, particularly when they are caring for a parent or significant family member. Healthcare professionals have a duty to familiarize themselves with the legislation applicable in the country where they work but the children's needs will be present even if appropriate legislation is not.

There are many children growing up in families as described above who are doing fine. The risk of health problems is at the group level [5, 10].

Despite law changes in the last decades, children who are caregivers are not adequately cared for. Many children:

- Do not receive sufficient information about their parents' illness and the consequences for everyday life
- Are often left to themselves
- Feel lonely
- Take responsibility for their parents
- Have so many care tasks at home that it affects their quality of life, school, and time with friends
- Take so much responsibility at home that it feels stressful and burdensome
- Experience traumas
- Experience dilemmas, difficult choices, and challenging loyalty conflicts
- Feel shame

Adults around the children believe that the children are doing better than they are [15, 17].

Support for Caregivers

In recent years, several reports have been written, and many have researched various aspects of being both child and adult caregivers. This chapter will highlight some of the knowledge available today, but a complete overview will be beyond the scope of the chapter.

Support for Children and Young People

Many children feel that they have no one to talk to about their situation, and most carefully consider whether they can trust that adults will really help if they are to tell about how they are at home. They consider how the adults will handle the information, whether they will care and what they will do. Children are afraid that adults may make the situation for the family worse. Children want to be involved and have their say when decisions are to be made. Children want to talk to adults who are honest and open, and who do not have a hidden agenda.

Children and young people want the parent who has SUD/MH to acknowledge their problem. It is easier for children to accept help from others when the parent with substance use problems is honest. An important and necessary part of the follow-up of children who are caregivers is to work with the parents, including the one who is sick. When help and support are to be planned and implemented, the whole family and the internal interaction in the family must be seen and considered. The children's situation improves when the couple's relationship and the parental role are addressed and worked on in treatment and follow-up [5].

Even though there are many risk factors for children growing up in families with SUD/MH, protective factors can also be present. In addition to working to reduce risk factors, healthcare professionals should contribute to strengthening such protective factors in families. Warm and sensitive parenting style, how parents monitor their children, and the quality of the relationship between parents and children are all factors of great importance [5]. Secure attachment, good interaction between parents, and family cohesion are others. For the children, it is important that the other parent protects them and keeps the family together. Therefore, it is important that the parent who is not sick receives good support and follow-up from the support system both for their own sake and for the sake of the children.

To thematize and work with parental role and parental functioning is thus important, even if addiction and mental illness are present. Both psychoeducation and interventions with elements from cognitive and behavioral approaches have an effect [13]. Working with parent–child interaction through family and parent training, for example, in the form of courses, can be a good measure. Meeting places for community between families in the same situation have been shown to be good, and both giving and receiving support from others in the same situation are experienced positively [5, 12, 17].

How to Meet Each Child

All children are different, and age, maturity, and other prerequisites mean that contact with children who are caregivers must be adapted to each child and each teenager. However, there will be some common elements that are important in all encounters.

Recognition

Children need to be seen as people who are affected by the situation. They need recognition that what happens to the sick/addicted person affects them.

Children need what happens in the family to be talked about. That adults are honest and show with words and actions that it is possible to talk about what is happening is crucial. It can also contribute to making it easier for the children to ask about things they are wondering about. Openness provides security and contributes to a sense of community even if the situation can be painful and difficult.

Children need to experience that they are involved in what is happening in the family. They must be included in conversations about the disease and the drug problem. In some situations, children can give their opinion and be heard when decisions are to be made. This does not mean that the children should have responsibility, but that they should experience that their opinions matter. The children can be involved in deciding what they should participate in and how they should have it in everyday life, such as what tasks they should have at home.

Information

Children need information about their parents' illness, treatment, and consequences for everyday life [5, 18, 19, 20]. The information must be concrete. Also, information about which reactions and feelings are natural to have in such a situation is important. The information must be adapted to the children's age and level of maturity. Not all details are necessary in all situations, but what is said must be true.

Adults Who Tolerate and Accept

Children need adults to have control over their own feelings and challenges so that it feels safe for the child to share theirs. Children will quickly stop asking if adults become angry or sad when the child asks questions. Children must be allowed to express their feelings and receive recognition for them without adults trivializing or comforting too quickly. Adults must be able to tolerate that children are sad and upset and recognize that such feelings are completely natural in a difficult life situation. Adults must be interested and explore children's experiences. It is nice to support children in that they are allowed to feel good, or let children understand that it is not their fault that there are difficulties in the family, but if children express such thoughts, one must not dismiss them but explore the child's thoughts first.

In Everyday Life

Knowing what is going to happen creates predictability. Predictability contributes to security and less worry. Some benefit from making family plans where all activities for adults and children are included. For the children, it can be good to know who will follow and pick up for school and leisure activities. Names and phone numbers of important adults in the child's life should be available to the children themselves. Routines for everyday life can provide structure in an otherwise chaotic existence and contribute to a greater degree of security.

For the children, it is a good thing that other adults, at school and in the neighborhood or leisure activities, know about the family's situation, that is, the disease/addiction. The children and the family can together plan who should know what. It is also of great help to the children that the family together talks about how it is okay to answer if someone asks about the home situation.

Adult children of people with addiction find it important to get away from the situation. When they no longer live in the situation, it is easier to seek help. Many types of interventions are helpful. It is more important to get support than what kind of support is offered [5].

A Checklist for All Who Are Going to Work with Children as Dependents

- Ensure that the department/unit has procedures/routines/guidelines for follow-up of children as dependents and see to it that everyone is familiar with these and follows them in meeting all patients/service users.
- Hang up posters on entrance doors and waiting rooms where it states that children and young people are expected and welcome.

- Talk to all adult patients who have children about how the parental role is affected by the disease and treatment. If it is a teenager who is a patient/user, talk to the parents about how the family and siblings are affected when one child is sick/has a substance use problem.
- Encourage all families to talk together about the disease, the treatment, and how family life is affected by one family member being sick and/or receiving treatment.
- Offer family and child counseling sessions.
- Document the work with children as dependents in an appropriate way in the patient's journal.
- If concerned about a child's care situation, consider contacting child welfare services for reporting and/or cooperation [19].

Support for Adult Caregivers

Recognition is also important for adult caregivers. Caregivers must be recognized as partners and be involved in the treatment and care for the sick person. In addition, caregivers need to receive support and guidance for their own sake [21–23]. Offers such as participation in support groups are also a good measure to gain better knowledge about the disease and situation and to reduce the feeling of being the only ones in this situation [24]. Peer support in groups with others in the same situation contributes to increased quality of life. In addition to increased understanding, participation in a network provides insight and help for processing [3].

It is a challenge that caregivers are not heard or given the possibility to contribute with information about the user and the user's situation to those who provide services. Caregivers are too rarely involved in planning, decisions and design of the services [22, 25–27]. Greater degree of collaboration and co-creation is necessary. The users of the services, including caregivers, must be involved both in defining the problem and how it should be worked with [6].

Interventions aimed at the whole family also mean something for the one who is sick and this person's risk of relapse and readmissions. Family interventions reduce such risk [28]. When offering counseling of both patient and family, it seems that this can increase understanding in the family in addition to reducing the risk of relapse and readmission [29]. In 2013, a research summary was published concluding that it can be said with certainty that family-based therapy in alcohol addiction treatment contributes to lower consumption and that the relationships in the family improve [30].

All types of psychological support to family and a partner have a positive effect on the family. Regardless of whether support is given individually or in group, which setting the support is given in and for how long, whether it is network support or help for self-help, all measures have an effect. It is the experience of support that is crucial [31].

Many caregivers spend a lot of energy trying to make everyday life as normal as possible by maintaining a facade outward. This means that they do not seek help [5].

This may mean that the support system must be available with a very low threshold, and to a greater extent actively approach caregivers.

For bereaved after drug-related deaths, it is recommended that support and offer of processing what has happened are given unsolicited. Caregivers should not have to ask for such offers themselves. The follow-up offer should be part of the municipality's procedures for taking care of the bereaved. The offer must of course be adapted individually, but both children and adults who are affected should be followed up [9].

As previously mentioned, there is a higher risk of violence in close relationships for caregivers of people with SUD/MH. Offers of counseling or therapy to the sick person and their partner together have a good effect. Such offers provide a reduction of violence in close relationships and a higher degree of satisfaction with the relationship [5].

Even though caregivers of people with SUD/MH experience lack of involvement and support, health workers believe it is important to involve caregivers in the work around patients and users. Both for the patient's recovery, for the caregivers' health and quality of life, and for the health workers' ability to understand, involvement with the caregivers is significant. Topics such as guilt and shame, boundary setting, understanding of disease and legislation are challenging, and counseling that includes legislation, confidentiality, and consent provisions is necessary [32, 33].

There is probably no contradiction between what caregivers want and what health personnel perceive that caregivers need. The reason why there is still not sufficient involvement of caregivers is a large and complex topic that will not be explored further in this chapter.

Available Support

Involvement of Caregivers

In some countries, involving family members in caregiving is mandatory by law, while in others, it is encouraged but not necessarily a legal obligation. Norway, for example, has strong regulations requiring the involvement of relatives in care processes, which ensures that caregivers are recognized and supported as an essential part of the care system [34–36]. In leading documents for the services in Norway, it is clearly stated that involvement of and support to caregivers is a natural and necessary part of good health care. The Health Directorate formulates the following recommendation about involvement of family and network in substance use treatment: "Family and network should be involved in the treatment in consultation with the patient/user" [34].

Other countries may have different approaches. For instance, in many EU nations, caregiving for older adults or individuals with disabilities often involves family members, but these responsibilities are typically not enforced by law. However, certain policies support caregivers through benefits and social services, which may vary significantly depending on national laws and welfare systems.

In some nations, such as Sweden, there are strong structures in place to support family caregivers, including children in some cases, where the law acknowledges their needs and provides access to services that may relieve the burden [37]. On the other hand, countries with less comprehensive welfare systems may have more informal caregiving roles for families, with less formal recognition and support [38].

Overall, while some countries, like Norway, mandate family involvement, the global landscape varies widely in terms of how family caregivers are supported, and whether their participation is legally required. The level of legal obligation and support provided to family caregivers often depends on the country's welfare model and healthcare policies.

Although not all countries have mandatory involvement of family members, family caregivers will largely have the same needs, and the guidelines described here may serve as inspiration for countries that do not have specific systems in place.

- Municipalities and hospitals should have systems for involving caregivers at all levels, municipalities should offer respite measures to alleviate the burden of care, and caregivers should receive training, guidance, and support.
- Health personnel should have competence in involving and supporting caregivers.
- Health personnel should have an overview of local support measures for caregivers.

Furthermore, caregivers should be involved in the assessment, treatment, and follow-up of the patient/user. Health personnel should be in dialogue with caregivers. For people who are subjected to coercion, caregivers should be involved to a particular degree.

Care for Children Who Are Caregivers

All health trusts should have personnel responsible for children as dependents, or childcare workers as such personnel may be called. In Norway, this is mandatory [36]. Childcare workers are meant to be responsible for promoting and coordinating health personnel's follow-up of children who are dependents to parents or siblings with mental illness, substance dependence, serious illness, or injury. Hospitals and municipalities are encouraged to appoint a coordinator for their child-responsible personnel.

Childcare personnel should [35]:

- Coordinate and promote the work in their own unit.
- Inform and guide colleagues (without taking over the responsibility; the responsibility should lie with each individual health personnel).
- Have an overview of relevant offers and assistance agencies internally and externally.
- Have good knowledge about the situation and needs of children as dependents.
- Have good knowledge about communication with children.

Coordinators for childcare personnel should:

- Be organized at a higher level in the hospital/municipality and report to management (local adaptations necessary).
- Coordinate and have an overview of the work of childcare workers.

- Be an advisor for childcare workers in the hospital or municipality.
- Organize training and guidance.
- Develop overviews of measures and assistance agencies/organizations.
- Interact with external agencies/organizations.
  The management at the hospital/municipality should:
- Develop procedures for working with children as dependents.
- Include children's needs in planning of health services.
- Include the work with children in strategic documents (such as cooperation agreements, treatment lines, and guides).
- Appoint a coordinator for childcare workers.
- Ensure relevant training and guidance for childcare workers.
- Provide basic training to all health personnel.
- Ensure that the units are adapted for children who are visiting.
- Ensure that information material is available for patients, caregivers, and employees.

Stories for Reflection

Supporting people in vulnerable situations and people with complex disorders and their caregivers is a competence that requires more than factual knowledge. As a professional practitioner, one needs to acquire "advanced knowledge, practical skills, values, and attitudes" [39, p. 2].

Using stories can facilitate a deeper understanding in the reader of themselves and others through the self-reflection the story stimulates. Stories also provide an opportunity to address sensitive topics that can otherwise be challenging to address [39]. Stories based on the reality that exists out in the field also make it possible to reflect on realistic ethical dilemmas [40]. It will also be easier to see the person behind symptoms and signs when reading about people's own experiences [39]. Such experiences can help to challenge prejudices and preconceptions. Developing attitudes and values is a vital part of competence enhancement [39].

People's own values, ethics, and intuition will influence the contact with caregivers in the clinical everyday life, and the ability for self-reflection must therefore be included in all competence enhancement. Stories and clinical examples can contribute to this. An important part of the education of healthcare workers is about the ability to establish good relationships with others. To achieve this, skills other than acquiring theoretical knowledge are needed [40].

Self-awareness, self-regulation, self-motivation, social awareness, and social skills are five key abilities in healthcare workers. To get the opportunity to develop these skills, emotional engagement is needed [40]. Using stories stimulates emotional engagement and can therefore be a tool in the development of necessary skills [39]. The reader will quickly encounter the characters in a story and can usually identify emotional reactions in themselves and in the story. By feeling their own and others' emotions, the reader can, in turn, be stimulated to analyze the complex situations, relationships, and events that take place in the story and that trigger the emotions they have identified. Thoughts and feelings that spring from stories will contribute to significant reflection [40, 41].

In encounters with caregivers, there is rarely one correct way to meet people. The most important thing is to always think about the caregivers, include and involve them in the situation.

In this section, you can read stories from real encounters with caregivers. They are meant for inspiration and reflection, and reflection questions are suggested under each story.

The examples are from a center for next of kin and carers in Norway that offers counseling to caregivers both in person, over the phone, and online. All stories are anonymized.

Carl and the Breach of Confidentiality

Suzannah works in a team in the municipality. One of the service users she follows up is a young man named Carl. There is suspicion that Carl has a possible schizophrenia disorder, but he has not been drug-free long enough for a thorough assessment to be carried out. He also has had several short stays in prison due to less serious drug-related crimes. He has a mixed-use problem that includes injecting heroin. Suzannah experiences Carl as depressed, and he occasionally expresses that it doesn't matter whether he lives or dies. After the last prison stay, Carl is without housing. He mostly stays with his mother, even though he also spends large parts of the time outdoors. He wants as little to do with his mother as possible. He thinks she is nagging and clingy. The mother herself has substance use problems with alcohol and various medications. She is on disability pension and lives in a municipal apartment.

One afternoon just before Suzannah is about to leave work, she receives a text message from Carl. Suzannah doesn't quite understand what the message is and tries both to call Carl and send a text without getting a response. She becomes worried. Even though the message itself does not say that Carl intends to take his own life, Suzannah gets a bad feeling. She knows that Carl does not want her to talk to his mother, but she calls her anyway. Maybe he is there, she thinks. Carl's mother answers immediately. He is not there. Both Suzannah and the mother know where Carl usually stays, and they agree on the mother going there immediately. After a few minutes, the mother calls back. She has found Carl but can't get in touch with him. Suzannah calls an ambulance, which arrives at the scene after a few minutes. Carl receives an injection of naloxone and comes to himself, but the ambulance workers assess him as hypothermic and in such poor condition that they take him to the emergency room.

A couple of days later, an angry Carl shows up at Suzannah's place of work. He is furious that she called his mother and threatens to report her for breach of confidentiality. Suzannah tries to explain why she called, but Carl doesn't want to listen.

Reflection Questions

- Did Suzannah do the right thing when she contacted Carl's mother?
- Could she have handled the situation differently?

Paul's Dad

Paul was 8 years old when he first encountered a center for caregivers. He lived with his mother and came with her to counseling sessions. Paul resented that he couldn't stay with his father overnight because his father was using drugs. Paul thought his mother's decision was unfair. At the same time, he was angry with his father who was using drugs when he knew Paul wasn't allowed to visit. He felt bad that his dad chose drugs over of being with him.

Paul's father worked for a voluntary organization for many years, but over time developed so much anxiety and depression that he couldn't be at work. He was diagnosed with (post-traumatic stress disorder (PTSD) but got little out of the first treatment he tried. After that, he didn't have the energy to seek further treatment. It became too difficult for the family to stay together, and the parents divorced when Paul was 5 years old. Pauls´ father gradually started to increase drug use. Paul's mother was clear that she thought dad was not able to take care of Paul during overnight stays. The father did not protest.

In the conversations, it was important to give Paul the opportunity to talk about what he was thinking and feeling. He received confirmation that his anger and frustration were understandable and natural. He also learned that there are many children who experience similar situations to his and that the feelings and reactions he experienced were shared by many others. With support from the professional at the center, his mother was able to accept and accommodate Paul's feelings without becoming defensive or resorting to "it's for your own good." In addition, Paul and his mother received thorough explanations of how drug addiction and PTSD can affect a person.

Paul returned to the center when he was 16 years old. At that time, his father had died.

The death was drug-related, probably not suicide. This time Paul came alone. He was again met with confirmation, recognition for what he was thinking and feeling, as well as information about normal reactions. In the conversations, he was able to understand and articulate his mother's decision from earlier in a new way. Now he was mostly glad that he had not been allowed to be with and stay overnight with his father during the periods of drug use. He received support for his feelings, which were a mix of grief, disappointment, and relief.

Reflection Questions

- Is there any information about a parent's illness and lifestyle that children should be shielded from?
- Is it unproblematic to relate to one parent's version in such a situation?

Omar Managed to Care for Himself

Omar, a man in his forties, wanted a conversation with someone in his partner's treatment team. His partner Bridget was hospitalized with severe kidney and liver failure after long-term drug use. They had met several years ago in a drug treatment institution and had been married for 5 years. He was desperate and said they had now been told that the prognosis was very poor. They had no children, so Omar was the sole relative. The parents had broken contact with Bridget many years ago.

Omar found it difficult to know how he could be helpful in the situation. He felt he was running out of strength and was afraid of getting sick himself. He struggled with painful thoughts and feelings, and was anxious about what the future would bring, preparing for a fatal outcome.

At the same time, he was worried about falling back into old drug habits himself.

He got to talk to Penny, Bridget's contact nurse. Both a human being and a nurse, she could recognize many of the feelings and thoughts that Omar described. The two of them had good talks about powerlessness, inadequacy, fear, and existential questions. These were conversations that largely did not deal with solutions but dealt with the vulnerability and pain of being human in the face of death. Silence and presence became the central elements in the contact between Omar and Penny. They collaborated on a project where trust and open questions helped Omar to understand more of what his wife's illness and their previous life experiences did to him. An important topic also became what he needed to be able to face death together with his partner.

Omar had trouble sleeping and stomach pains that came and went. Medical examinations had not revealed any physical cause, and Omar thought them to be stress related. He felt guilty of being tired and had thoughts about wanting to get away from everything. For Omar, it was good to get confirmation of such thoughts and reactions being normal.

In his youth, Omar played the violin. In the conversations with Penny, the topic of self-care came up. Omar could feel provoked when friends said, "you have to remember to take care of yourself." He understood that the statement was well-intentioned but found it very difficult to know how to do it. The violin playing came up in this context, and he found the instrument again. He played old music, but also created his own. He sometimes also played for his partner, but mostly he played for himself. He used the music to express his feelings, but at the same time, the music gave him strength.

In the last conversation between Omar and Penny, he was still desperate and afraid for Bridget, the future, and himself. Yet he felt stronger and less alone.

Reflection Question

- In life's big questions, it is easy to be unsure about the boundaries between supporting caregivers and becoming personal. What do you think about Penny's conversations with Omar?

How Is Anna Doing?

Anna's mom had periods of severe depression and confusion. During these periods, she drank a lot of alcohol. She was not able to take care of Anna and her siblings when she was like this, but the children's father Perry compensated as best he could. Anna's mom did not want help and did not want anyone outside the family to know about the situation.

Anna had a lot of nightmares and did not want to go to school. Perry's twin brother with whom he had close contact recommended him to contact a Family Support Center.

In the first conversation, many good pieces of advice were given about what could help the mother, but Perry did not think he would be able to get his wife to accept any of them. He expressed understanding of the situation not being good for the children. He was grateful for the advice he receives about what is good for Anna and her little sister and what he can do.

Perry did not show up for the next session.

Reflection Questions

- Most children who are dependents do not live in situations that can be characterized as neglect, but occasionally as a helper you may become very worried about a child's situation. What do you think about Anna's situation?
- Imagine that Anna comes back as a 25-year-old and asks you why you didn't do anything when you knew how much she was hurting. What could you answer then?

Laila Wants to Participate

Laila has a boyfriend who has SUD/MH. Laila herself has a social science background and is familiar with the treatment system. Perhaps her experience has contributed to her girlfriend deciding to check herself into a treatment institution. Laila is happy that Leni has made such a decision and is wholly positive about what awaits.

After a short time, Laila becomes frustrated. She feels completely cut off from what is happening around her girlfriend. She is not included in the treatment plan, and it is not easy to keep in touch with Leni, as she is in processes that require her full attention. They both request couple sessions, as they think it is important that they are together in the process that lies ahead.

They do not get it.

Was it the routines that were lacking? Concern for confidentiality? The questions were many, but Laila never got a proper answer.

Now she can only hope that their relationship can withstand the distance and the parallel processes they are in. Laila has little contact with her family after she came out as a lesbian. The family is deeply religious and cannot accept her relationship with Leni. Laila manages to get support for herself but keeps coming back to the question of why she should not be a natural part of the treatment plan around Leni.

Reflection Questions

- How could you as part of the treatment team around Leni have included Laila?
- Imagine that you are the only one in the team who is concerned with including spouses and other family members. What would you say to persuade the others in the team?

Always a Mother

Reyna's daughter Nancy has a severe mental illness, but lives by herself and manages well in everyday life. In periods she uses marihuana, and there is usually a worsening of her condition afterward.

Reyna and Nancy have a close relationship, and the daughter has consented to her team being able to contact her mother and vice versa.

Reyna is often worried about Nancy and anxious that she cannot handle all responsibilities in everyday life. Nancy is good at pulling herself together when she must, and Reyna believes that the team overestimates her. Reyna has time and again brought this up when she sees her daughter failing and consequently must handle defeats.

Reyna feels that her commitment is being questioned, and she believes the team talks behind her back about her being "over involved" and other unpleasant things. But Reyna cannot give up. For her daughter's sake, she continues to "nag." The situation wears on her, and she often feels despair over not being taken seriously.

In meetings and in phone contact, the team is polite and friendly, and often says things like "just call if there is anything." Reyna experiences that there always "is something" but feels like a nuisance if she calls too often.

Her wish is that she could have regular scheduled meetings with the team so that she could gather questions and topics for discussion, as well as being taken seriously as the one who knows her daughter best through 20 years.

Reflection Questions

- What could be the reasons that the team does not include the mother?
- If you were new in the team around the daughter, which questions would have been natural to ask the others about when it comes to caregiver involvement?

On the Same Team

A couple of parents have for several years done their best to follow up their son Max. He has both a drug addiction and major mental health challenges. They have at times been quite exhausted. After they got regular contact with a drug consultant and a therapist, they have experienced it to be better. They still find it painful when Max relapses, but the experience of not being alone has been of great help and support to them. The dialogue with the treatment team has also made them more confident in the choices they make toward their son. They have gained more peace of mind to occasionally say no to what Max suggests they should participate in, and they experience that they to a greater extent manage to take care of themselves. The fact that the parents set some limits also makes it clearer for the follow-up team what Max manages and what he needs help with. Previously, the parents have compensated to a significant degree. Both the team and the parents experience that this cooperation also makes Max take more responsibility for himself and his choices. The parents are of a different cultural background, but the treatment team has been very attentive to using the interpretation service in all important meetings and conversations, and spontaneous contact outside of these is conducted in English.

Reflection Questions

- What works in the contact between the follow-up team and the parents?
- What makes confidentiality not a problem in the collaboration around the son?

Summary

- Caregivers of people with SUD/MH are a group with great burdens. Young carers are particularly vulnerable. They need to be involved and supported by the health services.
- Involving the whole family in the work around people with SUD/MH is important and necessary and has a positive effect both for the person who is sick/ dependent, for adult caregivers, children, and health personnel.
- Recognition, information, inclusion, and cooperation are key words. Health personnel should identify both adults and children who are caregivers and ensure that they are involved and become a natural part of the work around the person who needs support and treatment.
- Caregivers also need support for their own sake. Health personnel should know about relevant services.
- Helpers need to know themselves and their own reactions in meeting with caregivers. And must seek support and guidance among colleagues and from experts in the field when necessary.

Recommended Literature and Online Resources

- Families affected by addiction. A handbook. (Springer Nature, 2025).
- The Carers Worldwide's website highlights the challenges carers face, such as financial strain and isolation, and emphasizes the organization's work in improving carers' physical, emotional, and social well-being. Website: carersworldwide.org
- The Embracing Carers´ website highlights partner organizations, provides valuable guides, and emphasizes the importance of family caregivers worldwide. For

professionals working with carers, this site offers insights into the experiences and challenges faced by caregivers across different countries, promoting better support systems and raising awareness about their vital role in health and social care. Website: embracingcarers.com/resources-for-carers-around-the-world

- The Eurocarers´ website offers resources on advocacy, healthcare, and practical tools for carers. Website: eurocarers.org
- The International Alliance of Carer Organizations website highlights best practices, supports the development of family carer organizations, and facilitates international advocacy for caregiving policies. Website: internationalcarers.org
- The Royal College of Psychiatrists' website provides guidance on treatments, wellbeing strategies, and support for families and caregivers. Website: rcpsych.ac.uk/mental-health/treatments-and-wellbeing.

Acknowledgments I would like to express my sincere gratitude to the staff at Pårørendesenteret [Relatives' center] for generously sharing their real-life experiences and stories. I am also deeply thankful to director Unn Birkeland for her support and for allowing me the time necessary to complete this writing.

References

1. Sælør KT, Biong S. «Å få lyset til å fortsette å brenne»: En fenomenologisk studie av håp hos pårørende i psykisk helsevern ["To keep the light burning": a phenomenological study of hope in family members involved in mental health care]. Scand J Psychol. 2017;4:e3.
2. Government. Regjeringens pårørendestrategi og handlingsplan [The Norwegian Government's CaregiverStrategyandActionPlan].[Internet].[2020-Dec-8;Retrieved2021-Sept-9].Availableat https://www.regjeringen.no/no/dokumenter/regjeringens-parorendestrategi-og-handlingsplan/id2790589/
3. Opinion AS. Nasjonal pårørendeundersøkelse [Norwegian National Caregiver Survey]. [Internet]. [2020-Jan; Retrieved 2021-Sept-9]. Available from https://www.helsedirektoratet.no/rapporter/nasjonal-parorendeundersokelse-2021-2022/%20Nasjonal%20p%C3%A5r%C3%B8rendeunders%C3%B8kelse%202021-2022.pdf/_/attachment/inline/c5685675-dee2-4406-b88b-1514158d767c:a2b63672e5e9a7af37d95aae93d0ca5b271c6d26/Nasjonal%20p%C3%A5r%C3%B8rendeunders%C3%B8kelse%202021-2022.pdf.
4. Pasient-og brukerrettighetsloven [The Norwegian Patient and User Rights Act]. 1999. Lov om pasient-og brukerrettigheter av 1999-07-02 nr 63.
5. Selbekk A, Faugli A, Kufås E, Løvås M, Ruud T. Kunnskapsoppsummering om situasjonen og hjelp til barn og partnere av personer med rusproblemer [Knowledge summary on the situation and support for children and Partners of Individuals with substance use problems]. Akershus: Akershus universitetssykehus; 2019.
6. Bjørkquist C, Hansen GH. Samproduksjon med pårørende til personer med ROP-lidelser [Co-production with relatives of people with concurrent substance use and mental health disorders (SUD/MH)]. Tidsskrift for omsorgsforskning; 2017; 03(3).
7. United Nations Office on Drugs and Crime. World drug report 2023. Vienna: UNODC; 2023. Available at https://www.unodc.org/res/WDR-2023/WDR23_Exsum_fin_DP.pdf
8. Titlestad KB, Mellingen S, Stroebe M, Dyregrov K. Sounds of silence. The "special grief" of drug-death bereaved parents: a qualitative study, Addict Res Theory 2020; 29:2.
9. Biong S, Sveipe EJ, Ravndal E. «Alt verker og alt har satt seg fast»: om pårørendes erfaringer med overdosedødsfall [Everything hurts and everything feels stuck': on relatives' experiences with overdose deaths]. Psykhelse rus. 2015;04(12)

10. Torvik FA, Rognmo K. Barn av foreldre med psykisk lidelse eller alkoholmisbruk. Oslo [Children of parents with mental illness or alcohol use disorder]. Oslo: Norwegian Institute of Public Health; 2011. Report No. 4
11. Meld. St. 30 (2011–2012) Se meg! En helhetlig rusmiddelpolitikk. Alkohol—narkotika—doping ['See Me! A Comprehensive Drug Policy. Alcohol—Drugs—Doping']. Oslo: Oslo: Ministry of Health and Care Services; 2012.
12. Broning S mfl. Selective prevention programs for children from substance-affected families: a comprehensive systematic review. Subst Abuse Treat Prev Policy 2012;7:23.
13. Siegenthaler E, Munder T, Egger M. Effect of preventive interventions in mentally ill parents on the mental health of the offspring: systematic review and meta-analysis. J Am Acad Child Adolesc Psychiatry 2012; Jan;51(1):8–17.e8.
14. Haugland B, Bugge KE, Trondsen MV, Gjesdahl S. Familier i motbakke. På vei mot bedre støtte til barn som pårørende [Families in adversity. On the way to better support for children as relatives]. Bergen: Fagbokforlaget; 2015.
15. Ruud T, Birkeland B, Faugli A, Hagen KA, Hellman A, Hilsen M, et al. Barn som pårørende. In: Resultater fra en multisenterstudie [Children as relatives. Results from a multicenter study]. Lørenskog: Akershus University Hospital, Lørenskog; 2015.
16. The Health Personnel Act. 1999. Lov om helsepersonell av 1999-07-02 nr 64.
17. Kufås E, Weimand B. "Når jeg ser han, får jeg sånn stikk i hjertet …" Barn og ungdom som har foreldre med rusmiddelproblemer—en kvalitativ levekårsstudie [When I see him, I get this sting in my heart … Children and adolescents with parents with substance use problems—a qualitative study of living conditions]. Oslo: The Norwegian Directorate of Health; 2015.
18. Helsenorge.no. Barn som pårørende trenger åpenhet om sykdom [Children as Relatives Need OpennessAboutIllness].[Internett].[Updated2018-Nov-19.Retrieved2021-Sept-11].Available from https://www.helsenorge.no/parorende/barn-psykisk-sykdom#hva-trenger-barn-og-unge
19. Bergem AK. Når barn er pårørende [When Children are Relatives]. Oslo: Gyldendal; 2018.
20. Bergem AK. Jeg skal passe på deg [I will look after you]. Oslo: Gyldendal; 2015.
21. Weimand BM, Hedelin B, B-Hall-Lord ML, Sallstrom C. Left alone with straining but inescapable responsibilities: relative's experiences with mental health services. Issues in Ment Health Nurs 2011; 32(11): 703–710.
22. Weimand BM. Experiences and nursing support of relatives of persons with severe mental illness [doktorgrad]. Karlstad: Karlstad University; 2012.
23. Kletthagen HS. Everyday life of relatives of persons suffering from severe depression: experiences of health, burden, sense of coherence and encounters with psychiatric specialist health services [doktorgrad]. Karlstad: Karlstad University; 2015.
24. Ewertzon M. Familjemedlem till person med psykossjukdom: bemötande och utanförskap i psykiatrisk vård [doktorgrad]. Örebro: Örebro University; 2012.
25. Bradley E. Carers and co-production: enabling expertise through experience? Ment Health Rev J. 2015;20(4):232–41.
26. Cree L, Brooks HL, Berzins K, Fraser C, Lovell K, Bee P. Carers' experiences of involvement in care planning: a qualitative exploration of the facilitators and barriers to engagement with mental health services. BMC Psychiatry. 2015;15(1):208.
27. Rowe J. Great expectations: a systematic review of the literature on the role of family carers in severe mental illness, and their relationships and engagement with professionals. J Psychiatr Ment Health Nurs. 2012;19(1):70–82.
28. Bird V, Premkumar P, Kendall T, Whittington C, Mitchell J, Kuipers E. Early intervention services, cognitive-behavioural therapy and family intervention in early psychosis: systematic review. Br J Psychiatry. 2010 Nov;197(5):350–6.
29. Okpokoro U, Adams CE, Sampson S. Family intervention (brief) for schizophrenia. Cochrane Database Syst Rev 2014 Mar 5;2014(3):CD009802.
30. Akram,Y, Copello A. Family-based interventions for substance misuse: a systematic review of reviews. Lancet 2013; 382: 24.
31. Templeton L, et al. Psychological interventions with families of alcohol misusers: a systematic review. Addict Res Theory. 2010;18(6):616–48.

32. Pettersen SE. Helsearbeideres erfaringer og tanker om ivaretakelse av pårørende til ROP-pasienter. En kvalitativ studie av erfaringer og tanker helsearbeider har om ivaretakelse av pårørende til ROP-pasienter [Healthcare Workers' Experiences and Thoughts on Caring for Relatives of Patients with SUD/MH. A Qualitative Study of Healthcare Workers' Experiences and Thoughts on Caring for Relatives of Patients with SUD/MH [Master's Thesis]. The University of Tromsø; 2017.
33. Kalsås ØR, Selbekk AS, Ness O. «Jeg får et helt annet innblikk»: Fagpersoners erfaringer med familieorientert praksis i rusbehandling ['I get a completely different insight': professionals' experiences with family-oriented practice in substance use treatment]. Nordisk Alkohol Nark. 2020;37(3):243–61.
34. The Norwegian Directorate of Health. Behandling og rehabilitering av rusmiddelproblemer og avhengighet. Psykososiale forhold i rusbehandling: Familie, bolig, økonomi, utdanning, arbeid og nettverk. Involvering av familie og nettverk i rusbehandling [Treatment and Rehabilitation of Substance use Problems and Addiction. Psychosocial Factors in Substance use Treatment: Family, Housing, Finances, Education, Work, and Social Networks. Involvement of Family and Social Networks in Substance use Treatment]. [Internet]. [Updated 2017-Jan-24; Retrieved 2021-Sept-24]. Available from https://www.helsedirektoratet.no/retningslinjer/behandling-og-rehabilitering-av-rusmiddelproblemer-og-avhengighet
35. The Norwegian Directorate of Health. Involvere pårørende i utredning, behandling og oppfølging av pasient eller bruker. I Pårørendeveileder [Involve Relatives in the Assessment, Treatment, and Follow-up of the Patient or User. In the Relatives' Guide]. [Internet]. [Updated 2018-Jan-16; Retrieved 2021-Sept.24]. Availble from https://www.helsedirektoratet.no/tema/parorende
36. The Norwegian Directorate of Health. Helseforetakenes og kommuners plikt til pårørendeinvolvering. I: Pårørendeveileder [The Duty of Health Enterprises and Municipalities to Involve Relatives. In: Caregives Guide]. [Internet]. [Updated 2018-Jan-18. Retrieved 2021-Sept-12]. Available from https://www.helsedirektoratet.no/veiledere/parorendeveileder/helseforetak-og-kommuners-plikter-overfor-parorende
37. Eurocarers. *Support for children as next of kin in Sweden*. Available from: https://eurocarers.org/support-for-children-as-next-of-kin-in-sweden/
38. United Nations Department of Economic and Social Affairs. *Caregiving in an ageing world*. UN DESA Policy Brief No. 143. Available from: https://www.un.org/development/desa/dspd/2020/04/caregiving-in-an-ageing-world/
39. Smeby JC, Mausethagen S. Profesjonskvalifisering [professional qualification]. I: Smeby JC, Mausethagen S. Kvalifisering til profesjonell yrkesutøvelse [in: Smeby JC, Mausethagen S. Qualification for professional practice]. Oslo: Universitetsforlaget; 2017.
40. Powell S, Scott J, Scott L, Jones D. An online narrative archive of patient experiences to support the education of physiotherapy and social work students in north East England: an evaluation study. Health Educ. 2013;26(1):25–32.
41. Lehmann J. Teaching professional health care practice: considering the elements of emotions and artistry. Aust Health Rev. 2008;32(1):127.

14 User Participation: Easier Said Than Done?

Ole Petter Askheim and Henning Pettersen

Abstract

Even though user participation has strong support and backing among both people with substance use and mental disorders (SUD/MH) and the service employees, much is lacking before the involvement is satisfactorily realized. The reasons can be linked to various conditions and levels. They are about both organizational and structural conditions, professional approaches, and tensions. Perhaps it can also be about attitudes toward the target group. People with SUD/MH are a complex and diverse group. Especially toward this group, both profession, morality, and politics can easily be mixed. To put the issues on the agenda and reflect on practice and what controls practice and decisions when user participation is to be realized becomes important.

Keywords

User participation · Co-production · Organizational conditions · Street-level bureaucrats · Professional approaches

O. P. Askheim (✉)
Department of Health and Social Sciences and Section for Mental Health and Rehabilitation, University of Inland Norway, Elverum, Norway
e-mail: ole-petter.askheim@inn.no

H. Pettersen
Department of Health and Social Sciences and Section for Child Protection, Social Work and Social Education, University of Inland Norway, Lillehammer, Norway
e-mail: henning.pettersen@inn.no

T. W. Lie, L. Lien (eds.), *Integrated Treatment of Co-occurring Substance Use and Mental Health Disorders*, https://doi.org/10.1007/978-3-032-20049-5_14

User participation is a fundamental goal in working with people with substance use and mental disorders (SUD/MH). The participation should take place through a close collaboration between the user and the services. Both users and service providers agree on the goal and the importance of user participation for a successful treatment result. At the same time, studies show that there is a long way to go before satisfactory user participation is realized. The chapter discusses issues related to user participation primarily from the services and service providers' perspective. The empirical background is experiences in services for persons with SUD/MH in the Norwegian welfare state, where several studies show that user involvement is pivotal both concerning service development and treatment outcome [1–3]. Thus, knowledge developed in the Norwegian context can have transfer value to other countries and contexts.

Both organizational conditions and different perspectives among service providers can impede user participation. This can have the form of tensions, dilemmas, or challenges and can be related to the lack of time and resources and to dilemmas between accepting the users' wishes and what the employees consider professionally justifiable. In daily practice, service providers find that the realization of the goals of user participation is filled with tensions, dilemmas, and challenges. Such tensions are related to the lack of time and resources, but also to dilemmas between accepting the users' wishes and what the employees consider professionally justifiable. In the tension between acceptance of a diversity of life choices and what can be considered acceptable, the services use management techniques that seek to steer users' choices in the "right" direction.

The mix of problems related to SUD/MH has a low status. The user group is quickly placed in the category of "unworthy needy" where problems are seen as caused by self-inflicted wrong choices. Whether such attitudes toward the target group are found among service providers is also a topic that should be included in the discussion about user participation for people with SUD/MH.

User Participation: A Central Goal for People with SUD/MH

In the Norwegian Directorate of Health's "National guidelines for assessment, treatment and follow-up of people with co-occurring substance use disorder and mental disorder - SUD/MH," user participation is a central area [4]. The guidelines in many ways represent a deepening and concretization of the patient or user's right to participation and information as it is established in the Patient and User Rights Act passed in 1999 [5]. An overarching goal as formulated in the guidelines is that users should have real influence on the design of the services, both on an individual and on a system level. User participation is seen as important from a humanistic perspective so that the users can gain control over important aspects of their life and in this way gain increased authority. The guidelines lead up to four concrete recommendations:

1. The treatment should be arranged so that the patient is able to make their own choices.
2. The treatment should be arranged so that the user receives information about self-help, an understanding of what self-help can imply and about eventual user-controlled measures in their local area.
3. An individual plan should be developed for each individual as a means of user participation.
4. The treatment plan and treatment goals should be developed in collaboration with the user. It is emphasized that the person's own resources must be supported throughout the entire treatment process in order to improve quality of life and to establish a working alliance on the users' own terms.

User participation is presented in a similar way in the Norwegian Health Directorate's "Guide to local mental health work and substance use work in the municipalities" [6]. Already in the preface, it is emphasized that health, care, and welfare services are increasingly focusing on the user's own contribution to change and mastery of health and life situations. User influence is seen as a fundamental value and a guideline for the services. The guide emphasizes more in depth that user participation implies that the user is considered an equal partner in discussions and decisions that concern his or her problem, and that user participation presupposes that the services actively work to develop cooperation with the users, so that the users' coping ability and engagement in the treatment are strengthened.

What Does User Participation Entail?

When user participation is emphasized as a fundamental goal and as a means to realize objectives such as resource development among the users, increased coping and quality of life, the SUD/MH field does not differ from other welfare areas. User participation is increasingly a general principle in politics and service development in the welfare field. What user participation should entail more precisely, however, often appears as unclear. The concept of user participation is not unambiguous. The uncertainty can firstly be linked to the degree of participation. A much-referred source in the literature is Shelley Arnstein's so-called ladder of user participation (ladder of participation) [7]. The ladder illustrates that the degree of user participation is about the degree of exercise of power and transfer of power. It operates with eight steps divided into three main groups, indicating the degree of participation from what is characterized as nonparticipation and symbolic participation at the lower steps to various degrees of user power indicated as partnership, delegated power, and citizen control at the top of the ladder.

The concept of user participation can also be linked to different "welfare discourses" that reflect different ways of viewing the relationship between individuals and the public. The discourse concept can simply be defined as an organization of knowledge and thought patterns that underlie how a phenomenon is defined and expressed linguistically, and which represents power. When a discourse takes hold, it will guide further development of the field of knowledge [8]. In the literature, a main distinction is often made between a "democratic" or "rights-oriented"- and a "consumer-oriented" user participation discourse [9]. The rights discourse springs from the individual's democratic right to influence his/her own life by virtue of being a citizen. In the consumer discourse, it is the individual user as a consumer of services that is central. The individual is seen as the one who best knows his/her needs and therefore is able to make the best choices about which services are needed. The discourse is linked to a market thinking where users should have the freedom to choose service providers who can best meet their needs and interests.

In recent years, various terms with the prefix "co" have gained increasing traction as an approach to user participation. In welfare and care politics, co-production and co-creation are concepts that are increasingly replacing the concept of user participation both internationally and in Norway [10, 11]. In literature, co-production is often used in a more narrow sense than co-creation. The term is linked to a collaboration to produce specific services and benefits. Co-creation also focuses on how co-production creates new relationships and common values between the actors [12]. Definitions of the terms co-creation and co-production, however, largely overlap, and they are used interchangeably in empirical studies [13]. As the wording indicates, it is the partnership, cooperation, and interaction between the service providers and the users that are in focus. The approaches mark opposition to both a hierarchical approach in service design, where the service provider is seen as the active expert and the user assumes a passive recipient role, and a market model, where the user's role is limited to being a consumer of services [14, 15]. Users are seen here as full-fledged and competent citizens with the right to influence services that concern them and have resources and competence that can improve these services. Instead of the user being seen as a "participant," they are seen as a co-producer or co-creator and an equal contributor with a complementary competence to the service providers. Through mutual relationships in welfare production, increased trust and cohesion between the actors will be created.

Primarily based on treatment and diagnostics, the term "shared decision-making" is used within the health service to describe the desired communication between the patient or user and the services [16]. The term was first used for patients in cancer treatment, who could consider the effect and side effects related to different treatment alternatives, but has been extended and is utilized in a couple of health areas. The basis for practicing shared decision-making is that none of the treatment alternatives appear to be obviously the best for the patients, but it becomes a question of how to weigh advantages and disadvantages against each other. Such a trade-off will in principle also depend on values and preferences [17].

In Norwegian welfare policy, the concept of user participation was introduced in the 1990s [18]. This does not mean that there was no attention to the users before. From the 1970s, there was an increasing emphasis on user groups' rights [19]. However, it was mainly about participation at the system level via interest organizations, through representation in councils and committees and through expressing opinions in hearings. Concepts such as "co-determination" and "influence" were applied. Alm Andreassen compares the development with the emergence of workers' rights to co-determination and influence in matters that concerned them as they were drawn into formal cooperation with state authorities. The cooperative principles were extended to a "general corporatism under the administration" [20, p. 89].

When the concept of "user participation" came into welfare policy in the 1990s, the users' rights were extended to the individual level. The users' individual right to influence and co-determination was affirmed as a fundamental democratic human right. The rights perspective is manifested by enshrining individual user rights in the legislation. In 1999, the act on patient and user rights was passed (amended to the Patient and User Rights Act in 2011) [5]. In 2001 in Norway, the right to have an individual plan drawn up for people with "long-term and coordinated services from the public aid services" was enshrined in the act. Later, the legal basis was extended to the Health and Care Services Act, the Mental Health Care Act, and the Specialist Health Services Act [21].

The concepts of co-production and co-creation had their breakthrough in the Norwegian public report "Innovation in Care" (2011) where the concepts are presented as fundamental principles for the development of the future care services [22]. The perspective is continued in policy documents across government constellations throughout the 2000s, not least in the health and care sector [18]. In many ways, the approach can also be seen as a continuation of the cooperation thinking from the system level to the individual level. Users and services are presented with common interests in cooperating trustfully to create good solutions.

As stated in the guidelines for assessment, treatment, and follow-up of people with SUD/MH and the guide in local mental health work and substance use work, user participation appears as a "co-project." Plans and objectives should be developed in cooperation between the users and the services. This should be done by taking the users' resources and wishes as a starting point and by providing the necessary information for them to make their choices.

Broad Support for a Collaborative User Participation Process

Research shows that a trustful interaction process is strongly emphasized by both users with SUD/MH and service providers. Studies among users confirm that positive collaborative relationships where service providers respect the users' perspectives and the partnership they are involved in are given decisive weight for a positive result [23, 24]. Respect for the users' autonomy, flexibility that permits choices, and partnership with the therapist are given decisive importance for achieving positive results. It is seen as crucial that users feel accepted and met with positive expectations and that they are seen as equal citizens of society. Furthermore, the importance of service providers expressing faith in them and not giving up, but going together with them also in situations where it is difficult, is emphasized. As Lauveng summarizes, it is about being seen as a unique human being and the difference between being treated and interacting [25, p. 136].

In Ness and colleagues' study [23], users also emphasize the importance of service providers being able to provide more practical help and not least to have the service employees as a discussion and conversation partner where they can get help to clarify their own situation and sort out what is important vs. less important problems. In this way, they can through the collaboration make their own reflected decisions and choices themselves. This also implies that service providers must have an understanding and respect for the fact that people can be different and prioritize their lives in different ways.

Users' perception of what is important in a participation process harmonizes well with how employees in the services for people with SUD/MH formulate the importance of user participation. Studies among municipal employees clearly show that for them, user participation appears meaningful and something they are keen to promote in service delivery [25, 26]. Statements like these are quoted in Krane Hanssen and Henriksen's study from municipal substance use measures [27, p. 146]: "We get nowhere unless the user is involved and participates in the processes that concern him"; "We make decisions together with the participants"; "I plan the days according to the users' needs." Service providers describe as particularly meaningful that they have a close relationship with the user and that the user should be involved in deciding what he or she needs. Øydgard and colleagues [28, p. 121] relate the employees' attitude to what Järvinen and Mik Meyer [29] describe as the ideal of strengthening citizens' autonomy and responsibility. By involving the users in the choice of solutions, their self-determination is strengthened, and the professional's role is to support the users in their positive development through supportive relational work. Employees are also concerned that they have an advocacy role for the users as caretakers of their rights and dignity, and that it is sometimes necessary for them to defend the users in encounters with other public agencies. In a similar way as the users in Ness and colleagues' study [23] pointed at the importance of service providers being able to contribute as a conversation partner in situations where life appears complicated, employees also emphasize the importance of them being able to function as "co-actors" in the user's life, to understand and find solutions.

Collectively, the employees clearly express a recovery perspective on their work. Recovery is an approach that has strongly entered local mental health work. In the Norwegian Directorate of Health's "Guide for local mental health work and substance use work for adults" [6], recovery appears as a central principle. Similarly to user participation, recovery is not a clear-cut concept [30]. The basic principle, however, is that coping on the users' terms should be facilitated for [31]. The users should participate in all decisions about their own life, and their own priorities should be the basis for treatment. Professionals have an important responsibility in helping users understand the consequences of their choices. A trust-based collaboration between users and employees thus becomes a fundamental foundation in the work. In line with this, the health authorities have launched several national strategies to incorporate the user perspective in treatment. These are all strategies that have been developed as a result of demands put forward by user and family organizations: the right to free treatment choice in specialist health services [32], medication-free treatment offers [33] and user-controlled admissions in mental health care [34]. Especially, user-controlled admissions have been shown to reduce the need for hospital admissions and give users strengthened autonomy, sense of responsibility, and increased daily coping [35].

Good Intentions: Failing Results

Despite positive attitudes among employees in services for people with SUD/MH, it still seems to be a long way to go before user participation is realized in a satisfactory way in practice. Lien summarizes that there are systematic deficiencies when it comes to how users in practice experience participation [36]. Many do not feel that their own resources have been asked for or that their own priorities and wishes have been in demand. In Thommesen's doctoral thesis on the experiences of people with SUD/MH, they tell that they have to work hard and long before they manage to get employees in the services to see the challenges from their perspective [37]. When the Ministry of Health and Care Services introduced a "standardized patient course" for mental health and substance use from January 1, 2019, an important goal was to increase user participation and user satisfaction and coherent and coordinated patient courses [38]. An evaluation of the scheme shows that users feel that they are not involved enough in the course and lack real influence over the service offers [39]. They experience a lack of communication and information between different therapists both within the same unit and between different services because they constantly have to repeat the same information to the services. Users fear that the standardized course, due to capacity problems, means that there is less time to develop relationships with service providers in different parts of the course and that it becomes more of an efficiency measure than a scheme that strengthens user influence.

Tensions, Dilemmas, and Challenges

The clear feedback from the users about the importance of participation and positive goodwill and good intentions among service providers, in other words, does not seem to result in user participation being realized in satisfactory ways. Counter mechanisms and tensions related to the implementation must be identified and given attention.

While the employees are committed to realizing user participation through a trustful collaboration with the users, they also portray the work as filled with tensions. The tensions can be linked to their role as what Michael Lipsky calls "street-level bureaucrats" [40]. The employees are the executors of the welfare policy goals. They interact directly with the users at the "ground level" and are supposed to take care of their interests, but at the same time, as street-level bureaucrats, they are part of an organization, a bureaucratic structure that sets guidelines and expectations for them.

The work of street-level bureaucrats is characterized by discretion. They are in "human-treating organizations" where each case must be assessed based on individual considerations. They thus have some freedom of action in their work. Through interpretations of rules and regulations and prioritization of resources, they gain significant influence. They become policy producers as much as executors of the approved policy [41]. At the same time, their work situation is filled with tension. Hjörne, Juhila, and van Nijnatten link the tensions to three main dilemmas [42]: between autonomy and control, between responsiveness to individual needs and standardization, and between supply and demand. Altogether, this means that street-level bureaucrats will inevitably experience difficult priority conflicts within limited resources, and they must maneuver between the wishes and expectations of the users and the demands and guidelines from the organization they are part of, and from the surroundings. Often some ideals must be abandoned for others to be realized [43].

In studies of how employees in services for people with SUD/MH seek to implement user participation, they highlight several issues as difficult and filled with conflicts [25, 26]. A field of tensions is linked to the tension between Hanssen and colleagues' distinction between "the users' perspective" and "a professional user perspective" [44], or between the users' wishes, and what the professionals consider to be in their best interest. These are dilemmas that arise in daily practice, or what Komesaroff characterizes as "microethics" [45]. The dilemmas are linked to the users' health or functional ability and to what extent they are seen as capable of making "right" or "good" choices from a professional point of view. As one employee at a housing facility for people with mental disorders put it:

> The dilemma in psychiatry in general is that it's often not so beneficial for them [the users] to be in control. They think they have a right to this and that, but often it's not so beneficial for them to control things themselves. There are constantly difficult ethical dilemmas in this field. They have a right to user participation, while at the same time they should not control everything. You have the concept that is so nice and great, but at the same time in practice it's a bit difficult [25, p. 177].

At the same time, there are many users who cannot participate in shared decision-making, because they are not capable of it [46]. Shared decision-making presupposes that there are choices, and that the users understand what different choices will entail. This is not always the case for many of those with SUD/MH.

The tensions will be present even if the employees work from a recovery perspective. Even though the basic perspective here is that one should work on the user's terms and accept and live with diversity and differences [30], dilemmas related to what are the limits of what employees can accept from a "professional user perspective" may arise in practice.

Another area of tension is related to the resources the employees have at their disposal and the organizational frameworks within which the employees operate. Contributing to making the residents independent and self-reliant is complicated by scarce resources and lack of staffing, and everyday life will easily be dominated by daily, routine activities. The employees feel that they neither have the time nor the resources to meet the expectations from both the authorities and the users [26, 27]. Especially toward people with such complex problems as SUD/MH, this is experienced as filled with conflicts. The daily work is thus characterized by constant dilemmas about what and who the employees should spend time and resources on.

The work is also greatly influenced by structural barriers related to legislation, economy, and professional power. This is made visible, among other things, through the closure of 24-hour treatment in mental health care, through the shift arrangements in health services, and by limited opening hours for the outreach teams that have been developed in recent years (read about ACT and FACT-teams in Chap. 12).

A tension that is highlighted here is the tension between the demands for systematic planning and documentation of the work, on the one hand, and the need to spend time with the users to build trust and relationships, on the other [27]. Karlsson and Borg [30] point out as a dilemma that health policy authorities have contributed to developing strategies and technologies to control, manage, and monitor the users through the use of professional guides and guidelines for mental health and substance use work, while the same authorities impose on professionals to work in line with the ideals of user participation, human rights, and recovery. However, these are not necessarily opposing strategies as health policy guidelines and advisors in the field in recent years have increased emphasis on services containing recovery-oriented practices and user participation. In Øydgard and colleagues' study about mental health work in the municipalities [28], service providers express, on the one hand, a resignation over the extent of the documentation they are required to do. But at the same time, some express frustration over the lack of documentation because this means that they do not know the users' history and cannot see what has been tried before or found earlier.

The tensions expressed here are focused in recent literature about the street-level bureaucrat role where it is shown that new documentation and control regimes like New Public Management reduce the possibilities for discretion by focusing on seemingly objective standardizations that the effects of the work are measured from [47]. Hjörne et al. [42] argue that the increasing management thinking in welfare work affects all three of the mentioned dilemmas (autonomy vs. control, responsiveness to individual needs vs. standardization and supply vs. demand) in a negative way. This management paradigm is expressed within the mental health and substance use field by the intention that everything and everyone can be measured and quantified. It involves a reductionist view of what is legitimate knowledge and treatment [48]. This can also be exemplified by the introduction of activity-based funding (ISF), which the national health authorities implemented in specialized somatic health care in 1997. This financing scheme was implemented in mental health care in 2016 following the model from the somatic hospitals, with the main purpose of stimulating cost-effective patient treatment [49].

Literature on street-level bureaucrats has recently also focused more specifically on how organizational conditions, professional norms, and cultural conditions influence the work of street-level bureaucrats and frame their opportunities for discretion [47]. To some extent, issues related to organizational conditions and professional attitudes are linked together. The point here is that different organizational forms and professional approaches will have consequences for the view the different sectors and professions have on user participation and what significance it has for how user participation is sought to be implemented. Furthermore, it is a challenge that recommended treatment approaches despite good intentions do not necessarily strengthen user participation. The evaluation of the mentioned standardized course for mental health and substance use shows that a great deal remains to be achieved concerning more user participation and coherent and coordinated courses. This applies especially to routines and measures that are directly aimed at patients, for example, involving patients in the preparation of treatment plans and active participation of a course coordinator [50].

People with SUD/MH are a complex and composite group that requires comprehensive approaches and good coordination between different parts of the services [51]. Bjørkquist and Hansen [52] characterize the challenges the services face in relation to this group as what in organizational literature is called "wicked problems" [53, 54]. These are problems that elude simple solutions and where better coordination between public agencies is highlighted as an important tool for handling the challenges.

A challenge is that measures for people with SUD/MH should be coordinated both within and between specialist health services and municipal services. In 2009, the so-called "Coordination reform" was passed in the Norwegian parliament [55]. The intention was to establish better coordination between the municipal services and the specialist care. The municipalities were given a greater responsibility for treatment and follow-up of patients within substance use and mental health, but the responsibility is still shared between the municipalities and the specialist health service linked to the regional health trusts. In the municipalities, the responsibility is distributed between different sectors.

Despite these coordination efforts, there still exist different cultures and different professional logics in the work with people with SUD/MH. At the state level, substance use care and psychiatry are partly retained as two different policy areas with very different histories and different status. At the service level, the tensions can be manifested both within organizations at the same administrative level and between levels, for example, between primary and secondary services. There are conflicts between medical and social work approaches and whether the problem should primarily be seen as a mental health problem or a substance use problem. The conflict between a medical approach and a recovery-oriented approach can illustrate the point [56, 57]. How the socialization of the professions that populate the services occurs will thus also have significance for their discretion [58]. Through professional socialization, service providers will adopt some values and attitudes that will shape professional practice and how they meet the tension between satisfying the users' desires and what the professionals believe is in their best [59]. In this context, the question becomes how a lack of coordination and different understandings of problems related to substance use and mental health affect how user participation is implemented in practice.

How the services are more specifically organized in the municipalities will also have an impact on the street-level bureaucrats' "room for maneuver" for user participation [60]. The street-level bureaucrats might experience conflicting institutional logics between the actors: On the one hand, realizing goals for cooperation based on equality and confidence; and on the other hand, a bureaucratic logic based on hierarchical organization, sectorization, and goal-oriented rationality [10, 61]. Wilkins and Wenger emphasize that street-level bureaucrats in less hierarchical organizations have greater opportunities for discretion and thus user participation than employees who work within strictly hierarchical structures [59]. Voorberg et al. point at the importance of organizational structures and processes that encourage and invite to good communication for how cooperation succeeds [13]. In a study on municipal implementation of user participation [26], employees in a housing arrangement for people with mental disorders with so-called "co-living shifts" highlight that such organization makes the work situation more flexible and that it becomes easier to be responsive to the residents' wishes and needs when they arise.

> We stay here more, we don't have to say that now I'm off duty, so now I can not take that talk, because now I have to report. We are allowed to sit down with one for two hours, if he needs you to be there for two hours, because then you can postpone other tasks until the evening, it can actually wait - the report that needs to be written or "whatever". So, in that sense it's not just that I have a lot of free time, but you see that the residents are so much more relaxed when they see that ... yes, now I have him here for two days. [26, p. 177]

People with SUD/MH: Not Worthy Needy?

In addition to coordination problems, lack of holistic approaches, and different professional perspectives and tensions as important reasons for lacking user participation, one might also ask if attitudes toward the target group are a contributing cause. Not least, people with extensive substance use problems are a group with low status both in the services and in the population more generally. Mental disorders are among the diseases medical practitioners rank with the lowest status next to fibromyalgia, and the trend has not changed in the period between 1990 and 2014 [62]. Leukemia, brain tumor, and heart attack are at the top of the list. Stigmatization might create substantial challenges for user participation if stereotypical perceptions of substance users lay premises for how the services are outlined and not the wishes and needs of the users [63]. What becomes particularly stigmatizing for people who are dependent on illegal drugs is that they, according to current legislation, are considered criminals while the addiction is also defined as a disease.

In welfare politics, a distinction is made between "worthy" and "unworthy needy" [64]. Worthy needy cannot be blamed for their problems. They are seen as victims of tragedies and deserve full sympathy and support. The unworthy needy, on the other hand, have themselves to blame for the difficult situation they are in. Not least, people with substance use disorders are perceived in such a category, and some experience being treated in a condemning way and with a lack of respect [65]. Fuller uses the term "rankism" as a term for various forms of discrimination that all have common roots [66]. They all have to do with the consideration of some people or groups to have greater dignity than others. "Rankism" will thus also have an impact on the extent to which different user groups are worthy to participate in their treatment or problem solving. To what extent such attitudes persist and can be found in parts of the services and in the population more generally is also a topic that belongs in the discussion about user participation for people with SUD/MH. If the stigma connected to persons with substance disorders also affects the involved services, the users' status and rights to involvement will be further reduced [63, 67].

However, there are signs that point in a different direction. Several stakeholders advocates for a new substance use reform with less focus on punishment and more treatment for those who use illegal substance This has been an ongoing debate among central politicians for several years, and recently the political parties in the parliament reached an agreement stating that the use of illegal substances shall still be punishable, but wish to legislate that persons having severe substance use problems shall not be punished [68].

Participation as Governance

Inspired by the French philosopher Michel Foucault, prevailing approaches to user participation have been criticized for representing a soft form of power exercise and control of the users [69, 70]. A fundamental starting point for Foucault is that the exercise of power in modern societies does not occur through an authoritarian and repressive use of power. On the contrary, it is exercised through exerting influence of formally free individuals, their actions, and self-perceptions. The power seeks to bring out certain perceptions and capacities in the individual and enable him or her to act in certain ways. The power thus becomes "productive" in the sense of creating or constructing. It makes people behave in certain ways rather than preventing them from behaving in others.

Foucault links such an exercise of power to the concept of discourse [71]. The discourse establishes "regimes of truth" where certain understandings of reality achieve status as self-evident. The power acts in this way as disciplining by setting the frames for what is considered normal, good, or healthy. The productive exercise of power is about bringing the individual toward a norm or a standard of normality as it is defined in the prevailing "regimes of truth." By getting people to apply these as a frame for reality and for themselves, people's thinking, attitudes, and actions will be influenced.

The sociologist Pierre Bourdieu used the term "doxa" or "the doxic field" to describe aspects of culture and society that most people take for granted and which they find no reason to question [72]. It is a "silent knowledge," something that is considered self-evident and not subject to discussion, but which frames the actions of individuals. Bourdieu also links such self-evident truths to the more invisible aspects of power in society. A fundamental starting point is that our practices, expressions, and interactions must be related to objective, structural conditions, often beyond the individual's consciousness. For those in power, one of the most important tools is to produce and implement categories of understanding that we immediately apply to various areas. The truths take on the character of doxa and appear so natural that those dominated submit to the silent knowledge.

In the field of welfare policy, such truths are taken for granted through positively charged concepts such as health, wellness, and a good and dignified life. Not least, the active, participating, and responsible individual today appears as an ideal that politics and services should strive to realize [73]. As stated in the White Paper "Future Care" from 2013 [74]:

> A vibrant welfare society should help citizens to make the best possible use of their own resources, and not make them passive service recipients. The greatest care resource therefore is located within the users themselves. Activation and self-help can contribute to better utilization of society's total resources. The development in health and care services has not sufficiently emphasized the opportunities users themselves have to participate in planning and production of service provision and actively contribute to restoring or improving their level of function. (p. 49)

For those who have difficulties in asserting their rights or participating in decisions about their own treatment, this can pose new challenges. As Lauveng points out, it can result in further stigmatization and some feeling of yet another failure in life [75].

The Professions as Performers of Productive Power

As mentioned, the street-level bureaucrats are the implementers of the welfare policy goals. In other words, they are the ones who should fill the goals of health, dignity, life mastery, and quality of life with content. They should interpret the welfare policy objectives, rules, and regulations, and prioritize resources. This work takes place in the tension between safeguarding the interests of the users and the demands and expectations of the organization they are part of and their environment. In this work, they exercise considerable discretion and thus also considerable power.

The street-level bureaucrats are portrayed as the central executors of what Foucault calls bio-power [76]. They should lead the population with the purpose of promoting truth, quality of life, and safety based on the intentions of the established "truth regime." They play a central role both in the production of knowledge that forms the basis for governing the population or specific groups and in that they are the ones who initiate and assist in the governance processes. Their task is to guide those who do not live somewhat in accordance with the ideas of how citizens in the welfare state should live their lives, in the "right direction" [77].

In this work, the professions use various "power technologies" [78, p. 23], that is, instruments, methods, and institutional procedures that seek to control the individual's behavior and subject it to certain goals and forms of discipline and control. A particularly important approach is what is referred to as "self-technologies," which is about how the individual makes himself the object of his/her own governance. The individual puts into use the socially created knowledge when understanding and defining him–/herself. This becomes the starting point for the individual's identity formation and self-understanding. Foucault characterizes the process with the concept "governmentality," which he emphasizes as a particularly significant form of governance in the modern, liberal society [79]. The governance will in principle always take place by directing the governance toward the individual's self-governance.

Foucault [79] characterizes the power that the professions (e.g., health and social workers, psychologists, and educators) exercise as "pastoral power" [80], which is not exercised through repressive control, but through guidance, counseling, and care [81, 82]. Just as the clergy offered salvation by possessing the religious truth, the professions guide individuals toward good health, wellness, quality of life, and happiness. The professionals' task becomes to provide the client with the necessary knowledge that enables him/her to make "independent" but at the same time correct, good, and healthy choices. Hessle [83] portrays the process as "invading with goodwill," while Villadsen describes the exercise of power as a "governance through clarification" [70, p. 215]. This is done partly through increased emphasis on evidence-based methods defined by researchers and professionals. From the professionals, it can be argued that what they do is to enrich the client with so much information that he/she is better able to make a conscious and independent choice. Service users are portrayed as individuals with resources, autonomy, and the right and ability to make independent choices. But at the same time, the choices should be responsible and made within frames that are perceived as acceptable and valued. They should be made within certain norms, rules, and boundaries, for example, the prevailing perceptions of what is seen as a good, responsible, and respectable life. If you have a substance use problem, the goal is to get you sober or at least limit the substance use and create opportunities to participate and master society and have a better and more dignified life as defined by the established truth regime. The moral divide between good and evil, sinful and pure, continues in new forms in the scientific divide between healthy and pathological, normal and deviant [78].

> It is this version of "freedom" that is strived for in the modern welfare state and not other and more anarchistic versions - for example, the freedom to believe that pension and free weekends are absolutely in preference to work and everyday life. The slogan "freedom under responsibility" is known by even the most maladjusted anti-citizen, and it is this kind of freedom that social workers and educators talk about when the users are to be involved. [77, p. 45–46]

The governance of pastoral power implies that not all choices and statements that the users come up with in the dialogue with the services without further ado are respected and accepted. As a professional, you can choose to continue the dialogue toward clarifications that bring the individual closer to what Villadsen calls his/her "real self" [70], but which is so far not realized due to, for example, social deviance, substance use, and apathy. By giving the client knowledge and information that increases his or her capacity for self-governance, the person is made better able to make "free choices." However, in this way the user's wishes are not "free." They do not exist in themselves, but are products of certain discursive processes, practical techniques, and power relations. Paternalism penetrates in a “soft” and “invisible” way.

The fact that user participation in practice can implicate a scant visible exercise of power applies especially where user participation is presented as a collaborative project as user participation appears in the guidelines for investigation, treatment, and follow-up of people with SUD/MH [4]. An awareness of such power processes is thus important for service providers who want to work from a recovery approach where the patient’s own wishes, goals, and visions should be leading for the treatment and which emphasizes the diversity and differences in what people perceive as good and dignified lives. At the same time, the therapists face various dilemmas. They should, on one hand, be loyal to their employer and at the same time offer treatment that is effective and which they consider is in the users’ best interest. Especially in our efficiency-oriented healthcare system, such different considerations can be difficult to reconcile. The awareness among professionals must therefore also include an awareness of how they relate and maneuver in such fields of tension.

Critics also point out that in the literature on co-creation and co-production, the power perspective is glaringly absent [84, 85]. There is a basic harmony perspective underlying the co-creation and co-production thinking. Without being questioned, the participating actors are presented as having the same goals and a common interest in achieving the good holistic solutions. Torfing and colleagues present it as both researchers and practitioners see the co-creation process as a pragmatic, problem-solving process that is free of power and politics [86]. Similarly, Lund and Hole point out that challenges and potential interest conflicts between patient and healthcare professionals within a shared decision-making thinking are little discussed [87]. Healthcare professionals may experience challenges in accepting or understanding that the patient has other values and preferences than what prevails in the health services.

In summary, the contributions from Foucault and Bourdieu together provide a clear picture of how the emphasis on participation and collaboration with the users in practice can involve a refined governance. Through health and social workers’ notions of what is normal and abnormal, right and wrong, often appears as unconscious, or what Bourdieu calls “doxic,” a governance of the users toward these values can appear as a consciousness raising of the user. The process will appear as one where the users gain insight into and become aware of what is in their own best interest. At the same time, such processes take place through what Foucault referred to as productive power processes. Through the use of various power technologies used by the professionals, certain perceptions and attitudes are brought forward that make the service users act in certain ways. And it happens as the individuals seemingly freely decide and choose these actions and forms of behavior. Such a realization implies not that the professions can and should avoid governing and exercising power in interaction with the users. The relationship between the users and the service providers is by definition asymmetric. And the relationship is initiated because the users need help that is both right and necessary to govern. The point is primarily to be aware of how the invisible power impacts both users and service providers.

Summary

- User participation in the SUD/MH area has broad support both among service users and employees.
- In practice, the users often experience systematic shortages of participation.
- Lacking participation can be attributed to both legislation, organizational and cultural conditions, lacking resources, public attitudes, and professional judgments.
- In their daily practice, employees experience dilemmas between accommodating to the users' wishes and what they as professionals think are the best for the users.
- Collaborative user participation can cover up professional governance.
- Reflections among the employees over what directs their practice and decisions are of utmost importance.

Reflection Questions

- Are there certain challenges and dilemmas in practicing user involvement among people with SUD/MH—if so, which ones, and why?
- To what degree and in which way can various professional approaches to SUD/MH have impact on how user involvement is practiced?
- To what degree and in which way can attitudes to people with SUD/MH influence the degree of user involvement?
- Which tools can the professionals apply in order to guide the service users in the "right direction" and at the same time can be viewed as user involvement?
- What are the challenges, dilemmas, and possibilities for establishing shared decision-making for persons with SUD/MH?

Recommended Literature and Online Resources

- Askheim OP, Christensen K, Fluge S, Guldvik I. User participation in the Norwegian welfare context. An analysis of policy discourses. J Soc Policy. 2017;46(3):583–601. https://doi.org/10.1017/S0047279416000817.
- Beecher B, Young JA, Carbajal B, Fair B, Guarino JE. Perceptions of mental health and substance use services by individuals experiencing homelessness. Soc Sci J. 2023:1–14. https://doi.org/10.1080/03623319.2023.2229163.
- Liu P, Currie S, Adamyk-Simpson J. What are the most important dimensions of quality for addiction and mental health services from the perspective of its users? Patient Exp J. 2018;5(1):106–14. https://doi.org/10.35680/2372-0247.1244.
- Neech SGB, Scott H, Priest HM, Bradley EJ, Tweed AE. Experiences of user involvement in mental health settings: user motivations and benefits. J Psychiatr Ment Health Nurs. 2018;25:327–37. https://doi.org/10.1111/jpm.12466.
- Pettersen H, Landheim A, Skeie I, Biong S, Brodahl M, Benson V, Davidson L. Helpful ingredients in the treatment of long-term substance use disorders: a

collaborative narrative study. Subst Abuse: Res Treat. 2019;13:1–9. https://doi.org/10.1177/1178221819844996.

- Sheikhan NY, Kuluski K, McKee S, Hiebert M, Hawke LD. Exploring the impact of engagement in mental health and substance use research: a scoping review and thematic analysis. Health Expect. 2023;26:1806–19. https://doi.org/10.1111/hex.13779.

References

1. Brekke E, Lien L, Davidson L, Biong S. First-person experience of recovery in co-occurring mental health and substance use conditions. Adv Dual Diagn. 2017;10(1):13–34.
2. Pettersen H, Landheim A, Skeie I, Biong S, Brodahl M, Benson V, Davidson L. Helpful ingredients in the treatment of long-term substance use disorders: a collaborative narrative study. Subst Abuse: Res Treatment. 2019;13:1–9.
3. Semb R, Sælør KT, Borg M. Resist or adapt? A narrative analysis of endeavors for belonging among young adults with co-occurring substance use and mental health problems. J Psychosoc Rehabil Ment Health. 2021;8:273–85.
4. Helsedirektoratet [Norwegian Directorate of Health]. Nasjonal faglig retningslinje for utredning, behandling og oppfølging av personer med samtidig ruslidelse og psykisk lidelse – ROP-lidelser. [National professional guideline for assessment, treatment and follow-up of people with co-occurring substance use and mental disorder – SUD/MH]. Oslo: Norwegian Directorate of Health; 2012.
5. Lov om pasient- og brukerrettigheter (pasient- og brukerrettighetsloven) [Act on Patient and User Rights (Patient and User Rights Act)]. Oslo: Ministry of Health and Care Services; 1999.
6. Helsedirektoratet. Psykisk helse- og rusarbeid for voksne. Nasjonal veileder. [Guide in local mental health and substance use work for adults]. Oslo: Norwegian Directorate of Health; 2025. https://www.helsedirektoratet.no/veiledere/psykisk-helse-og-rusarbeid-for-voksne
7. Arnstein SR. A ladder of citizen participation. J Am Inst Planners. 1969;35(4):216–24.
8. Jørgensen MW, Phillips L. Diskursanalyse som teori og metode. [Discourse analysis as theory and method]. Fredriksberg: Roskilde Universitetsforlag; 1999.
9. Braye S. Participation and involvement in social care: an overview. In: Kenshall H, Littlechild R, editors. User involvement and participation in social care. Research informing practice. London: Jessica Kingsley Publishers; 2000.
10. Røiseland A, Sørensen E, Torfing J. Advancing co-creation in local governance. The role of coping strategies and constructive hybridization. Edward Elgar Publishing; 2024.
11. Torfing J, Sørensen E, Røiseland A. Transforming the public sector into an arena for co-creation: barriers, drivers, benefits, and ways forward. Adm Soc. 2019;51(5):795–825.
12. Brandsen T, Steen T, Verschure B. Co-production and co-creation: engaging citizens in public services. New York: Routledge; 2018.
13. Voorberg WH, Bekkers VJ, Tummers LG. A systematic review of co-creation and co-production. Embarking on the social innovation journey. Public Manag Rev. 2015;17(9):1333–57.
14. Hunter S, Ritchie P. Co-production and personalisation in social care. London & Philadelphia: Jessica Kingsley Publishers; 2007.
15. Pestoff V. Citizens and co-production of welfare services. Public Manag Rev. 2006;8(4):503–19.
16. Kienlin S, Eiring Ø, Kasper J. Samvalg [Shared decision-making]. Michael. 2020;17(24):127–43.
17. Peterson M. An introduction to decision theory. New York: Cambridge University Press; 2009.

18. Askheim OP, Christensen K, Fluge S, Guldvik I. User participation in the Norwegian welfare context. An analysis of policy discourses. J Soc Policy. 2017;46(3):583–601. https://doi.org/10.1017/S0047279416000817.
19. St. meld. [White paper] no. 25 (1996–97) Åpenhet og helhet [Openness and wholeness] Oslo: Norwegian Ministry of Social Affairs and Health; 1996.
20. Andreassen TA. Brukermedvirkning, politikk og velferdsstat [User participation, politics, and welfare state]. Oslo: Arbeidsforskningsinstituttet [Work Research Institute]; 2004.
21. Lov om kommunale helse- og omsorgstjenester m.m. (helse- og omsorgstjenesteloven). Act on municipal health and care services, etc. (Health and care services act). Act 201106-24-30. Lov om etablering og gjennomføring av psykisk helsevern (psykisk helsevernloven) [Act on establishment and implementation of mental health care (Mental Health Care Act)]. Act 2019-06-21-48. Lov om spesialisthelsetjenesten m.m. (spesialisthelsetjenesteloven) [Act on specialist health services, etc. (Specialist Health Services Act]. Act 2020-12-04134.
22. NOU [Norwegian Public Report] 2011:11 Innovasjon i omsorg [Innovation in care services]. Oslo: Ministry of Health and Care Services; 2011.
23. Ness O, Kvello Ø, Borg M, Semb R, Davidson L. Sorting things out together: Young adults' experiences of collaborative practices in mental health and substance use care. Am J Psychiatr Rehabil. 2017;20(2):126–42.
24. Pettersen H, Lofthus A-M. Brukererfaringer med psykiske helsetjenester. Hva viser oppsummert forskning? [User experiences with mental health services. What does summarized research show?]. Tidsskrift for psykisk helsearbeid [Journal of Mental Health Work]. 2018;15(2–3):112–23.
25. Lauveng A. Vi må slutte å behandle samtidig rus og psykisk lidelse—vi skal behandle mennesker [We must stop treating simultaneous substance use and mental illness – we should treat people]. In: Landheim A, Wiig FL, Brendbekken M, Brodahl M, Biong S, editors. Et bedre liv. [A better life]. Oslo: Gyldendal; 2016.
26. Askheim OP. Brukermedvirkning – fra politikk til praksis. Hvordan implementeres de politiske målsettingene på bakkenivå? [User participation – from politics to practice. How are the political objectives implemented at the grassroots level?]. Tidsskrift for velferdsforskning [J Welf Res]. 2020;23(3):170–86.
27. Krane Hanssen J, Henriksen Ø. Politikk og tjenester innen rusomsorg [Politics and services in substance use care]. In: Anvik CH, Sandvin JT, Breimo JP, Henriksen Ø, editors. Velferdstjenestenes vilkår. Nasjonal politikk og lokale erfaringer [Conditions of Welfare Services. National politics and local experiences]. Oslo: Universitetsforlaget; 2020.
28. Øydgard GW, Moen HB, Sjåfjell L. Psykisk helsearbeid i kommunene. [Mental health work in the municipalities]. In: Anvik CH, Sandvin JT, Breimo JP, Henriksen Ø, editors. Velferdstjenestenes vilkår. Nasjonal politikk og lokale erfaringer [Conditions of Welfare Services. National politics and local experiences]. Oslo: Universitetsforlaget; 2020.
29. Järvinen M, Mik-Meyer N, editors. At skabe en professionell [Creating a professional]. Copenhagen: Hans Reitzels Forlag; 2012.
30. Biong S, Borg M. Hva handler recovery om? [What is recovery about?]. In: Landheim A, Wiig FL, Brendbekken M, Brodahl M, Biong S, editors. Et bedre liv [A better life]. Oslo: Gyldendal; 2016.
31. Karlsson B, Borg M. Recovery. Tradisjoner, fornyelser og praksiser, 2. utg. [Recovery. Traditions, renewals and practices, 2nd ed.]. Gyldendal: Oslo; 2023.
32. Helsedirektoratet [Norwegian Directorate of Health]. Rett til valg av behandlingssted. [The right to free choice of treatment]; n.d. Accessed 03.04.25 https://www.helsedirektoratet.no/lov-og-forskrift/rett-til-valg-av-behandlingssted.
33. Helse- og omsorgsdepartemenet [Ministry of Health and Care Services]. Medikamentfrie tilbud I psykisk helsevern – oppfølging av oppdrag 2015 [Drug-free offers in mental health care – follow-up of assignment 2015]. Available at https://www.regjeringen.no/no/dokumenter/medikamentfrie-tilbud-i-psykisk-helsevern%2D%2D-oppfolging-av-oppdrag-2015/id2464239/.

34. Helse- og omsorgsdepartementet [Ministry of Health and Care Services]. Oppdragsdokument fra Helse Sør-Øst. [Assignment document from Health South-East]; 2014. Available at https://www.regjeringen.no/globalassets/upload/hod/sha/oppdragsdokumenthso.pdf.
35. Strand M, von Hausswolff-Juhlin Y. Patient controlled hospital admission in psychiatry: a systematic review. Nord J Psychiatry. 2015;69(8):574–856.
36. Lien L. Hva kan leger og psykologer lære av historiene? [What can doctors and psychologists learn from the stories?]. In: Landheim A, Wiig FL, Brendbekken M, Brodahl M, Biong S, editors. Et bedre liv [A better life]. Oslo: Gyldendal; 2016.
37. Thommesen H. Hverdagsliv, selvforståelse og dobbeltdiagnose – om mennesker med uvanlige erfaringer [Everyday life, self-understanding and dual diagnosis – about people with unusual experiences]. (Doctoral dissertation). Bodø: Bodø University College; 2009.
38. Helse- og omsorgsdepartementet [Ministry of Health and Care Services]. [Nye pakkeforløp for psykisk helse og rus: Bedre behandling og mer forutsigbarhet] New package courses for mental health and substance use: Better treatment and more predictability. 2018. Available at https://www.regjeringen.no/no/dokumentarkiv/regjeringen-solberg/aktuelt-regjeringen-solberg/hod/nyheter/2018ny/nye-pakkeforlopene-for-psykisk-helse-og-rus-bedre-behandling-og-mer-forutsigbarhet/id2610736/.
39. Ådnanes M, Høiseth JR, Magnussen M, Thaulow K, Kaspersen SL. Pakkeforløp forpsykisk helse og rus – brukere, pårørende og fagfolks erfaringer [Package courses for mental health and substance abuse – experiences of users, relatives and professionals]. SINTEF Health Serv Res. 2021;00090.
40. Lipsky M. Street-level bureaucracy. Dilemmas of the individual in public services. New York: Russel Sage Foundation; 1980.
41. Meyers KM, Vorsanger S. Street-level bureaucrats and the implementation of public policy. In: Peters BG, Pierre J, editors. The handbook of public administration. London: Sage Publications; 2007.
42. Hjörne E, Juhila K, Van Nijnatten C. Negotiating dilemmas in the practices of street-level welfare work. Int J Soc Welf. 2010;19(3):303–9.
43. Vabø M. Bakkebyråkratiet – der emosjonelt arbeid blir politikk [The Street-level Bureaucracy – where emotional work becomes politics]. In: Vabø M, Vabo SI, editors. Velferdens organisering [The Organization of Welfare]. Oslo: Universitetsforlaget; 2014.
44. Hanssen H, Humerfelt K, Kjellevold A, Norheim A, Sommerseth R. Faglig skjønn i utøvelse av profesjonelt helse- og sosialfaglig arbeid [Professional discretion in the practice of professional health and social work]. In: Hanssen H, editor. Faglig skjønn og brukermedvirkning [Professional Discretion and User Participation]. Bergen: Fagbokforlaget; 2010.
45. Komesaroff P. From bioethics to microethics: Ethical debate and clinical medicine. In: Komesaroff P, editor. Troubled bodies: critical perspectives on postmodernism, medical ethics and the body. Melbourne: Melbourne University Press; 1995.
46. Joseph-Williams N, Elwyn G, Edwards A. Knowledge is not power for patients: a systematic review and thematic synthesis of patient-reported barriers and facilitators to shared decision making. Patient Educ Couns. 2014;94(3):291–309.
47. Hupe P, Hill M, Buffat A. Introduction: defining and understanding street-level bureaucracy. In: Hupe P, Hill M, Buffat A, editors. Understanding street-level bureaucracy. Bristol: Policy Press; 2016.
48. Karlsson B, Borg M, Samarbeidsbasert forskning. Demokratisk kunnskapsutvikling i psykisk helse- og rusarbeid [Collaborative Research. Democratic knowledge development in mental health and substance use work]. Oslo: Gyldendal; 2021.
49. Norwegian Directorate of Health. Innsatsstyrt finansiering [Activity-based funding], IS-2568; 2017.
50. SINTEF. Pakkeforløp for psykisk helse og rus – brukere, pårørende og fagfolks erfaringer. Rapport 2. [Package course for mental health and substance use – experiences of users, relatives and professionals. Report 2]. SINTEF Digital – Health Services Research; 2021.

51. Evjen R, Øiern T, Kielland KB. Dobbelt opp. Om ruslidelser og psykiske lidelser (4. utgave). [Double up: on substance use disorder and mental disorders (4th ed.)]. Oslo: Universitetsforlaget; 2018.
52. Bjørkquist C, Hansen GV. Coordination of services for dual diagnosis clients in the interface between specialist and community care. J Multidiscip Healthc. 2018;11:233–43.
53. Fimreite AL, Lango P, Lægereid P, Rykkja LH. Organisering, samfunnssikkerhet og krisehåndtering [Organization, societal security and crisis management]. Oslo: Universitetsforlaget; 2011.
54. Vabø M, Vabo S, editors. Velferdens organisering [The Organization of Welfare]. Oslo: Universitetsforlaget; 2014.
55. Helse- og omsorgsdepartementet [Ministry of Health and Care Services]. St. meld [White paper] No. 47 (2008–2009) Samhandlingsreformen. Rett behandling – på rett sted – til rett tid. [The Coordination Reform. Right treatment – at the right place – at the right time]. 2009.
56. Landheim A, Wiig FL, Brendbekken M, Brodahl M, Biong S, editors. Et bedre liv [A Better Life]. Oslo: Gyldendal; 2016.
57. Kolstad A, Kogstad R. Medikalisering av psykososiale problemer [Medicalization of psychosocial problems]. Oslo: Abstrakt Forlag; 2019.
58. Evans T. Street-level bureaucracy, management and the corrupted world of service. Eur J Soc Work. 2016;19(5):602–15.
59. Wilkins VM, Wenger JB. Street-level bureaucrats as public actors. In: Hupe P, Hill M, Buffat A, editors. Understanding street-level bureaucracy. Bristol: Policy Press; 2016.
60. Andersen J. The scope of possibilities for User Influence in Norwegian Municipal Care Services. J Soc Policy. 2020:1–19.
61. Røiseland A. For all seasons? Exploring the policy-context for co-creation. Public Money Manag. 2023:1–9.
62. Album D, Johannesen LEF, Rasmussen EB. Stability and change in disease prestige: a comparative analysis of three surveys spanning a quarter of a century. Soc Sci Med. 2017;180:45–51.
63. Corrigan P, Schomerus G, Shuman V, Kraus D, Perlick D, Harnish A, Kuleza M, Kane-Willis K, Qin S, Smelson D. Developing a research agenda for understanding the stigma of addictions Part I: lessons from the mental health stigma literature. Am J Addict. 2017;26(1):59–66.
64. Midré M. Bot, bedring eller brød? Om bedømming og behandling av sosial nød fra reformasjonen til velferdsstaten [Punishment, recovery or bread? On the assessment and treatment of social distress from the Reformation to the welfare state]. Oslo: Universitetsforlaget; 1990.
65. Lloyd C. The stigmatization of problem drug users: a narrative literature review. Drugs Educ Prev Policy. 2013;20(2):85–95.
66. Fuller R, All rise. Somebodies, nobodies and the politics of dignity. San Francisco: Berret-Koehler Publishers; 2006.
67. Sheehan L, Corrigan P. Stigma of disease and its impact on health. In: Richards CS, Cohen LM, editors. The Wiley encyclopedia of health psychology. Wiley; 2020. p. 5765.
68. Norwegian Ministry of Justice and Public Security. Prop. 112 L [White Paper]. Endringer i straffeloven og legemiddelloven mv. [Changes in the Criminal Code and the Medical Devices Act]. Oslo: Norwegian Ministry of Justice and Public Security; 2025.
69. Cruikshank B. The will to empower. Democratic citizens and other subjects. Ithaca: Cornell University Press; 1990.
70. Villadsen K. Det sociale arbejdes genealogi [The genealogy of social work]. Copenhagen: Hans Reitzels Publishing; 2004.
71. Foucault M. The order of discourse. In: Young R, editor. Untying the text: a post-structuralist reader. Boston: Routledge; 1981.
72. Bourdieu P. Outline of a theory of practice 16. Cambridge: Cambridge University Press; 1977.
73. Jensen Ph, Pfau-Effinger B. Active' citizenship: the new face of face of welfare. I Goul Andersen, Guillemard, A-M, Jensen, P. & Pfau-Effinger (eds.), The changing face of welfare. Policy Press; 2005. p. 1–14.
74. Norwegian Ministry of Health and Care Services. Meld St [White Paper] no. 29 (2012–2013) Morgendagens omsorg [Future Care]. 2013.

75. Lauveng A. Veibok for ingenmannsland – et reisebrev [Roadmap for no man's land – a travel letter]. In: Eriksson BG, Beston G, Holte JS, Hummelvoll JK, editors. Det nødvendige brukerperspektivet i psykisk helsearbeid [The Necessary user perspective in mental health work]. Report no. 8. Karlstad: Karlstad University; 2005.
76. Foucault M. The history of sexuality. New York: Pantheon Books; 1978.
77. Bjerge B. Empowerment og brugerinddragelse i praksis: Mellem forestillinger og det muliges kunst. [Empowerment and user involvement in practice: Between imaginations and the art of the possible]. Aarhus: Center for Substance Abuse Research. Aarhus University; 2005.
78. Mik-Meyer N, Villadsen K. Magtens former [The Outlines of power]. Copenhagen: Hans Reitzel's Publishing; 2007.
79. Foucault M. Governmentality. In: Foucault M, editor. Power. Essential works of Foucault 1954–1984. Volume 3. London: Penguin Books; 2002.
80. Dean M. Governmentality. Power and Rule in Modern Society. London: Sage Publications; 2006.
81. Foucault M. The Subject and power. Crit Inq. 1982;12(2):219–45.
82. Holmes D. Police and pastoral power: governmentality and correctional psychiatric nursing. Nurs Inq. 2002;9(2):84–92.
83. Hessle S. Att invadera med välvilja. [Invading with goodwill]. Lund: Studentlitteratur; 2018.
84. Askheim OP. Samproduksjon som velferdssektorens kinderegg [Co-production as the welfare sector's kinder egg]. J Care Res. 2016;2(1):24–36.
85. Jenhaug L. Samskaping og brukerdrevet innovasjon i offentlige omsorgstjenester i et maktperspektiv [Co-creation and user-driven innovation in public care services from a power perspective] (Doctoral dissertation). Inland Norway University of Applied Sciences; 2020. Available at https://brage.inn.no/inn-xmlui/handle/11250/2688845.
86. Torfing J, Peters GB, Pierre J, Sørensen E. Interactive governance – advancing the paradigm. Oxford: Oxford University Press; 2012.
87. Lund J-Å, Hole T. Samval og den autonome pasienten – er konfliktar underkommuniserte? [Co-decision and the autonomous patient – are conflicts undercommunicated?]. Michael. 2020;17:145–52.

Kintsugi: The Art of Repairing in Gold 15

Ruth Marie Donovan

Abstract

The chapter invites the reader to reflect about humanity, values, and attitudes, related to how the healthcare system on system and individual level can and do approach people with substance use and mental disorders (SUD/MH), with the authors' personal recovery journey as a starting point. Further, the chapter reflects on how traumatic experience could be transformative in creating new life repairing past wounds if mental health care is looking for the resources and opportunities in every human.

Keywords

User perspective · User involvement · User-centered communication · Recovery · Lived experience · Empowerment · Shared decision-making · Relational competence

Insanity in individuals is something rare
but in groups, parties, nations and epochs, it is the rule. —Friedrich Wilhelm Nietzsche, 1886

The sky is also above me. The earth I walk on is also under my feet.

If I pay close attention, I can feel the wind hitting me. The sun can feel warm. For I also know what is cold. I round a corner of the gravel road. Wonder for a

R. M. Donovan (✉)
Public Speaker, Author, and Campaign Strategist, Bergen, Norway
e-mail: ruthdonovan@me.com

T. W. Lie, L. Lien (eds.), *Integrated Treatment of Co-occurring Substance Use and Mental Health Disorders*, https://doi.org/10.1007/978-3-032-20049-5_15

moment if I'm asleep. Hope that I have put on clothes. Look down at my legs. Thankfully. Training tights. Running shoes. Everything checks out. Music in my ears. "Once I was seven years old" ... The words hit me. Tears behind the lenses. Don't know why. I walk along the gravel road. With shoes. With tights. With tears behind the lenses. I know I'm not asleep. But I also don't know if I'm awake. Back in the car. The song is over. The tears behind the lenses are forgotten. The car starts and I drive away from the gravel road. I leave no trace. I was not here (Ruth Marie Donovan, 2015).

People who struggle with addiction and mental issues often have traumas in their past and have often experienced abuse, harmful relationships, mistrust, and rejection, which implies several questions: How to create a relationship built on safety and trust? How can courage, dignity, suffering, empathy, and creativity show the way?

In Search of Courage, Vulnerability, and Power

Psychiatry has not been easy to shake and is still characterized by an ideology and a view of humanity that carries the legacy after we handed over the art of mastering the mind and heart to DSM-5 and ICD-11. It is therefore important to continue the discussion about ideology, view of humanity, ethics, and use of coercion. But that is not my job to do in this chapter. My wish with the next pages is only to make you think. Really think. And invite you into my reflections, my dreams, thoughts, my hope, but also my frustration. And through that, maybe be able to ignite a spark in you and that you become part of a new and optimistic approach to how we want to treat people who struggle. That you will dare to step out of your comfort zone. That you have the courage to stand up against injustice. Courage to speak when others are silent. Courage to protect people against condescension and violations. Courage to use your knowledge and your competence and your creativity to promote the potential in your fellow human beings.

> Have the courage to use your own reason – That is the motto of enlightenment. —Immanuel Kant, 1785

How can you challenge the existing and be part of drawing up a new reality? For the future within mental health care will in no way resemble the past. Thank God for that. It is not the system that will be the cause of the obvious changes we will see and experience. The answer lies in technology and the revolution we are facing. The digital transformation is a reality and changes the way we interact, receive services, but also how we participate and use our knowledge and competence in. For many users, the digital transformation can mean greater freedom, more flexibility, and less experience of asymmetric power relations. But it can also mean a digital class divide if users do not have the digital maturity that is a prerequisite for keeping pace with the digital changes. So to all you leaders in mental health: Fasten your seatbelts! We are about to take off! Because that's the way it is, actually. The development we are experiencing now is a huge upheaval that we only sense the contours of. The digital patient is here, and now this new patient expects an equal encounter with the digital health services. Before the pandemic, there were many psychologists who were not allowed to meet their patients digitally. After 2020, psychology sessions on Zoom have become the norm. And to quote Nietzsche, it is not the mentally ill who are the problem. It is rather the structures and the system around that do not always understand the need to combine knowledge and competence with creativity and creative power. Who do not dare to surrender to the magic of a timely Kairos, who forgot the old philosophers, and who every day, unfortunately, contribute to suppressing the art of being human.

So what do you think so far? Want to join? Am I triggering your curiosity? No passport needed! You just need a ticket to get onboard! Before we take our seats and get ready, I want to tell you a little more about me.

I: A Broken Bowl. Repaired in Gold

I myself have a mental disorder. Or as my psychologist would have said, a mental injury. An injury can fortunately be repaired. Disease and suffering can be treated and sometimes cured. My injuries occurred as a result of severe traumas inflicted on me. Traumas that shook my body, my soul, and my mind. Traumas that wiped out all naivety and changed the untouched and the vulnerable forever.

The word trauma means wound and a psychological trauma is therefore a wound in the soul and in the mind. Wounds can heal, but will often leave scars. I like the philosophy of repairing and rehabilitating.

In Japan, a damaged or broken bowl is repaired. It is not thrown away. Instead, it is glued together with gold, precisely because something that is damaged should not be seen as something that is destroyed, but something that becomes stronger and more beautiful when it is put together and repaired. This art is called Kintsugi, to repair in gold. We have something to learn from this philosophy. To see people who struggle with mental disorders and injuries as people who in various ways have stood in experiences and challenges that have overwhelmed them. We should equip mental health care with gold and glitter in the therapy room. To remind broken souls of their dignity and help them piece together a damaged and fragmented interior.

My injuries were severe, and for a long time I believed that I was destroyed forever. A person without meaning, without prospects for improvement, doomed to an eternal existence behind the plexiglass separating reality from unreality, an invisible membrane separating the living from the dead. According to the diagnostic system, I have complex PTSD with a moderate to severe degree of dissociation. This means that I have lived in an inner fragmented world for most of my life.

Where abuse, violence, and wickedness live in my body more than in important files in my memory bank. Consequence? Chronic pain. Emotional unavailability. The experience of unreality. The experience of being disconnected from feelings.

The Experience of Only Existing. Chronic Pain, Tinnitus, and Suicidality

Go back to the first paragraph of this chapter. What do you think of me now? Am I the same? Has your trust in my thoughts changed? Do you still believe I can influence you to think? To be brave? And am I worthy of your time?

I ask you because I am afraid. Afraid of stigma. My own and yours. I am good at talking myself down. Telling myself that I do not deserve love. That I do not deserve life. That's why I'm afraid of people in health services. Those who have read about disease, diagnoses, and symptoms. I'm afraid they're going to label me. Define me. Trap me. And ally themselves with my inner dark demons. And that's scary. Because then I will become a little powerless. Do you understand me?

But you, I also want to tell you about the gold that fills my scars. Because what makes me more beautiful today are the opportunities and the qualities that suffering and trauma have paved the way for. It is indeed demanding and complicated to build an inner dissociative structure. The Australian psychiatrist George Blair-West has stated that there is nothing wrong with the minds of people who have dissociative disorders, but that these people manage to come up with extraordinary, smart, and sophisticated strategies when trauma captures and one cannot escape. As a result of having lived large parts of my life in a fragmented inner world, I have developed the ability to see complex relationships more quickly. Developed heightened alertness. Deeper empathy. Stronger cognitive abilities. As well as reduced anxiety and fear of the unknown. I take chances both privately and professionally, I am brave and I dare to stand in my own and others' vulnerability. Because nothing has taught me more about life than what traumas have done. When you live with death breathing down your neck as a paralyzing fear of the unknown, the final, and the gruesome, then death actually tells you about surrender. A surrender to life and an acceptance that you cannot control death, but that you can take greater control over your own emotions and reactions by understanding and recognizing your own needs.

However, it is important to emphasize that I in no way wish to trivialize or romanticize life as injured, for it has been a life I would not wish anyone to experience. An existence on the fringes of where one would think it was possible to exist. But here I am, indeed. Very much alive with my disabilities that are invisible to everyone. I have a high work capacity, juggle many balls in the air and succeed both professionally and privately. But I still struggle with insecurity and inner conflicts and have to live with chronic pain, tinnitus, and excessive observation. Nevertheless, it is motivating to experience that after many years of inner struggle and therapy, I am able to experience life and the surroundings as real. Experiencing the world and oneself as living can be both overwhelming, emotionally difficult, and intellectually challenging. This summer, for example, I thought the grass was very green and the flowers on the trees unusually beautiful. They have probably always been like that.

It's Just That I Haven't Seen It

I never knew the stars could shine so bright? You could not see them. Your eyes were blurred by grief and disturbing images. —Ruth Marie Donovan, 2011

So what do you say to join me in a little thought experiment? Let's imagine the following: That people with injuries, traumas and complex mental disorders can, if given the opportunity, increase their potential to be greater than their actual starting point? I challenge this hypothesis because I often experience it to be the opposite for people with SUD/MHD. Does it have to be like this? Can our services prevent people from achieving their potential because they are characterized by a reductionist view of humanity? Where people are broken down into smaller and more understandable parts and thereby see the whole?

Shouldn't we rather put together the parts to then explain the whole? Can more people achieve more? Can we as a society and as health services dare to dream bigger? Aim higher? Everything can't be low threshold. Some must also be mid-threshold, and some must be high-threshold.

The game of science is, in principle, without end. He, who decides one day that scientific statements do not call for any further test, and that they can be regarded as finally verified, retires from the game. —Karl R. Popper, 1959

Arne, Aaron, and the Butterfly

The butterfly has been used countless times as a metaphor for personal change. And it's not so strange. The butterfly is for most the image of metamorphosis. From a gray and gloomy caterpillar body to a moth with a color play that can take the breath away from most. And the beautiful thing is that the caterpillar body contains everything needed to develop into a magnificent specimen of itself. But it depends on the caterpillar getting protection, that no one tears it down from its habitat, and that it gets the opportunity to spread its wings and take off into life. That's how it is with us humans too. Today I thank my psychologist Arne and the sociologist Aaron for their contributions in allowing me to become my butterfly. That I discovered my own color plays in line with my own boundaries with respect and with dignity. Now I live as a whole. The past is my history, the present is my experienced moment, and the future is tomorrow for which I make plans today.

We are coming to understand health not as the absence of disease, but rather as the process by which individuals maintain their sense of coherence (i.e., sense that life is comprehen-

> sible, manageable, and meaningful) and ability to function in the face of changes in themselves and their relationships with their environment. —Aaron Antonovsky, n.d.

The User Perspective and the Helper Role: Who Is the Victim?

Is the sociocultural context in which psychiatry exists sustainable and health-promoting? What do you think if you were to evaluate this context in light of Pierre Bourdieu's theories? Wouldn't we easily be able to argue that systems, regardless of their utility, can be maintained due to internalized and accepted structures of ideas, perceptions, traditions, and thus worldview? And that within these structures a reality of what is considered sick or healthy is maintained, even if it is stigmatizing and at worst limiting and dangerous? And shouldn't we therefore critically evaluate any context that aims to repair, cure, and care, to also be able to act destructively if we do not consider the danger and possibility of destructive habitats? Read Bourdieu. Be enlightened. Be wise.

> Every established order tends to produce the naturalization of its own arbitrariness. —Pierre Bourdieu, 1977

But at the other extreme, we can also, in our obvious intentions to help, contribute to victimization and maintenance of the victim role. And by triggering the victim role in presumptive vulnerable groups, it contributes to creating asymmetry and an artificial us and them. How do we then balance our helper role in a sea of established practices? And how can we best navigate to avoid the danger of maintaining misery, and thus suffering?

Nursing theorist Katie Eriksson writes about three different forms of suffering [1]:

1. Life as suffering. For life will inflict pain and suffering on us. We can lose our job, our house, get divorced and experience loss when the children move out, or when a close relative dies.
2. Disease as suffering. Disease can strike us in life and create suffering. Many people get cancer, rheumatic diseases, or mental disorders. Disease and injury that occur can therefore be seen as suffering.
3. The suffering of care. This is a form of suffering inflicted on patients and users by healthcare personnel. That is, contact with healthcare personnel increases the suffering or inflicts unnecessary pain, loss, and violations on the patient. This form of suffering we should talk more about within SUD/MH care. How much unnecessary suffering do healthcare personnel inflict on their patients through unnecessary use of coercion, through definitional power, and through a language that is charged and full of inherent powerlessness?

Nora Jacobson [2] studied human perceived dignity among the homeless and drug addicts on the streets of Toronto. Her findings were strong narratives about people who perceive themselves as second-class citizens where they were spat on, harassed, and ignored. This experience removes inherent dignity and is replaced with a perceived indignity that again feels like dehumanization of oneself. In comparison, nearly 900 OAT users participated in a user survey in Norway and were asked about their experience of the OAT system [3]. The responses and feedback are disheartening and show almost a systemic contempt for humanity. Many of the users feel powerless and feel that the therapists do not wish them well. As many as one in five experience no participation in their own treatment, and many of the users doubt whether the system is there to help them. As many as seven out of ten feel powerless toward the system and many do not trust their OAT doctor. How can this happen? And what is it about this system that creates so little trust and such a lack of feeling heard? The Danish psychologist Dorthe Birkemose says that powerlessness among employees can contribute to "brutalization," which is a term that refers to attitudes and actions of employees that gradually become harsher, more blunt, passive, or thoughtless and lead to violations of other people [4].

The user perspective is not something new that people have come up with. People have known about the importance of participation and empowerment for thousands of years. Likewise, our autonomy and our tendency to be defiant are known phenomena. If you threaten a person's autonomy and control over their own life, even people with sophisticated intellectual resources will resist and be defiant. And no matter how much we agree with what is being said, it will be dismissed, and we will resist, and unwanted negative behavior can be reinforced. This can be confirmed through Brehm's theory [5] of reactance from 1966. An underrated theory in all interaction with our fellow human beings. You will never go wrong if you meet your fellow human beings with trust, empathy, curiosity, generosity, magnanimity, and the belief in everyone's inherent resources.

Then an important birthplace is created. Namely the birthplace for change, joy, trust, and faith. The belief that what I am experiencing now can get better one day.

> Learn from the people
> Plan with the people
> Begin with what they have
> Build on what they know
> Of the best leaders
> When the task is accomplished
> The people will remark
> We have done it ourselves. —Lao Tzu, n.d.

The Art of Communicating in Gold

When I was invited to write a chapter in a book about SUD/MH, I didn't quite understand the meaning of the acronym itself. For what is it about the system that has led to an inflation in the meaningless use of silly acronyms? This is also important to have a real debate or discussion about. For acronyms are a form of power technique put into a system by people with definitional power. The words we use create images and images create associations and associations create attitudes and therefore affect the way we treat each other. We should learn from marketing and those who sell products we like and that we want. They respond to needs, desires, and they try through communication and means to create attraction, fulfill dreams, create a longing, or a belief that this product can give me what I need or can fulfill a need or solve a problem I have.

Health services within SUD/MH often do the opposite. Namely to maintain stigma, exclusion, and give an experience of something that both smells and tastes bad. What do you think about these offers: "ATIS = alternative to inpatient stay," "leisure with assistance," or welcome to "the department for psychosis?" Also taste these words: Living skills. Residual work capacity. Measures. Treatment resistant. Beyond pedagogical reach. Drug abuser. Who on earth came up with this? Condescending and dehumanizing. Imagine if it was you. How can you use a health-promoting language that contributes to relation, closeness, love, and that brings out the power and color play in your fellow human beings? Use the language. Color it in gold. Words can repair. Words can heal—in gold.

> Words have a magical power. They can bring either the greatest happiness or deepest despair. —Sigmund Freud, 1900

The CREAM Model: The DNA of Creativity

Creativity needs to have a larger role in mental health work. And by that, I don't mean patients who paint and engage in various forms of artistic expression. But employees must use creativity and improvisation when dealing with people who are struggling. Most problems in this world are open. That is, there is no simple recipe that can solve the problem. Sometimes problems are closed and all we need is a procedure or recipe. It could be assembling Ivar shelves from Ikea or knitting a Marius sweater in medium size. But now, most problems in this world are open, and therefore it is a paradox to me that we believe that checklists and package courses are the solution to complex problems that have neither a beginning nor an end. Here comes creativity and the ability to improvise. It is an art in itself. In the book *Kreativitet og innovasjon. Fem sider av nesten samme sak* [Creativity and innovation—five sides of almost the same thing], the author launched *KREM-modellen* (the CREAM model) to solve open problems [6]:

- **K**—stands for creative competence that invites more than thinking outside the box. An encouragement for people with different perspectives to come together and challenge each other.
- **R**—stands for relational competence because creativity is not created inside the heads of individuals, but rather in the interaction between people. And creativity as a collective achievement requires relational competence in creative and safe relationships.

- **E**—stands for expertise and emphasizes the importance of subject and competence. You cannot be a creative math teacher if you don't know math.
- **M**—stands for motivation because motivation is a prerequisite for those who want to solve an open problem. People with SUD/MH need our creative power and our creativity. So, in addition to gold and glitter, the therapy room also needs a good portion of CREAM (KREM). To restore people by releasing the potential in the creative action space.

It's not the notes you play, it's the notes you don't play. —Miles Davis, n.d.

Summary: A Human Encounter in Harmony and Rhythm

Everyone has something intact in them. Address the intact and acknowledge what works, what the person masters, and what the person cares about. Who can stand to be pointed out everything you cannot do? How addicted you have been? How messy your place is, or how many times you have been late to pick up the OAT medicine? Why is there still so much moralizing and paternalism in this field? Why should we educate the patients and force them into a reality they cannot master or want to be a part of? Put on different glasses and look again. Who is the butterfly sitting in front of you? Maybe you discover the color play that your eyes do not immediately see.

Everyone needs predictability, community, activities, the experience of mastering, and feeling a sense of belonging. But we also need to feel significant. That someone needs us. That I am important. That I as a person have a value and that I am of significance. No one can survive with only coffee, marble cake, and a SUD/MH measure.

Take Miles Davis with you in the next human encounter. Don't think about the words you say. But what you say in your silence. In the words between the lines. In the sound between the notes. What your body language expresses. And how your eyes can create a connection. Think of yourself as an instrument. Where you determine your tones and invite to a collaboration with the patients you have in front of you. Music is created between people. SO, dance in human encounters. Let the improvisation lead you into the unknown. Because it is precisely when we allow creative power and the room for possibilities to emerge, that we can really make a difference. The art of improvisation is not about stupidity. But about RAW knowledge. About wild knowledge. And about a surrender to the art of being human.

References

1. Eriksson K. The suffering human. Oslo: Tano AS; 1995.
2. Jacobson N. A taxonomy of dignity: a grounded theory study. BMC Int Health Hum Rights. 2009;9:3.
3. proLARNett. 861 brukere—om LAR i Norge. Hvordan opplever brukerne LAR-behandlingen de mottar, og i hvilken grad medvirker de i egen behandling? ProLAR Nett sin brukerunder-

søkelse 2021 [861 users—about OAT in Norway. How do users experience the OAT treatment they receive, and to what extent do they participate in their own treatment? ProLAR"s user survey 2021]. 2021. Available at https://prolarnett.no/wp-content/uploads/2023/06/Endelig-rapport-MASTER-proLAR-Nett-des-21.pdf
4. Birkemose D. Når gode mennesker handler ondt. Forråelse som mestringsstrategi [When good people act evil. Betrayal as a coping strategy]. Bergen: Fagbokforlaget; 2024.
5. Brehm JW. A theory of psychological reactance. New York: Academic Press; 1966.
6. Oddane T, Kreativitet og innovasjon. Fem sider av nesten samme sak [Creativity and innovation. Five sides of almost the same thing]. Bergen: Fagbokforlaget; 2017.

Promoting Recovery and Social Inclusion 16

Linda Nesse

Abstract

People with co-occurring mental health and substance use problems face significant barriers to well-being, participation, and involvement. In this chapter, we will explore the concepts of recovery and social inclusion. Within the fields of mental health and substance use, recovery and social inclusion are rights-based concepts that originate in the survivor movement and are increasingly considered relevant for health and social services. We will then consider how recovery and social inclusion can be interpreted, developed, approached, and applied in practice.

Keywords

Personal recovery · Social recovery · Recovery capital · Social inclusion · Social exclusion · Citizenship · Community · Belonging · Mattering · Human rights

According to the Declaration of Human Rights [1, 2], everyone has the right to mental health and social inclusion. This includes "*the right to liberty, independence and inclusion in the community,*" as well as "*the right to available, accessible, acceptable and good quality care*" [3]. However, there are substantial social

L. Nesse (✉)
Research Centre for Substance Use Disorders and Mental Illness, Innlandet Hospital Trust, Hamar, Norway
e-mail: linda.nesse@sykehuset-innlandet.no

T. W. Lie, L. Lien (eds.), *Integrated Treatment of Co-occurring Substance Use and Mental Health Disorders*, https://doi.org/10.1007/978-3-032-20049-5_16

inequalities in the degree to which people have access to opportunities for well-being, participation in the community, and satisfactory support and services.

Compared to the population at large, people with co-occurring mental health and substance use problems face disproportionate barriers to well-being, such as housing instability, poverty, inadequate opportunities for employment and engagement in activities, limited social support, somatic health disparities, reduced life expectancy, and discrimination. In addition, the organization of health and social services is often complex, thus reducing the accessibility of coordinated and tailored support related to substance use, mental health, and social or other basic needs [4]. Some have claimed that in the context of mental health and substance use problems, the biggest barrier to overcome is exclusion [5].

In this chapter, the concepts of recovery and social inclusion will be introduced as relevant rights-based frameworks when working with people with co-occurring mental health and substance use problems. Next, various approaches anchored in recovery and social inclusion will be discussed, along with how these can be interpreted, developed, and applied in practice.

What Is Recovery?

Recovery is a word that is used in a wide variety of everyday contexts, often referring to the restoration of or return to a previous state following an injury, illness, challenge, or crisis. In the context of co-occurring mental health and substance use problems, the term *recovery* may have multiple and sometimes contradictory connotations. Within mental health and substance use, recovery may refer to processes or outcomes and to clinical, personal, or social changes in life. It is often considered elusive, confusing, and difficult to describe.

The sections below will separately outline some main conceptual ways of understanding recovery, in addition to some common criticisms. In practice, these perspectives may intersect, and recovery may take different shapes and forms across individuals and life stages.

Clinical Recovery

The word recovery has often been considered synonymous with what we can label *clinical recovery*. The concept of clinical recovery stems from the medical model of health. This term primarily refers to improvements in functioning and symptomatology or recovery *from* substance use and mental health problems [6]. Clinical recovery is generally considered observable and measurable and may, for instance, be expressed through reduced substance use and reduced symptoms of psychopathology. When a set of observed symptoms are considered to no longer exceed the established clinical threshold, a person can be considered in remission and clinically recovered. In this way, clinical recovery corresponds well with the common understanding of recovery as the restoration of normalcy and functioning.

Historically, mental health systems typically adopted a pessimistic view of recovery. Recovery for people with serious mental health problems was considered unlikely, as serious mental health problems were viewed as chronic in nature. However, emerging research on clinical recovery in the 1970s and 1980s contributed to reducing the then-widespread systemic clinical pessimism embedded within psychiatry, thus enhancing hope and optimism that people with serious mental health problems could find ways to lead satisfying and fulfilling lives, despite having experienced struggles and despair [7]. This gradually had implications for service provision, with increased emphasis on the potential for rehabilitation.

Today, one of the common criticisms of clinical recovery is its illness- or problem-orientation. In the clinical perspective, health is understood through illness and the absence of illness. A potential risk is that the clinical perspective on recovery fails to recognize the role of personal and social resources, resilience, and solutions in people's everyday lives, beyond any previous or persisting struggles with mental health and/or substance use [8]. Another related criticism is that everyday life outside the scope of treatment and services is often insufficiently acknowledged as the context in which recovery happens [8]. Furthermore, it may be argued that the person's subjective perceptions of their recovery and active efforts toward creating positive change in their own lives are typically inadequately recognized within clinical recovery [6]. As a result of these criticisms, two other perspectives that at least partially diverge from clinical recovery have emerged as a call for more person-centered and rights-based approaches. Below we will look at these perspectives, as well as their underlying principles and implications.

Personal Recovery

Personal recovery stems from the social movements that are often labeled "the survivor movement." Starting in the 1960s, the survivor movement fought for the right to recognition, agency, and participation for people with mental health problems, both within psychiatric services and in society [9]. This movement developed alongside other social movements, such as the civil rights movement. Advocates for the rights of people with lived experience of mental health problems have criticized the way mental health systems perceive people, as illustrated by this quote by Patricia Deegan [10, p. 92]: "*Those of us who have been diagnosed are not objects to be acted upon. We are fully human subjects who can act, and in acting, change our situation. We are human beings, and we can speak for ourselves.*"

Relatedly, one of the early and most impactful definitions of personal recovery, made by William Anthony, was recovery as "*a deeply personal, unique process of changing one's attitudes, values, feelings, goals, skills and/or roles. It is a way of living a satisfying, hopeful, and contributing life even with limitations caused by illness. Recovery involves the development of new meaning and purpose*" [11, p. 15]. Personal recovery is focused on the voice, agency, and capabilities of the individual in recovery, beyond struggles and symptoms [12]. As such, personal recovery is a process that involves living life on one's own terms. In contrast to clinical recovery, *personal recovery* may thus be understood as recovery *in* mental health and substance use problems, or recovery *outside of or beyond* mental health and substance use problems [5].

Personal recovery has represented a vital shift from illness to well-being and quality of life, focusing on the person rather than the problem experienced [9]. Today, however, there is growing concern that this perspective is frequently applied in services without sufficient consideration of social and relational dimensions, as well as structural issues that negatively impact mental health and substance use problems—such as poverty, homelessness, or discrimination [13]. In this way, personal recovery can become decontextualized, as well as individualized, or "outsourced" to the person. The concept of personal recovery can thus, for instance, be used to make individuals responsible for their own processes, including any challenges and difficulties, or to justify a reduction in service provision or the fragmentation of services. This may be considered an exploitation of personal recovery as originally intended when brought forward in the fight for equal rights by people with lived experience [14].

Social Recovery

Social recovery, like personal recovery, originated in the survivor movement, and its role has been increasingly emphasized since the turn of the century. The social recovery perspective situates recovery processes in everyday life, in relationships, and in the community rather than merely within the individual. It was developed as a critical response to individualistic adaptations of personal recovery in health and social services [6].

A reworked version of Anthony's original definition suggests that social recovery is "*a deeply social, unique, and shared process in which our living conditions, material surroundings, social relations and sense of self evolve. It is about striving to live satisfying, hopeful and reciprocal lives, even though we may still experience threats, stressful social situations, and distress*" [15, p. 11]. This new definition seeks to contextualize the process of recovery, as well as our distress, within our social realities and the societies we belong to.

Not only is recovery about changing one's relationship with mental health and substance use—but often perhaps more so about recovering from or despite difficult life circumstances and living conditions. Furthermore, recovery in a social perspective is understood as an interpersonal and relational process, heavily affected by social determinants of health on the community and societal levels [16, 17].

Research on recovery related to substance use has shown that the resources available to us may play a positive or negative role in our opportunities for making changes. This may include social relationships and support from family, friends, peers, and health and social workers. It may also include opportunities for participating in meaningful activities and social settings, and satisfactory material living conditions and financial resources. In addition, the social and material realities of our lives are closely linked to our possibilities for experiencing a sense of safety, stability, and security—all of which are components in personal recovery.

Dimensions of Recovery

The authors of a seminal literature review, Mary Leamy and colleagues, identified five essential dimensions in recovery through an analysis of empirical studies, resulting in the acronym CHIME: connectedness, hope, identity, meaning, and empowerment [18]. In this framework, *connectedness* refers to the experience of having access to support, engaging in mutual and rewarding relationships with others, and being part of the community and society. *Hope* refers to the experience of having possibilities, opportunities, and aspirations for the future. *Identity* refers to the development of a positive sense of self, of new roles, and of overcoming barriers such as internalized stigma. *Meaning* refers to the experience of purpose through spirituality, social connections, goals, and activities, to name a few. Finally, *empowerment* refers to the experience of enhanced personal agency, and personal strengths and resources. Each of these five dimensions has personal and social underpinnings, and connectedness, identity, and empowerment have been particularly highlighted as inherently relational [19]. Recovery can be argued to involve the dynamic interplay between these dimensions.

Another group of authors, Larry Davidson and colleagues, developed an integrated model of dimensions in recovery explicitly related to co-occurring mental health and substance use problems [20]. Several relevant personal and social dimensions were identified, including the significance of initiating change, developing self-acceptance, self-compassion, and a sense of personal agency, nurturing hope and optimism for the future, connecting or reconnecting with others, and engaging with or participating in the community [20]. This model has been referred to as the "hopscotch" model of recovery to signify that the various identified components are common elements that we dynamically move between at different stages in our recovery processes [20]. Recovery will look somewhat different for each person, across the lifespan, and depending on our life circumstances and living conditions.

Facilitators of and Barriers to Recovery

There are a variety of facilitators and barriers that may play a role in enabling recovery. Such facilitators and barriers have often been labeled *recovery capital*. This concept stems from qualitative research with individuals who experienced positive change related to substance use without ever receiving support from health or social services [21]. This was originally called *natural recovery*, or *spontaneous recovery*, to indicate the lack of formal interventions involved in facilitating such change.

William Cloud and Robert Granfield, who originally developed the concept of recovery capital, noticed that a shared characteristic among many people who experienced recovery without any formal intervention, such as outpatient or inpatient substance use treatment, was their relatively strong access to resources, or capital [21]. Those who experienced natural recovery were typically more socially privileged in terms of their overall life circumstances and living conditions, and the authors' interpretation was that access to resources appeared to play a vital role in accounting for the difference observed in recovery outcomes.

Cloud and Granfield [21] outlined recovery capital as consisting of four main categories of components: social capital, physical capital, personal capital, and cultural capital. *Social capital* has to do with the social resources available to us, such as social networks, interpersonal relationships, community, and social support. *Physical capital* may encompass financial and material assets, such as a steady income and satisfactory housing conditions. *Personal capital* may include personal skills and knowledge, and educational or occupational resources. Finally, *cultural capital* has to do with our knowledge of norms, systems, structures and useful social and community information. In combination, the availability of resources within each of these domains may have implications for our possibilities for recovery. Furthermore, access to these forms of recovery capital may reduce barriers to treatment or other forms of formal support. Consequently, recovery capital is both an explicitly and implicitly relevant concept also within treatment and services, and health and social workers may play an important role in strengthening recovery capital [22].

In terms of recovery capital, structural factors appear to be of great importance in exacerbating or sustaining co-occurring mental health and substance use problems, as well as in hindering recovery. This includes poverty, neglect, violence, discrimination due to gender identity or sexual orientation, racism, incarceration, and fragmented service provision [23]. As such, arguments have been made that recovery capital should be addressed within an intersectional analysis to best understand the differential ways in which various aspects of our social and material realities and identities interact [24]. This brings us to the related issue of social inclusion.

What Is Social Inclusion?

Social inclusion refers to the social integration of individuals and groups [25, 26]. Social inclusion can, for instance, be defined as "*the process of improving the terms of participation in society*" [27]. By contrast, the antonym *social exclusion* may be viewed as "*a state in which individuals are unable to participate fully in economic, social, political, and cultural life, as well as the process leading to and sustaining such a state*" [28]. As such, both social inclusion and exclusion are social processes and emphasize the extent to which we feel we have opportunities for participation and belonging in society. Processes of social inclusion and exclusion are dynamic, and people may have enhanced or reduced opportunities for participation in certain life domains or periods of life.

Social inclusion implies the right to be included and the right to involvement [29]. Social inclusion can thus entail participation and belonging in one's local community or communities, opportunities to make a difference, to have an influence and use one's voice, possibilities for being an equal fellow citizen along with others, and recognition, equity and autonomy. Some core components include relationships, activities, employment, and personal economy [30]. Experiences of social inclusion may rely on subjective meaningfulness and can thus not merely be assessed based on objective, standardized criteria [31]. Consequently, there may be a gap between experienced inclusion, from the point of view of the person themselves, and observed inclusion, as regarded by others.

Social inclusion both refers to the person's experiences of social integration, as well as societal and communities' practices to secure social integration [32]. Social inclusion can occur in different domains—in close relationships with family, friends, and peers, in interactions with other community members, through informal social recognition in the community, and through more formal or structured initiatives [31, 32]. The promotion of social inclusion for people with mental health and substance use problems can entail efforts to support involvement in personally meaningful relationships and activities, efforts to facilitate access to essential resources and information, and efforts to support the development of skills and interests [32].

Citizenship

Social inclusion is used as an umbrella term to describe concepts and frameworks that address issues of social justice. One specific framework for social inclusion is the citizenship framework developed by Michael Rowe and colleagues [33]. The notion of citizenship is embedded in social sciences as well as in the civil rights movement [34]. In this framework, citizenship can be defined as community membership gained through access to essential rights and resources, responsibilities, constructive social roles, and reciprocal relationships with others [33]. Citizenship affirms people's subjective sense of belonging and experienced connectedness and requires social recognition as a valued member of the community [33]. It thus relies on the interaction between internal experiences and perceptions, and external issues, systems, and practices.

There are several ways to accomplish a sense of citizenship, or exercise citizenship [32]. However, although individuals can make personal efforts to gain access to it, there are systems and structures that need to be in place to secure citizenship equally for all citizens, regardless of any individual differences. This societal responsibility especially targets formal dimensions of citizenship, meaning dimensions such as the right to vote and access to suitable housing. Formal dimensions of citizenship are interconnected with experiencing a sense of belonging and a sense of community. Citizenship may have an influence on overall well-being [35].

Citizenship can be experienced to different extents or degrees, depending on structural factors, such as civil rights and living conditions, as well as participation in everyday arenas and activities [36, 37]. It has been argued that some persons and groups experience partial citizenship, which is understood as a form of social inclusion that is conditional and limited, and others experience full citizenship, allowing them to enjoy the range of privileges associated with being acknowledged as a community member on the same level as everyone else. The experience of limited citizenship has been cited as heavily affecting people in socially marginalized positions, including and perhaps especially people with co-occurring mental health and substance use problems [38].

Citizenship and recovery have been argued to be complementary concepts, with citizenship focusing mostly on social factors, and recovery more on subjective experiences [13]. The term *recovering citizenship* has been developed to signify that often, the issue that needs recovering for people with co-occurring mental health and substance use problems is full recognition as members of the community and society, rather than the problems at hand [13].

Mattering

Mattering is another relevant framework to make social inclusion more tangible [39]. Mattering concerns the basic human need to experience a sense of belonging in the world. Isaac Prilleltensky [39] defined mattering as "*the experience that you are valued and that you can add value*" (p. 1). In other words, mattering is intertwined with citizenship in the sense that it captures the need for recognition from others and the need to contribute. When we feel like we matter to ourselves and others and that others matter to us, we can experience connectedness, meaning, and well-being. Conversely, any deprivation of opportunities for mattering can cause harm both to individuals and to communities [39]. Experiences of being deprived of mattering may accelerate, produce, or sustain mental health and substance use problems.

Mattering is created through relationships with family, friends, community members, peers, service providers, and strangers. It can emerge through formal and informal activities, such as employment or community sports teams, and in defined or less defined contexts, such as in supported housing settings or in the broader neighborhood. It entails access to resources and opportunities, as well as opportunities to develop skills and to exercise one's personal agency [39]. Mattering can be promoted to transform well-being on the personal, relational, and community levels [40].

Experiences of mattering may develop when we have somewhere to be or something to do, and thus get to participate and be involved [41]. It is closely tied to having social roles and responsibilities. A quote by a service user in a study on the impact of meaningful activities illustrates how existential this is: "*Unless you have some kind of occupation you don't really exist at all, do you, in society or as an individual*?" [38, p. 201]. In this sense, participation relies on the subjective feeling that we matters in the world, which also touches upon issues of justice and human rights.

Experiences of Social Inclusion

There are several studies that can give us an insight into the accumulated cost of social exclusion and the positive difference that social inclusion can make. In one study of social inclusion, service users who had experiences with life disruptions due to mental health or substance use described a continuous loop of exclusion. They felt that they were viewed as different, less valued, and less capable than other people due to their struggles [4]. This came from external reactions and previous experiences of being stigmatized by others, as well as internalized stigma. For these participants, external and internal stigma took a toll on their health and well-being and produced a feeling of being socially excluded—one participant even used the word *ostracized* to describe the severity of this experience [4]. To avoid further experiences of stigma, several participants chose to isolate to protect themselves, as illustrated by this quote: "*I isolated myself from a lot of people, I try and stay out of people's road.*" [4, p. 361]. This isolation was also associated with feelings of shame and self-criticism, thus making it even more difficult to escape the negative loop of ongoing exclusion.

Relatedly, in another study, young adults with co-occurring mental health and substance use problems who received municipal services described their attempts to navigate their feelings of difference [42]. Navigation was done through balancing between being on the margins and being part of mainstream society. Among these young individuals, the struggle of relating to others who lived more ordinary lives was a common experience, often attributed to a lack of resources and shared references. One of the participants described it this way: "*It seems that it's about looking for belonging anywhere, really... (...) I feel like a tortoise without a shell, like I don't have a house to crawl into*" [42, p. 9, my translation]. However, some wanted to live differently and outside of the norm, and some felt that they were gradually becoming more anchored within mainstream society as time went on, and in this way deepening their sense of belonging [42]. Receiving unconditional acceptance and support from others were perceived as important puzzle pieces in the process of becoming more personally and socially anchored.

In terms of belonging, access to arenas that facilitate social inclusion can make a difference. In one study of exploring participation in a low-threshold community sports team, the team was found to be an essential arena for promoting social inclusion [41]. The study participants, who were involved in a range of different sport activities, felt that regardless of their current or past experiences, they could show up to activities and be well received by others. They were included and felt like a part of the team—like they mattered on the same level as everyone else. Through the community sports team, they were viewed as resourceful, could see themselves as resourceful, recognized the resources in others, and got access to various forms of resources [41]. The participants were recognized as team members and players, were supported to take on responsibilities on the team, and thus held valued social roles. One participant described the significance of doing activities with others in the process of establishing a positive identity: "*You need to get some time off from being ill. Because that is a small part of you, but it takes over every part of you*" [41,

p. 10]. Finally, being on the team created a sense of belonging that for some functioned as a bridge to mainstream society, or as a safe haven away from everyday emptiness and social isolation, from services, or from society.

In relation to mental health and substance use, social inclusion is often described as complex and difficult to navigate or balance in practice [43]. Barriers and facilitators that are structural may manifest in people's everyday lives and social realities [44], thus reminding us of the need for integrated efforts and initiatives when seeking to promote social inclusion in practice.

Promoting Recovery and Social Inclusion

As we have seen above, recovery and social inclusion can be considered complementary and partially overlapping frameworks. These frameworks can inspire health and social services for people with co-occurring mental health and substance use problems to focus on the right to self-determination, participation, and involvement. In practice, the provision of relevant support involves the promotion of personal and social recovery processes, as well as citizenship and mattering [45].

Recovery-oriented practices can be used as an umbrella term for describing efforts to promote recovery and social inclusion, encompassing practices that health and social workers engage in to support people who are in recovery [12]. There is no clearly defined way to engage in recovery-oriented practices—it can instead be considered a flexible approach informed by core values and principles. Recovery-oriented practices imply supporting the person in recovery in their everyday context and collaboratively striving to find satisfactory and relevant solutions to their everyday problems [46]. This requires responsiveness and can involve providing tangible support, including practical, material, and informational aid, or intangible support, such as emotional and relational care. Recovery-oriented practices are inherently personalized, highlight strengths and resources, and involve shared decision-making. Human rights, service user rights, and citizenship are important priorities in recovery-oriented practices [45].

The content of recovery-oriented practices will differ depending on the role of health and social workers within their organization and in relation to service users, and depending on the type and structure of services provided. Recovery-oriented practices can entail assistance with identifying and accessing housing options, relevant housing support, and developing a sense of home and belonging, guided by subjective preferences and needs. It can also involve exploring activity options and opportunities for engagement, including employment, leisure activities, and social arenas, with personal priorities, interests, skills, and resources in mind. Next, and related to both issues above, recovery-oriented practices can include assessing personal economy if experiencing financial challenges, and, if needed, reviewing available opportunities for financial aid that can improve stability, predictability, and possibilities for community participation. Further, it can include navigating contact with family members or friends following any relational challenges, and conflicts and supporting the formation of new social connections, depending on what matters to the person in recovery.

In addition to multifaceted tangible support in everyday life, recovery-oriented practices also imply expressions of empathy, care, trust, confidence, and understanding. Health and social workers may play a vital role through carrying hope for positive change on behalf of and with the person in recovery [47], especially through continued presence and availability over time. Promoting reasonable hope, meaning hope for change that requires small steps and is concrete and within reach, is essential [48, 49]. Furthermore, expressions of micro affirmations, or small expressions of recognition, acknowledgment, and acceptance, for instance, through kind words or helpful gestures, are vital [50].

Recovery-oriented practices may have their relevance in municipal services as well as specialized mental health and substance use treatment, in integrated services, in low-threshold services, and in nonprofit and voluntary organizations. There are, however, differences between services and systems in terms of their institutional conditions and cultures, and thus in their readiness to adopt a recovery-oriented approach to health and social work [6, 51]. In services that originate within the medical model, it may be more difficult to integrate recovery-oriented practices due to competing paradigms, priorities, and logics [51]. Similarly, in services that are well established, the willingness to adopt approaches that differ from previous practices may be lower. Often, the work of promoting recovery is juxtaposed to navigating and minimizing risk [52].

Overall, recovery-oriented practices are more likely to be successfully integrated in services if anchored with managers [48]. Put differently, managers need to prioritize recovery-oriented values and principles, provide supportive and flexible working conditions, and facilitate collaboration, dialogue, and reflection, for such practices to have the best chances at being successfully integrated. For individual health and social workers, receiving support from managers and colleagues may also make a positive difference when seeking to adopt a recovery-oriented approach. This allows for shared reflections and perspectives on what works and what can be done differently.

On the individual level, health and social workers can assess service users' experiences of recovery and citizenship, as well as engage in discussions of their current needs, priorities, and wishes [53]. Health and social workers can seek to assess the forms of recovery capital that are available to or can be made available to each service user, including potential gaps between their current situation and their hopes for the future. Furthermore, health and social workers can provide information about rights and opportunities for strengthening citizenship. By extension, health and social workers can strive to engage in acts of citizenship, namely acts to strengthen citizenship in dialogue with and on behalf of service users [54].

On the system level, services can participate in making nuanced and updated knowledge about recovery and social inclusion available. It may also be relevant to reflect on ways in which current practices can contribute to facilitating or hindering recovery and social inclusion. In addition, it may be meaningful to reflect on how routines can be adjusted to best support recovery and social inclusion. This can be approached individually, as well as with colleagues, both in informal and more formal or structured settings. It may finally be useful to explore relevant topics related to recovery and social inclusion in dialogue with service users.

Summary

- People with co-occurring mental health and substance use problems face significant community- and system-level barriers to well-being, participation, and inclusion, including barriers related to housing, employment and activities, social support, discrimination, and access to services.
- Recovery and social inclusion are rights-based conceptual frameworks with origins in the survivor movement that can be applied in health and social services for people with co-occurring mental health and substance use problems.
- Recovery processes involve positive subjective changes in connectedness, hope, identity, meaning, and empowerment. Life circumstances, living conditions and the availability of various personal, relational, and material resources, or recovery capital, may have positive or negative implications for recovery.
- Social inclusion can be strengthened through promoting mattering and citizenship. Mattering refers to the experience of adding value and being valued. Citizenship requires recognition and creates a sense of belonging through rights, responsibilities, roles, resources, and relationships.
- Health and social workers can engage in individual or shared reflections on how to promote recovery and citizenship in the settings and services they work within. Managers can facilitate the integration of recovery-oriented practices on the organizational level.

Reflection Questions

- What am I/are we already doing to promote recovery and social inclusion? What works, and why and how does it work?
- What are the potential barriers I/we face when attempting to promote recovery and social inclusion? What can we change or adjust?
- How can I/we work to provide information about relevant available resources? How can I/we work to promote access to relevant forms of recovery capital?
- What can I/we emphasize to facilitate experiences of mattering and citizenship?

Recommended Literature and Resources

- Citizenship and Mental Health (Oxford University Press, 2014).
- Handbook of Social Inclusion: Research and Practices in Health and Social Sciences (Springer Nature, 2022).

- Housing, Citizenship, and Communities for People with Serious Mental Illness: Theory, Research, Practice and Policy Perspectives (Oxford University Press, 2017).
- Partnering for Recovery in Mental Health: A Practical Guide to Person-Centered Planning (Wiley, 2014).
- The Handbook of Recovery Capital (Bristol University Press, 2025).
- The Routledge International Handbook of Human Significance and Mattering (Routledge, 2025).

References

1. United Nations. Special Rapporteur on the right of everyone to the enjoyment of the highest attainable standard of physical and mental health (A/HRC/41/34). United Nations Human Rights Council; 2020. Available from: https://www.ohchr.org/en/documents/thematic-reports/ahrc4134-right-everyone-enjoyment-highestattainable-standard-physical.
2. World Health Organization. Mental health action plan 2013–2020. 2021. https://apps.who.int/iris/bitstream/10665/89966/1/9789241506021_eng.pdf?ua=1.
3. Ness O, Borg M, Davidson L. Facilitators and barriers in dual recovery: a literature review of first-person perspectives. Adv Dual Diagn. 2014;7(3):107–17. https://doi.org/10.1108/ADD-02-2014-0007.
4. Cogan NA, MacIntyre G, Stewart A, Tofts A, Quinn N, Johnston, et al. "The biggest barrier is to inclusion itself": the experience of citizenship for adults with mental health problems. J Ment Health. 2021;30(3):358–65. https://doi.org/10.1080/09638237.2020.1803491.
5. Davidson L, Roe D. Recovery from versus recovery in serious mental illness: one strategy for lessening confusion plaguing recovery. J Ment Health. 2007;16(4):459–70. https://doi.org/10.1080/09638230701482394.
6. Borg M, Karlsson B, Stenhammer A. Recoveryorienterte praksiser: En systematisk kunnskapssammenstilling [Recovery-oriented practices – a systematic review]. Drammen: Napha, Nasjonalt kompetansesenter for psykisk helsearbeid; 2013. Available from: https://www.napha.no/multimedia/4281/NAPHA-Rapport-Recovery-web.pdf.
7. Slade M. Mental illness and well-being: the central importance of positive psychology and recovery approaches. BMC Health Serv Res. 2010;10(1):1–14. https://doi.org/10.1186/1472-6963-10-26.
8. Borg M, Davidson L. The nature of recovery as lived in everyday experience. J Ment Health. 2008;17(2):129–40. https://doi.org/10.1080/09638230701498382.
9. Frese FJ, Davis WW. The consumer–survivor movement, recovery, and consumer professionals. Prof Psychol Res Pract. 1997;28(3):243–5. https://psycnet.apa.org/doi/10.1037/0735-7028.28.3.243.
10. Deegan P. Recovery as a journey of the heart. Psychiatr Rehabil J. 1996;19(3):91–7. https://psycnet.apa.org/doi/10.1037/h0101301.
11. Anthony WA. Recovery from mental illness: the guiding vision of the mental health service system in the 1990s. Psychosoc Rehab J. 1993;16(4):11–23.
12. Deegan PE. Recovery: The lived experience of rehabilitation. Psychosoc Rehab J. 1988;11(4):11–9. https://psycnet.apa.org/doi/10.1037/h0099565.
13. Rowe M, Davidson L. Recovering citizenship. Isr J Psychiatry Relat Sci. 2016;53(1):14–21.
14. Slade M, Amering M, Farkas M, Hamilton B, O'Hagan M, Panther G, Perkins R, Shepherd G, Tse S, Whitley R. Uses and abuses of recovery: implementing recovery-oriented practices in mental health systems. World Psychiatry. 2014;13(1):12–20. https://doi.org/10.1002/wps.20084.

15. Topor A, Boe TD, Larsen IB. The lost social context of recovery psychiatrization of a social process. Front Sociol. 2022;7:1–14. https://doi.org/10.3389/fsoc.2022.832201.
16. Price-Robertson R, Obradovic A, Morgan B. Relational recovery: beyond individualism in the recovery approach. Adv Ment Health. 2017;15(2):108–20. https://doi.org/10.1080/18387357.2016.1243014.
17. Topor A, Borg M, Di Girolamo S, Davidson L. Not just an individual journey: social aspects of recovery. Int J Soc Psychiatry. 2011;57(1):90–9. https://doi.org/10.1177/0020764009345062.
18. Leamy M, Bird V, Le Boutillier C, Williams J, Slade M. Conceptual framework for personal recovery in mental health: systematic review and narrative synthesis. Br J Psychiatry. 2011;199(6):445–52. https://doi.org/10.1192/bjp.bp.110.083733.
19. Tew J, Ramon S, Slade M, Bird V, Melton J, Le Boutillier C. (2012). Social factors and recovery from mental health difficulties: A review of the evidence. Br. J Soc Work. 2012;42(3):443–60. https://doi.org/10.1093/bjsw/bcr076.
20. Davidson L, Andres-Hyman R, Bedregal L, Tondora J, Frey J, Kirk TA Jr. From "double trouble" to "dual recovery": Integrating models of recovery in addiction and mental health. J Dual Diagn. 2008;4(3):273–90. https://doi.org/10.1080/15504260802072396.
21. Cloud W, Granfield R. Conceptualizing recovery capital: expansion of a theoretical construct. Subst Use Misuse. 2008;43(12-13):1971–86. https://doi.org/10.1080/10826080802289762.
22. Vanderplasschen W, De Meyer F, De Ruysscher C, Pouille A, Sinclair DL. The role of specialist substance use and addiction treatment in building recovery capital. In: Cloud W, Best D, editors. The handbook of recovery capital. London: Routledge; 2019. p. 169–92.
23. Padgett DK, Tiderington E, Tran Smith B, Derejko KS, Henwood BF. Complex recovery: Understanding the lives of formerly homeless adults with complex needs. J Soc Distress Homeless. 2016;25(2):60–70. https://doi.org/10.1080/10530789.2016.1173817.
24. Hennessy EA. Recovery capital: a systematic review of the literature. Addict Res Theory. 2017;25(5):349–60. https://doi.org/10.1080/16066359.2017.1297990.
25. O'Donnell P, O'Donovan D, Elmusharaf K. Measuring social exclusion in healthcare settings: a scoping review. Int J Equity Health. 2018;17:1–16. https://doi.org/10.1186/s12939-018-0732-1.
26. Wright N, Stickley T. Concepts of social inclusion, exclusion and mental health: a review of the international literature. J Psychiatr Ment Health Nurs. 2013;20(1):71–81. https://doi.org/10.1111/j.1365-2850.2012.01889.x.
27. United Nations. Leaving no one behind: The imperative of inclusive development. Report on the World Social Situation 2016. New York: United Nations; 2016. Available from: https://www.un.org/esa/socdev/rwss/2016/full-report.pdf.
28. Davey S, Gordon S. Definitions of social inclusion and social exclusion: the invisibility of mental illness and the social conditions of participation. Int J Cult Ment Health. 2017;10(3):229–37. https://doi.org/10.1080/17542863.2017.1295091.
29. Schormans AF. Social inclusion. In: Michalos AC, editor. Encyclopedia of quality of life and well-being research. Dordrecht: Springer; 2014. p. 6082–6.
30. Repper J, Perkins R. Recovery and social inclusion. In: Callaghan P, Playle J, editors. Mental health nursing skills. Oxford: Oxford University Press; 2009. p. 85–95.
31. Ball CM, Eiroa-Orosa FJ. A meta-synthesis of qualitative studies on citizenship and mental health. Ir J Psychol Med. 2024:1–8. https://doi.org/10.1017/ipm.2024.66.
32. Vandekinderen C, Roets G, Roose R, Van Hove G. Rediscovering recovery: reconceptualizing underlying assumptions of citizenship and interrelated notions of care and support. Sci World J. 2012;1:1–7. https://doi.org/10.1100/2012/496579.
33. Rowe M, Clayton A, Benedict P, Bellamy C, Antunes K, Miller R, Pelletier JF, Stern E, O'Connell MJ. Going to the source: creating a citizenship outcome measure by community-based participatory research methods. Psychiatr Serv. 2012;63(5):445–50. https://doi.org/10.1176/appi.ps.201100272.
34. Ponce AN, Rowe M. Citizenship and community mental health care. Am J Community Psychol. 2018;61(1-2):22–31. https://doi.org/10.1002/ajcp.12218.

35. Clayton A, O'Connell MJ, Bellamy C, Benedict P, Rowe M. The citizenship project part II: impact of a citizenship intervention on clinical and community outcomes for persons with mental illness and criminal justice involvement. Am J Community Psychol. 2013;51(1-2):114–22. https://doi.org/10.1007/s10464-012-9549-z.
36. Harper A, Kriegel L, Morris C, Hamer HP, Gambino M. Finding citizenship: what works? Am J Psychiatr Rehabil. 2017;20(3):200–17. https://doi.org/10.1080/15487768.2017.1338036.
37. Hamer HP, Finlayson M, Warren H. Insiders or outsiders? Mental health service users' journeys towards full citizenship. Int J Ment Health Nurs. 2014;23(3):203–11. https://doi.org/10.1111/inm.12046.
38. Blank AA, Harries P, Reynolds F. 'Without occupation you don't exist': occupational engagement and mental illness. J Occup Sci. 2015;22(2):197–209. https://doi.org/10.1080/14427591.2014.882250.
39. Prilleltensky I. Mattering at the intersection of psychology, philosophy, and politics. Am J Community Psychol. 2020;65(1-2):16–34. https://doi.org/10.1002/ajcp.12368.
40. Prilleltensky I, Scarpa MP, Ness O, Di Martino S. Mattering, wellness, and fairness: psychosocial goods for the common good. Am J Orthopsychiatry. 2023;93(3):198–210. https://doi.org/10.1037/ort0000668.
41. Nesse L, Borg M, Karlsson B. There are no thresholds here: social inclusion among the participants of a community sports initiative. Soc Incl. 2025;13:1–19. https://doi.org/10.17645/si.9284.
42. Semb R, Borg M, Ness O. Tilpasning eller tilbaketrekning? Tilhørighetsstrategier blant unge voksne med rus- og psykiske helseproblemer. [Adaptation or withdrawal? Belonging strategies among young adults with substance use and mental health problems]. Nord Welf Res. 2016;19(3):204–20. https://doi.org/10.18261/issn.2464-3076-2016-03-01.
43. Nord-Baade S, Ness O, Jensen CB, Rowe M, Opheim E, Landheim A. Barriers and facilitators for social inclusion among people with concurrent mental health and substance use problems. A qualitative scoping review. PLoS One. 2024;19(12):1–26. https://doi.org/10.1371/journal.pone.0315758.
44. Ogundipe E, Sælør KT, Biong S, Gonzalez MT. Core dimensions of social inclusion for residents with mental health and/or substance use challenges: a qualitative meta-synthesis. J Psychosoc Rehabil Ment Health. 2024:1–20. https://doi.org/10.1007/s40737-024-00415-1.
45. Le Boutillier C, Leamy M, Bird VJ, Davidson L, Williams J, Slade M. What does recovery mean in practice? A qualitative analysis of international recovery-oriented practice guidance. Psychiatr Serv. 2011;62(12):1470–6. https://doi.org/10.1176/appi.ps.001312011.
46. Slade M. Everyday solutions for everyday problems: how mental health systems can support recovery. 2012;63(7):702–4. https://doi.org/10.1176/appi.ps.201100521.
47. Sælør KT, Ness I, Borg M, Biong S. You never know what's around the next corner: Exploring practitioners' hope inspiring practices. Adv Dual Diagn. 2015;8(3):141–52. https://doi.org/10.1108/ADD-05-2015-0010.
48. Sælør KT, Carlsen SEL, Fadnes LT, Lorås L. Experiences of hope after treatment of Hepatitis C infection—a qualitative study. Int J Environ Res Public Health. 2022;19(23):1–13. https://doi.org/10.3390/ijerph192315732.
49. Weingarten K. Reasonable hope: construct, clinical applications, and supports. Fam Process. 2010;49(1):5–25. https://doi.org/10.1111/j.1545-5300.2010.01305.x.
50. Topor A, Bøe TD, Larsen IB. Small things, micro-affirmations and helpful professionals' everyday recovery-orientated practices according to persons with mental health problems. Community Ment Health J. 2018;54(8):1212–20. https://doi.org/10.1007/s10597-018-0245-9.
51. Speyer H, Roe D, Slade M. Recovery-oriented psychiatry: oxymoron or catalyst for change? Lancet Psychiatry. 2025;12(10):795–802.
52. Tickle A, Brown D, Hayward M. Can we risk recovery? A grounded theory of clinical psychologists' perceptions of risk and recovery-oriented mental health services. Psychol Psychother Theory Res Pract. 2014;87(1):96–110. https://doi.org/10.1111/j.2044-8341.2012.02079.x.
53. Medborgerskap i psykisk helsearbeid [Citizenship in mental health work]. In: Gonzalez MT, editor. Psykiske lidelser – Faglig forståelse og terapeutisk tilnærming [Mental disorders –

Professional understanding and therapeutic approach]. 2nd ed. Oslo: Gyldendal Akademisk. p. 522–6.
54. Hamer HP, Rowe M, Seymour CA. 'The right thing to do': fostering social inclusion for mental health service users through acts of citizenship. Int J Ment Health Nurs. 2019;28(1):297–305. https://doi.org/10.1111/inm.12533.

GPSR Compliance

The European Union's (EU) General Product Safety Regulation (GPSR) is a set of rules that requires consumer products to be safe and our obligations to ensure this.

If you have any concerns about our products, you can contact us on ProductSafety@springernature.com

In case Publisher is established outside the EU, the EU authorized representative is:

Springer Nature Customer Service Center GmbH
Europaplatz 3
69115 Heidelberg, Germany

Batch number: 10726060

Printed by Printforce, the Netherlands